Neurocritical Care in Neurosurgery

Editors

PAUL A. NYQUIST
MAREK A. MIRSKI
RAFAEL J. TAMARGO

NEUROSURGERY
CLINICS OF NORTH AMERICA

www.neurosurgery.theclinics.com

July 2013 • Volume 24 • Number 3

ELSEVIER

1600 John F. Kennedy Boulevard • Suite 1800 • Philadelphia, Pennsylvania, 19103-2899

http://www.theclinics.com

NEUROSURGERY CLINICS OF NORTH AMERICA Volume 24, Number 3
July 2013 ISSN 1042-3680, ISBN-13: 978-1-4557-7600-9

Editor: Jessica McCool

Neurosurgery Clinics of North America (ISSN 1042-3680) is published quarterly by Elsevier Inc., 360 Park Avenue South, New York, NY 10010-1710. Months of issue are January, April, July, and October. Business and Editorial Offices: 1600 John F. Kennedy Blvd., Suite 1800, Philadelphia, PA 19103-2899. Customer Service Office: 11830 Westline Industrial Drive, St. Louis, MO 63146. Periodicals postage paid at New York, NY, and additional mailing offices. Subscription prices are $360.00 per year (US individuals), $552.00 per year (US institutions), $393.00 per year (Canadian individuals), $674.00 per year (Canadian institutions), $502.00 per year (international individuals), $674.00 per year (international institutions), $177.00 per year (US students), and $243.00 per year (international students). International air speed delivery is included in all *Clinics* subscription prices. All prices are subject to change without notice. **POSTMASTER:** Send address changes to *Neurosurgery Clinics of North America*, Elsevier Periodicals Customer Service, 11830 Westline Industrial Drive, St. Louis, MO 63146. **Customer Service: 1-800-654-2452 (US and Canada). From outside the US and Canada, call: 1-314-453-7041. Fax: 1-314-453-5170. E-mail: JournalsCustomerService-usa@elsevier.com (for print support) and journalsonlinesupport-usa@elsevier.com (for online support).**

Reprints. For copies of 100 or more, of articles in this publication, please contact the Commercial Reprints Department, Elsevier Inc., 360 Park Avenue South, New York, NY 10010-1710. Tel. (212) 633-3812; Fax: (212) 462-1935; E-mail: reprints@elsevier.com.

Neurosurgery Clinics of North America is covered in *MEDLINE/PubMed (Index Medicus)*, *EMBASE/Excerpta Medica*, and *Current Contents/Clinical Medicine (CC/CM)*.

Printed and bound by CPI Group (UK) Ltd, Croydon, CR0 4YY

Transferred to digital print 2012

Contributors

EDITORS

PAUL A. NYQUIST, MD, MPH, FCCM, FAHA, FANA
Associate Professor of Neurology and Anesthesiology and Critical Care, Division of Neurocritical care, Departments of Anesthesia/ Critical Care Medicine, Neurology and Neurosurgery, The Johns Hopkins Hospital, The Johns Hopkins School of Medicine, Baltimore, Maryland

MAREK A. MIRSKI, MD, PhD
Associate Professor of Anesthesiology and Critical Care Medicine, Neurology, Neurosciences Critical Care Unit, Director, Division of Neurosciences, Critical Care, The Johns Hopkins Medical Institutions,
Director, The Johns Hopkins Hospital; Vice-Chair, Professor of Neurology, Anesthesiology, and Neurosurgery, Departments of Neurology, Anesthesiology and Critical Care, Johns Hopkins Hospital, Baltimore, Maryland

RAFAEL J. TAMARGO, MD
Walter E. Dandy Professor of Neurosurgery, Professor of Neurosurgery and Otolaryngology-Head and Neck Surgery, Director of Cerebrovascular Neurosurgery, Neurosurgical Co-Director, The Johns Hopkins Neurocritical Care Unit, Department of Neurosurgery, The Johns Hopkins University School of Medicine, Baltimore, Maryland

AUTHORS

JOSEPH G. ADEL, MD
Department of Neurological Surgery, McGaw Medical Center, Northwestern University Feinberg School of Medicine, Chicago, Illinois

SALAH G. AOUN, MD
Department of Neurological Surgery, University of Texas Southwestern Medical Center, Dallas, Texas

ROCCO A. ARMONDA, MD
Walter Reed National Military Medical Center, Bethesda, Maryland

NEERAJ BADJATIA, MD, MS, FCCM
Associate Professor of Neurology, Neurosurgery, Anesthesiology, University of Maryland School of Medicine, Chief, Section of Neurocritical Care, R Adams Cowley Shock Trauma Center, University of Maryland Medical Center, Baltimore, Maryland

PERRY A. BALL, MD
Section of Neurosurgery; Department of Anesthesiology, Dartmouth-Hitchcock Medical Center, Lebanon, New Hampshire

BERNARD R. BENDOK, MD, MSCI, FACS, FAANS, FAHA
Department of Neurological Surgery, McGaw Medical Center, Northwestern University Feinberg School of Medicine, Chicago, Illinois

ROSS BULLOCK, MD, PhD
Department of Neurosurgery, Lois Pope LIFE Center, Miller School of Medicine, University of Miami, Miami, Florida

JUSTIN M. CAPLAN, MD
Resident, Department of Neurosurgery, Johns Hopkins University School of Medicine, Baltimore, Maryland

WAN-TSU W. CHANG, MD
Departments of Neurology, Anesthesiology and Critical Care Medicine, and Neurosurgery, The Johns Hopkins School of Medicine, Baltimore, Maryland

GEOFFREY P. COLBY, MD, PhD
Assistant Professor of Neurosurgery, Department of Neurosurgery, Johns Hopkins University School of Medicine, Baltimore, Maryland

ALEXANDER L. COON, MD
Assistant Professor of Neurosurgery,
Neurology, and Radiology, Department of
Neurosurgery, Johns Hopkins University
School of Medicine, Baltimore, Maryland

MARC R. DAOU, BA
Department of Neurological Surgery, McGaw
Medical Center, Northwestern University
Feinberg School of Medicine, Chicago, Illinois

TAREK Y. EL AHMADIEH, MD
Department of Neurological Surgery, McGaw
Medical Center, Northwestern University
Feinberg School of Medicine, Chicago, Illinois

NAJIB E. EL TECLE, MD
Department of Neurological Surgery, McGaw
Medical Center, Northwestern University
Feinberg School of Medicine, Chicago, Illinois

LINTON T. EVANS, MD
Section of Neurosurgery, Dartmouth-Hitchcock
Medical Center, Lebanon, New Hampshire

IVAN ROCHA FERREIRA DA SILVA, MD
Cerebrovascular Center, Cleveland Clinic,
Cleveland, Ohio

ANTHONY R. FRATTALONE, MD
Clinical Fellow, Division of Neurocritical Care,
Department of Anesthesiology and Critical
Care Medicine, Johns Hopkins Medical
Institutions, Baltimore; Assistant Professor
of Neurology, Department of Neurology,
Uniformed Services University of the Health
Sciences, Bethesda, Maryland

EMILY J. GILMORE, MD
Assistant Professor, Department of Neurology,
Yale-New Haven Hospital, Yale University
School of Medicine, New Haven, Connecticut

DAVID M. GREER, MD, MA, FCCM, FAHA
Zimmerman and Spinelli Professor of
Neurology and Neurosurgery, Vice Chairman,
Department of Neurology, Yale-New Haven
Hospital, Yale University School of Medicine,
New Haven, Connecticut

JUDY HUANG, MD
Associate Professor of Neurosurgery,
Co-Director, Neurosurgery Residency
Program, Department of Neurosurgery,
Johns Hopkins University School of Medicine,
Baltimore, Maryland

DAVID Y. HWANG, MD
Assistant Professor, Department of
Neurology, Yale-New Haven Hospital, Yale
University School of Medicine, New Haven,
Connecticut

ATUL KALANURIA, MD
Division of Neurocritical care, Departments of
Anesthesia/Critical Care Medicine, Neurology
and Neurosurgery, The Johns Hopkins School
of Medicine, Baltimore, Maryland

RYAN KITAGAWA, MD
Department of Neurosurgery, Lois Pope LIFE
Center, Miller School of Medicine, University of
Miami, Miami, Florida

PETER D. LE ROUX, MD, FACS
Department of Neurosurgery, University of
Pennsylvania, Philadelphia, Pennsylvania

GEOFFREY S.F. LING, MD, PhD, FAAN
Attending Physician, Division of Neurocritical
Care, Department of Anesthesiology and
Critical Care Medicine, Johns Hopkins
Medical Institutions, Baltimore; Professor
of Neurology, Department of Neurology,
Uniformed Services University of the Health
Sciences, Bethesda; Professor of Neurology,
Colonel, Medical Corps, US Army, Bethesda,
Maryland

STUART SCOTT LOLLIS, MD
Section of Neurosurgery, Dartmouth-Hitchcock
Medical Center, Lebanon, New Hampshire

EDWARD MICHAEL MANNO, MD
Cerebrovascular Center, Cleveland Clinic,
Cleveland, Ohio

MANJUNATH MARKANDAYA, MBBS
Divisions of Surgical/Trauma Critical Care,
Neurosciences Critical Care, and Pulmonary/
Critical Care Medicine, Cowley Shock Trauma
Center, University of Maryland, Baltimore,
Maryland

SCOTT A. MARSHALL, MD
Neurology and Critical Care, Department of
Medicine, San Antonio Military Medical Center,
Fort Sam Houston, Texas

ANNA T. MAZZEO, MD
Department of Anesthesia and Intensive Care, San Giovanni Battista Hospital, University of Turin; Department of Anesthesia and Critical Care, Azienda Ospedaliera Città della Salute e della Scienza di Torino-Presidio Molinette, University of Turin, Turin, Italy

MAREK A. MIRSKI, MD, PhD
Associate Professor of Anesthesiology and Critical Care Medicine, Neurology, Neurosciences Critical Care Unit, Director, Division of Neurosciences, Critical Care, The Johns Hopkins Medical Institutions, Director, The Johns Hopkins Hospital; Vice-Chair, Professor of Neurology, Anesthesiology, and Neurosurgery, Departments of Neurology, Anesthesiology and Critical Care, Johns Hopkins Hospital, Baltimore, Maryland

ALLAN D. NANNEY III, MD
Department of Neurological Surgery, McGaw Medical Center, Northwestern University Feinberg School of Medicine, Chicago, Illinois

PAUL A. NYQUIST, MD, MPH, FCCM, FAHA, FANA
Associate Professor of Neurology and Anesthesiology and Critical Care, Division of Neurocritical care, Departments of Anesthesia/Critical Care Medicine, Neurology and Neurosurgery, The Johns Hopkins Hospital, The Johns Hopkins School of Medicine, Baltimore, Maryland

MAURO ODDO, MD
Maître d'Enseignement et de Recherche, Faculty of Medicine and Biology, Service de Médecine Intensive Adulte, Medico-Surgical ICU, Centre Hospitalier Universitaire Vaudois - CHUV, University of Lausanne, Lausanne, Switzerland

JOSE JAVIER PROVENCIO, MD
Cerebrovascular Center; Neuroinflammation Research Center, Cleveland Clinic, Cleveland, Ohio

ALEXANDER RAZUMOVSKY, PhD, FAHA
Sentient NeuroCare Services, Hunt Valley, Maryland

MARIANNA V. SPANAKI, MD, PhD, MBA
Department of Neurology, Henry Ford Hospital; Associate Professor of Neurology, Wayne State University School of Medicine, Detroit, Michigan

RAFAEL J. TAMARGO, MD
Walter E. Dandy Professor of Neurosurgery, Professor of Neurosurgery and Otolaryngology-Head and Neck Surgery, Director of Cerebrovascular Neurosurgery, Neurosurgical Co-Director, The Johns Hopkins Neurocritical Care Unit, Department of Neurosurgery, Johns Hopkins University School of Medicine, Baltimore, Maryland

PANAYIOTIS N. VARELAS, MD, PhD
Director NICU, Departments of Neurology and Neurosurgery, Henry Ford Hospital; Professor of Neurology, Wayne State University School of Medicine, Detroit, Michigan

SHOJI YOKOBORI, MD, PhD
Department of Neurosurgery, Lois Pope LIFE Center, Miller School of Medicine, University of Miami, Miami, Florida; Department of Emergency and Critical Care Medicine, Nippon Medical School, Tokyo, Japan

Contents

Traumatic brain injury (TBI) is a serious disorder that is all too common. TBI ranges in severity from mild concussion to a severe life-threatening state. Across this spectrum, rational therapeutic approaches exist. Early identification that TBI has occurred in a patient is paramount to optimal outcome. Proper clinical management should be instituted as soon as possible by appropriately trained medical providers. More seriously injured patients must be triaged to advanced care centers. It is only through this rational approach to TBI that patients may expect to achieve optimal clinical and functional outcome.

Patients with aneurysmal subarachnoid hemorrhage who survive the initial hemorrhage require complex interventions to occlude the aneurysm, typically followed by a prolonged intensive care unit and hospital course to manage the complications that follow. Much of the morbidity and mortality from this disease happens in delayed fashion in the neurocritical care unit. Despite progress made in the last decades, much remains to be understood about this disease and how to best manage these patients. This article provides a review of current evidence and the authors' experience, aimed at providing practical aid to those caring for patients with this disease.

Acute spinal cord injury (SCI) is associated with widespread disturbances not only affecting neurologic function but also leading to hemodynamic instability and respiratory failure. Traumatic SCI rarely occurs in isolation, and frequently is accompanied by trauma to other organ systems. Management of individuals with SCI is complex, requiring aggressive monitoring and prompt treatment when complications arise. Typically this level of care is provided in the neurocritical care unit. This article reviews the pathophysiology of the neurologic, cardiovascular, and pulmonary derangements following traumatic SCI and their management in the critical care setting.

Intracerebral hemorrhage (ICH) is a significant cause of morbidity and mortality. With the aging population, increased use of anticoagulants, and changing racial and ethnic landscape of the United States, the incidence of ICH will increase over the next decade. Improvements in preventative strategies to treat hypertension and atrial fibrillation are necessary to change the trajectory of this increase. Advances in the understanding of ICH at the vascular and molecular level may pave the way to new treatment options. This article discusses the epidemiology, pathophysiology, and current treatment options for patients with ICH. Differences in outcome and treatment between patients taking and not taking anticoagulant therapies are considered.

Management of intracranial pressure in neurocritical care remains a potentially valuable target for improvements in therapy and patient outcomes. Surrogate markers of increased intracranial pressure, invasive monitors, and standard therapy, as well as promising new approaches to improve cerebral compliance are discussed, and a current review of the literature addressing this metric in neuroscience critical care is provided.

Surgical techniques that address elevated intracranial pressure include (1) intraventricular catheter insertion and cerebrospinal fluid drainage, (2) removal of an intracranial space-occupying lesion, and (3) decompressive craniectomy. This review discusses the role of surgery in the management of elevated intracranial pressure, with special focus on intraventricular catheter placement and decompressive craniectomy. The techniques and potential complications of each procedure are described, and the existing evidence regarding the impact of these procedures on patient outcome is reviewed. Surgical management of mass lesions and ischemic or hemorrhagic stroke occurring in the posterior fossa is not discussed herein.

The cause of seizures in the neurosurgical intensive care unit (NICU) can be categorized as emanating from either a primary brain pathology or from physiologic derangements of critical care illness. Patients are typically treated with parenteral antiepileptic drugs. For early onset ICU seizures that are easily controlled, data support limited treatment. Late seizures have a more ominous risk for subsequent epilepsy and should be treated for extended periods of time or indefinitely. This review ends by examining the treatment algorithms for simple seizures and status epilepticus and the role newer antiepileptic use can play in the NICU.

Mechanical ventilation in neurologically injured patients presents unique challenges. Patients with acute neurologic injuries may require mechanical ventilation for reasons beyond respiratory failure. There is also a subset of pulmonary pathologic abnormality directly associated with neurologic injuries. Balancing the need to maintain brain oxygenation, cerebral perfusion, and control of intracranial pressure can be in conflict with concurrent ventilator strategies aimed at lung protection. Weaning and liberation from mechanical ventilation also require special considerations. These issues are examined in the ventilator management of the neurologically injured patient.

Microdialysis in the Neurocritical Care Unit   417

Ryan Kitagawa, Shoji Yokobori, Anna T. Mazzeo, and Ross Bullock

Effective monitoring is critical for neurologically compromised patients, and several techniques are available. One of these tools, cerebral microdialysis (MD), was designed to detect derangements in cerebral metabolism. Although this monitoring device began as a research instrument, favorable results and utility have broadened its clinical applications. Combined with other brain monitoring techniques, MD can be used to estimate cerebral vulnerability, to assess tissue outcome, and possibly to prevent secondary ischemic injury by guiding therapy. This article reviews the literature regarding the past, present, and future uses of MD along with its advantages and disadvantages in the intensive care unit setting.

Parenchymal Brain Oxygen Monitoring in the Neurocritical Care Unit   427

Peter D. Le Roux and Mauro Oddo

Patients admitted to the neurocritical care unit (NCCU) often have serious conditions that can be associated with high morbidity and mortality. Pharmacologic agents or neuroprotectants have disappointed in the clinical environment. Current NCCU management therefore is directed toward identification, prevention, and treatment of secondary cerebral insults that evolve over time and are known to aggravate outcome. This strategy is based on a variety of monitoring techniques including use of intraparenchymal monitors. This article reviews parenchymal brain oxygen monitors, including the available technologies, practical aspects of use, the physiologic rationale behind their use, and patient management based on brain oxygen.

Use of Transcranial Doppler (TCD) Ultrasound in the Neurocritical Care Unit   441

Atul Kalanuria, Paul A. Nyquist, Rocco A. Armonda, and Alexander Razumovsky

Transcranial Doppler (TCD) is a portable device that uses a handheld 2-MHz transducer. It is most commonly used in subarachnoid hemorrhage where cerebral blood flow velocities in major intracranial blood vessels are measured to detect vasospasm in the first 2 to 3 weeks. TCD is used to detect vasospasm in traumatic brain injury and post-tumor resection, measurement of cerebral autoregulation and cerebrovascular reactivity, diagnosis of acute arterial occlusions in stroke, screening for patent foramen ovale and monitoring of emboli. It can be used to detect abnormally high intracranial pressure and for confirmation of total cerebral circulatory arrest in brain death.

Hypothermia in Neurocritical Care   457

Neeraj Badjatia

Hypothermia has long been recognized as an effective therapy for acute neurologic injury. Recent advances in bedside technology and greater understanding of thermoregulatory mechanisms have made this therapy readily available at the bedside. Critical care management of the hypothermic patient can be divided into 3 phases: induction, maintenance, and rewarming. Each phase has known complications that require careful monitoring. At present, hypothermia has only been shown to be an effective neuroprotective therapy in cardiac arrest survivors. The primary use of hypothermia in the neurocritical care unit is to treat increased intracranial pressure.

This article reviews current guidelines for death by neurologic criteria and addresses topics relevant to the determination of brain death in the intensive care unit. The history of brain death as a concept leads into a discussion of the evolution of practice parameters, focusing on the most recent 2010 update from the American Academy of Neurology and the practice variability that exists worldwide. Proper transition from brain death determination to possible organ donation is reviewed. This review concludes with a discussion regarding ethical and religious concerns and suggestions on how families of patients who may be brain dead might be optimally approached.

NEUROSURGERY CLINICS OF NORTH AMERICA

RELATED INTEREST

Critical Care Clinics, January 2013 (Vol. 29, Issue 1)
Enhancing the Quality of Care in the ICU
Robert C. Hyzy, MD, *Editor*
http://www.criticalcare.theclinics.com/

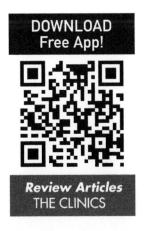

NOW AVAILABLE FOR YOUR iPhone and iPad

Preface
Neurocritical Care in Neurosurgery

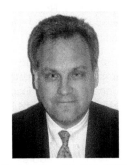

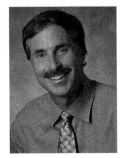

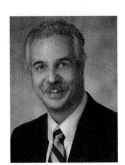

Paul A. Nyquist, MD, MPH, FCCM, FAHA, FANA

Marek A. Mirski, MD, PhD

Rafael J. Tamargo, MD

Editors

Neurosurgery is a technologically sophisticated interdisciplinary specialty. Neurologic centers of excellence incorporate multidisciplinary approaches, including physicians and medical professionals having diverse expertise. In response, the neurocritical care unit (NCCU) has quickly become the point of care for all patients with severe neurologic injury in the tertiary Neuroscience center. Patients treated in the NCCU include not only ventilated patients but also neurologic patients requiring specific neurologic interventions such as ICP monitoring and hypothermia. This has resulted in a body of knowledge that distinguishes Neurocritical care as a distinct field within critical care, with specialty-trained, neuroscience-focused physicians operating in multidisciplinary teams. As the terrain in clinical neurosciences becomes more complex, the issues surrounding the care of neurosurgical patients becomes more challenging. The proliferation of NCCUs and a still-palpable lack of detailed understanding of the medical management concerns of these patients have fueled the need for a variety of educational forums on this topic.

In this issue of the *Neurosurgery Clinics of North America*, we have focused on Neurologic Critical Care. We have chosen a variety of topics that are essential to the care of patients in the NCCU. Clinicians who work in the NCCU must master both general and neurologic ICU technologies that often

are the focus of other subspecialties. We have included sections that meet these challenges. Neurosurgeons and clinicians working in the NCCU need to understand the appropriate management of ventilators and the proper use of devices to monitor intracranial pressure. We have provided comprehensive reviews designed to update knowledge about these devices as well as new devices, including microdialysis and parenchymal brain oxygen sensors. These new technologies increasingly allow for more optimal management of physiologic parameters affecting the metabolic state of the brain. Knowledge about the use and interpretation of transcranial Dopplers (TCD) has long been an NCCU mainstay. TCDs are used for the diagnosis of intracranial disorders such as vasospasm. New studies have clarified the appropriate use of TCD in the NCCU. We have included commentary from some of the leading international experts on TCDs. Hypothermia is now used in cardiac ICUs as well as neuro ICUs. In addition to improving outcomes in cardiac arrest, it is frequently used in patients to reduce refractory ICP and has potential efficacy in other types of brain injury. We have included information focused on its present applications in the NCCU including techniques and strategies based on the practical experiences of leaders in the field.

The care of critically ill patients with neurosurgical and neurologic diagnoses can be quite

Neurosurg Clin N Am 24 (2013) xiii–xiv
http://dx.doi.org/10.1016/j.nec.2013.02.006
1042-3680/13/$ – see front matter © 2013 Published by Elsevier Inc.

challenging and we hope this issue enables the reader to apply current concepts to care for this interesting and challenging group of patients. We wish to thank our colleagues in the field of Neurosurgery and Critical Care Neurology who made this issue possible. It is through their dedication to academic and clinical pursuits that we were able to complete this issue of the *Neurosurgery Clinics of North America*. We would also like to thank Jessica McCool for her expert editorial skills, administrative efficiency, and good humor. We also thank the publishers at Elsevier for their support and interest in producing this volume.

Paul A. Nyquist, MD, MPH, FCCM, FAHA, FANA
The Johns Hopkins Hospital
Department of Neurology
Meyer 8-140
600 North Wolfe Street
Baltimore, MD 21287, USA

Marek A. Mirski, MD, PhD
Neurosciences Critical Care Unit
Division of Neurosciences
Critical Care
The Johns Hopkins Medical Institutions
The Johns Hopkins Hospital
Meyer Building, Room 8-140
600 N. Wolfe Street
Baltimore, MD 21287, USA

Rafael J. Tamargo, MD
Department of Neurosurgery
The Johns Hopkins Hospital
Zayed Tower 6115G
1800 Orleans Street
Baltimore, MD 21287, USA

E-mail addresses:
pnyquis1@jhmi.edu (P.A. Nyquist)
mmirski@jhmi.edu (M.A. Mirski)
rtamarg@jhmi.edu (R.J. Tamargo)

Moderate and Severe Traumatic Brain Injury
Pathophysiology and Management

Anthony R. Frattalone, MD[a,b],
Geoffrey S.F. Ling, MD, PhD[a,b],*

KEYWORDS

- Traumatic brain injury • Clinical practice guidelines • Head injury • Concussion • Coma
- ICP (intracranial pressure) • CPP (cerebral perfusion pressure)

KEY POINTS

- Traumatic brain injury (TBI) is a treatable condition.
- Early diagnosis of TBI is critical.
- Clinical practice guidelines (CPGs) are available to help clinical management across the spectrum of TBI severity.
- Optimal outcome depends on proper care beginning prehospital and continuing in an advanced clinical care setting by appropriately trained medical providers.

INTRODUCTION

TBI is pervasive and is a leading cause of death and disability, particularly in young people. Despite widespread use of preventative devices, such as helmets, seatbelts, and airbags, moderate to severe TBI disables 80,000 persons per year. A significant percentage of these patients require intensive neurologic management, including neurosurgery. Several CPGs have been written to help guide physicians in managing these complex patients. The most widely used are the Brain Trauma Foundation CPGs. Despite lack of evidence from randomized clinical trials (RCTs) to support every recommendation, CPGs provide a rational approach for treating this complicated group of patients. Moreover, there is emerging evidence that suggests improved outcomes when these CPGs are followed and specialized neurocritical care teams are providing the primary clinical care.[1–4]

PATHOPHYSIOLOGY

TBI is understood to be the result of 2 phases: initial neuronal injury followed by secondary insults. Initial neuronal injury occurs immediately and is due to the inciting traumatic event, whereas the second or late phase occurs from multiple neuropathologic processes and evolves over a period of minutes to days.

Because the primary injury phase is immediate, it is not easily treatable. In the most severe cases, this phase of injury may be deadly. Direct impact of parenchymal tissue against the bony vault of the skull leads to both neuronal and vascular

Disclaimer: The opinions expressed herein belong solely to the authors. They should neither be interpreted as belonging to nor endorsed by the Uniformed Services University of the Health Sciences, the US Army, the Department of Defense, or any other agency of the US federal government.
[a] Division of Neurocritical Care, Department of Anesthesiology and Critical Care Medicine, Johns Hopkins Medical Institutions, 600 N. Wolfe St, Baltimore, MD 21287, USA; [b] Department of Neurology, Uniformed Services University of the Health Sciences, 4301 Jones Bridge Rd, Bethesda, MD 20814, USA
* Corresponding author. US Army, 4301 Jones Bridge Road, Bethesda, MD 20814.
E-mail address: geoffrey.ling@usuhs.edu

Neurosurg Clin N Am 24 (2013) 309–319
http://dx.doi.org/10.1016/j.nec.2013.03.006
1042-3680/13/$ – see front matter Published by Elsevier Inc.

injuries. Lesions may be identified at both the side of collision as well as the opposite side, causing coup-contrecoup lesions. Moreover, rotational forces may lead to additional injuries, including diffuse axonal injury. Diffuse axonal injury is shearing of axons in cerebral white matter, causing neurologic deficits, such as encephalopathy. The consequences of this type of injury can be delayed by up to 12 hours after initial trauma. In cases of penetrating brain injury, skull fracture is present in addition to an injury tract. If the penetration is due to a high-velocity fragment, such as a bullet, there is superimposed tissue cavitation and possibly ricochet injury. Finally, diffuse microvascular damage occurs and is due to an early loss of cerebral vascular autoregulation and a loss of blood-brain barrier integrity.

Several types of bleeding complications are possible after TBI and often coexist, including subdural hematoma, epidural hematoma, intra-parenchymal hemorrhage, contusion, and traumatic subarachnoid hemorrhage. Subdural hematoma is the most common reason for ICU admission for head injury and constitutes approximately 50% of all TBI admissions; epidural hematoma accounts for approximately 3%. Skull fracture, especially in the temporal or parietal region, is an important cause of epidural hematoma, usually in association with laceration of the middle meningeal artery.

Focal injuries occur at the site of impact, often identified by neuroimaging as contusion or hematoma. The orbitofrontal and anterior temporal lobes are most commonly affected. Neurologic deficits are typically (but not exclusively) referable to the functions of those areas. The development of delayed hematoma formation may take up to several days after the initial injury.

The delayed nature of secondary injuries allows for medical and surgical intervention and has become a major focus of TBI treatment.[5,6] Injury at this level involves both neurons and glia. Many cellular processes are implicated in this phase, ultimately resulting in neuronal suicide. These mechanisms include hypoxia, ischemia, effects of free radicals, excitatory amino acids, certain ions (eg, calcium), ischemia, metabolic crisis, and inflammation.[7]

Inflammation has proved a critical element of the secondary TBI process. Within the central nervous system, the inflammatory process is activated almost instantaneously and undergoes a series of events, including expression of adhesion molecules, cellular infiltration, and additional secretion of inflammatory molecules and growth factors, causing either regeneration or cell death. Most likely, this inflammatory cascade is both helpful and deleterious to an injured brain and thus remains a critical area for research.[8]

Hypoxic and hypoperfusion injury is well recognized as a leading contributor to secondary brain injury. The injured brain is more susceptible to hypoxic-ischemic states, with changes in cerebral autoregulation exacerbating injury. Delayed neurologic deterioration is often caused by ischemic injury. Finally, posttraumatic vasospasm is thought a common occurrence and may worsen ischemic burden.[9]

Despite the advances made in understanding mechanisms of TBI, no single specific treatment has been shown to halt or reverse the chain of events leading to neuronal death. Thus, the clinical emphasis in severe TBI treatment remains supportive based on an understanding of intracranial anatomy and pathophysiology.

INTRACRANIAL DYNAMICS

The intracranial volume is relatively fixed and surrounded by an inelastic skull. The contents of the intracranial vault that contribute to intracranial pressure (ICP) are the brain (1300 mL), blood (110 mL), and cerebrospinal fluid (CSF) (65 mL).[10] Normal ICP in healthy adults is approximately 10 mm Hg.[11] The Monro-Kellie doctrine states that the intracranial contents are encased in a rigid skull and the components are relatively inelastic, so change in the volume of one component must be compensated for by reduction in the volume of another component of the system or ICP increases. Although this is a simplification of the complex pathophysiology involved, the Monro-Kellie doctrine provides a conceptual framework for understanding increased ICP causes and treatments in the context of TBI.

The brain parenchyma is made up largely of water, which is not compressible.[12] CSF, which contributes 10% of the intracranial volume, is produced predominantly by the choroid plexus, with a small amount produced as interstitial fluid from brain capillaries.[13] Approximately 10 mL/h to 20 mL/h of CSF is produced normally, and this amount is not significantly reduced by increased ICP.[14] CSF is taken up into the cerebral venous sinuses and drained through the arachnoid villi.[15] Intracranial blood volume, approximately 10% of the volume within the skull, is approximately two-thirds venous and one-third arterial. Flow of arterial blood is regulated largely by change in arteriolar caliber, which adjusts in response to systemic arterial pressure, Po_2, and Pco_2. When brain injury occurs and space-occupying lesions develop, the body must adjust its volumes of blood, CSF, and brain to compensate. In states of poor compliance, however, a seemingly insignificant increase in intracranial volume can result in a dramatic increase in ICP. Ultimately, if ICP increases beyond mean arterial pressure (MAP), arterial blood is unable to enter the skull, and global ischemia and cerebral ensue.

TRIAGE

When evaluating patients with known or suspected TBI, one must be able to effectively perform triage and assess quickly for proper initial management. Patients may be stratified as at low risk, moderate risk, or high risk for intracranial injury, using several criteria. Those with mild and nonprogressive headache and dizziness without loss of consciousness and normal neurologic examinations may be managed safely without neuroimaging. Close clinical monitoring with frequent neurologic examinations suffice. Under these conditions, it is imperative to withhold medications that may impair consciousness and responsiveness and thus interfere with clinical examinations. Examples of medications to avoid are central-acting analgesics and sedatives.

For patients with moderate risk to high risk for intracranial injury, CT head without contrast is recommended. This group of patients includes those with a history of a change in consciousness, alcohol or drug intoxication, posttraumatic seizure, vomiting, amnesia, or unreliable history.[16] Moreover, these patients should be transferred to a hospital with neurocritical care and neurosurgical services.

Most commonly, TBI patients are classified according to severity scores, such as the Glasgow Coma Scale (GCS). Using this scale, a score of 13 to 15 is considered mild injury, 9 to 12 moderate, and 8 or less severe TBI.[17] Although easy to use, the GCS is limited by its inability to take into account sedation, paralysis, intubation, or intoxication and may overestimate injury severity in these patients.[18] A newer scoring system, the Full Outline of Unresponsiveness Score, was developed to improve on these problems. Unlike the GSC, the Full Outline of Unresponsiveness Score includes a brainstem examination and is better performed on intubated patients.[19–21]

All TBI patients with persistent impairment of consciousness should be admitted to an ICU. A brief but thorough neurologic examination should be performed, with emphasis on level of arousal and orientation, GCS score, pupils and other cranial nerves, and basic language and motor function. Afterwards, these patients should promptly receive a noncontrast CT scan of the head. While reading the CT, special attention should be given for the presence of parenchymal abnormalities, such as contusion or edema, as well as skull or facial fractures. Contusions are often detected in areas of the brain that make contact with bony prominences, such as the frontal, temporal, and occipital poles. Additionally, small contusions may evolve into hemorrhages, which should be considered if clinical deterioration occurs because it might lead to herniation. A normal CT scan does not preclude a severe neurologic injury; if a patient's neurologic examination is abnormal, it must be assumed that a severe brain injury has occurred until proved otherwise. Repeat imaging should be strongly considered with any neurologic changes.

EMERGENCY DEPARTMENT AND NEUROCRITICAL CARE UNIT MANAGEMENT

Both neurologic and functional outcomes may be improved by first avoiding hypoxemia, hypercapnia, and hypovolemia.[1,16,22] In severe TBI, advanced trauma life support and brain resuscitation for TBI principles merge. Hypoxia, defined as Pao_2 less than 60 mm Hg, and hypotension, defined as systolic blood pressure less than 90 mm Hg, are common in general trauma and in TBI. Hypoxia and hypotension are present in 50% and 30% of severe TBI patients, respectively. Management must focus on correcting these problems immediately to optimize outcome.[23–25]

All trauma patients with severe TBI should be placed in a rigid cervical collar. There are 2 reasons for this. The first is to protect the cervical spinal cord and column until it is ascertained that neither is injured. Between 2% and 6% of TBI patients who reach the emergency department have cervical spine fracture. Surprisingly, iatrogenic damage to the spinal cord is estimated as high as 25% of those suffering from combined TBI and cervical cord injury. The other reason for the collar is to optimize cerebral venous drainage by maintaining the head in a midline position to minimize exacerbation of any intracranial hypertension. Caution should be used to not overtighten the collar because this impairs venous drainage.[26,27] Finally, the head of the bed should always be maintained at 30°, again to optimize venous drainage.

Endotracheal intubation by well-trained personnel in the emergency department or ICU setting is recommended for patients with a GCS score of 8 or less. The potential benefit of prehospital intubation for such patients remains controversial after conflicting results of 2 major studies.[28,29] The presence of an intact gag reflex should not deter from intubation. Intubation may have a deleterious effect on a TBI patient's ICP. Even simply laryngoscopy has been shown to cause a reflex sympathetic response, releasing catecholamines and thus increasing systemic blood pressure, which may worsen ICP.[30,31]

Many experts prefer rapid sequence intubation as a technique to secure the airway in TBI patients, but no RCT has been done to support this practice. Potential advantages of rapid sequence intubation are blunting of the sympathetic response, preoxygenation, and possibly a lower risk of aspiration. Because most comatose patients have intact gag reflexes, sympathetic responses occur and may have harmful effects.[32] A common practice is to use lidocaine to blunt the gag response to intubation but it has not been conclusively shown either good or bad.[33,34] A single dose of a very short-acting opioid, such as fentanil or sufentanil, in select cases may prove helpful minimize the response but this benefit must be weighed against the potential for worsened hypotension or premature respiratory depression.

Once definitive airway control is obtained, hypercarbia can be managed. A clear goal is to treat hypercarbia immediately, which is achieved by properly controlling minute ventilation. Continuous end-tidal carbon dioxide monitoring can be helpful in guiding mechanical ventilator adjustments. If there is increased ICP, then hyperventilation may be tried. Although widely used, this treatment option has potential for worsening the clinical state. Hyperventilation leads to cerebral vasoconstriction, which potentially exacerbates ischemia.[35,36] If used, the goal should be hyperventilation to Pco_2 34 mm Hg to 36 mm Hg as a temporary measure while arranging for more definitive therapies, such as hyperosmotic therapy or neurosurgical intervention. Hyperventilation without evidence of increased ICP or impending herniation should not be done. It has been shown that prophylactic hyperventilation worsens outcomes, possibly by lowering cerebral blood flow (CBF) and worsening ischemia.

After intubation, a portable chest radiograph should be obtained to confirm appropriate endotracheal tube placement and evaluate for signs of aspiration. Aspiration is a common problem in TBI patients and may lead to poor oxygenation or acute respiratory distress syndrome.

Positive end-expiratory pressure (PEEP) should be used judiciously in TBI patients. If needed to improve oxygenation, then the lowest level should be used that achieves clinical goals. High PEEP, however, can impair cardiac venous return, which may decrease cerebral venous drainage and thus worsen ICP. Studies on PEEP have shown that the impact of PEEP on ICP and cerebral perfusion

pressure (CPP) varies greatly among TBI patients, necessitating close monitoring and individual tailoring of this therapy.[38]

In cases of suspected elevated ICP, central venous access is needed. This catheter can be used to deliver hypersomolar saline solutions that are 3% or higher because these solutions can cause venous phlebitis. Also, vasopressors may be needed to meet CPP goals. Finally, a central venous catheter allows measurement of central venous pressure. Central venous pressure is important for providing a measurement of intravascular volume state. Volume management is an important aspect of trauma care.

Many experts recommend avoiding internal jugular catheters because compression or clot of this vessel may increase ICP. Also, placing this line requires putting patients in the Trendelenburg position. In this head-down position, ICP increases due to cerebral venous congestion. The femoral vein approach is safer than the subclavian but has a higher likelihood of infection. Thus, the subclavian approach is preferable.

Other accesses recommended are an arterial catheter and gastric tube. A radial arterial catheter should be inserted to allow optimal cerebral perfusion pressure management and frequent blood sampling. A feeding tube is needed. For this purpose, an orogastric tube should be used rather than a nasogastric tube until skull base and facial fractures are safely ruled out.

As discussed previously, hypotension must be prevented and treated aggressively. Studies reveal a direct correlation between negative fluid balance and worse neurologic outcome in TBI patients.[39] On admission, unless there is clinical evidence to the contrary, patients should be treated as though they are intravascularly depleted. Hypotension should be considered the result of hypovolemia or acute blood loss rather than a manifestation of TBI. In spinal cord injury, however, hypotension is frequently the result of compromised sympathetic tone. Fluid resuscitation using isotonic crystalloids is generally recommended to meet intravascular volume goals. Prehospital hypertonic saline resuscitation has been effective in some settings, such as the battlefield, but studies do not support its use in the civilian setting.[40,41] A randomized study of albumin for volume resuscitation suggests increased mortality and thus is not recommended.[42,43] In cases of elevated ICP, hypertonic saline solutions are considered. Hypotension in these cases is defined as a systolic blood pressure less than 100 mm Hg or, in cases of intracranial hypertension, a cerebral perfusion pressure less than 70 mm Hg.

At the other extreme, severe hypertension is dangerous in this patient population. It has been shown to be predictive of mortality and pneumonia.[44] Under these circumstances, blood pressure should be quickly lowered with agents, such as intravenous (IV) labetalol, nicardipine, or enalaprilat, because these agents have not been shown to cause elevations in ICP.

A thorough laboratory work-up, including complete blood cell count, electrolytes, glucose, coagulation parameters, blood alcohol level, pregnancy test (when appropriate), and urine toxicology, should be sent as soon as possible because these factors may dramatically influence a patient's treatment plan. Electroencephalography (EEG), either intermittent or continuous, is highly recommended because nonconvulsive seizures have been detected in 23% of moderate to severe TBI patients and are associated with the development of hippocampal atrophy.[45]

ADDITIONAL IMAGING

Initial neuroimaging that is normal does not preclude development of delayed lesion, such as edema or hemorrhage. Frontal or temporal contusions often worsen a day or 2 after the initial event. This is commonly caused by edema formation or hemorrhage, both of which can lead to fatal brainstem compression. Temporal contusions classically enlarge and cause uncal herniation.

It is recommended to repeat neuroimaging after several hours if there is any clinical deterioration or if a coagulopathy is present. Close attention should be paid for subarachnoid blood, which may be traumatic or due to aneurysmal rupture. A patient found down and thought to have suffered a TBI may have had a spontaneous subarachnoid hemorrhage from a ruptured cerebral aneurysm. Thus, if clinically suspicious, angiography should be considered in select cases to evaluate for underlying vascular malformation, such as aneurysm.

Although MRI provides much higher fidelity brain and spinal cord images than CT, these additional data are rarely helpful in guiding initial resuscitation. For this reason, CT is adequate. Once stable, however, the patients should undergo MRI. Typically, this is a day or 2 after admission. MRI may clarify and highlight regions of edema, microhemorrhages, or infarction. Newer sequences, such as gradient-recalled echo, susceptibility-weighted imaging, diffusion-weighted imaging, and diffusion tensor imaging, provide greater sensitivity for specific types of injury and hold potential for better prognostic tools in the future.[46] Either CT or MRI of the cervical spine should be considered in all severe TBI patients based on clinical suspicion.

INTRACRANIAL HYPERTENSION AFTER TBI

Most severe TBI patients develop intracranial hypertension as defined as ICP greater than 20 mm Hg. Consequently, TBI patients with GCS score of 8 or less after resuscitation should be considered as having this condition until direct ICP measurement proves otherwise. Because these patients typically have severely compromised neurologic examinations, thus limiting an examiner's ability to detect deterioration, ICP monitoring becomes a tool for assessing clinical worsening. Sustained elevations in ICP generally herald ongoing secondary injury, such as cerebral edema, hemorrhage, hydrocephalus, or ischemia, and, as a consequence, the management of ICP has become a foundation of neurocritical care. Several studies provide evidence that there is a correlation between the extent and duration of ICP elevation and poor outcomes after TBI.[47] Despite this association, evidence is lacking that supports the notion that ICP management improves clinical outcome. Because the brain is anatomically compartmentalized, herniation syndromes may occur without associated changes in global ICP. An example is after posterior fossa hemorrhage, there may be brainstem herniation without changes in ICP above the tentorium.

CPP, which is the difference of ICP and mean arterial pressure, is generally used to understand the connection between systemic circulatory function and CBF. CPP has become a surrogate for determining adequacy of brain perfusion. CPP is a global measure and does not provide any insight into regional differences in perfusion. Normal subjects autoregulate CBF. In an uninjured state, CBF is constant at 50 mL/100 g tissue/min across a wide range of MAP. At least one-third of TBI patients, however, have abnormal cerebral autoregulation. When this occurs, such patients have pressure passive perfusion. CBF varies directly with changes in MAP. With increased MAP, CBF increases leading to increased cerebral blood volume and, thus, increased ICP. Conversely lower MAPs may cause hypoperfusion and ischemia.[48,49] For this reason, a goal CPP between 50 mm Hg and 70 mm Hg is usually targeted. This value has been chosen because it allows sufficient pressure to overcome the elevated ICP while avoiding problems with hypertension.

CPGs recommend ICP monitoring in patients with severe TBI who are comatose (GCS score <9) after resuscitation and who either have abnormalities on CT scan or meet at least 2 of the following 3 criteria: age greater than 40 years, systolic blood pressure less than 90 mm Hg, or motor posturing.[50] Optimally, ICP is measured by devices placed inside the brain—intraventricular or intraparenchymal monitors. Intraventricular catheters or extraventricular drains are favored by most neurocritical care specialists because these devices allow for therapeutic drainage and sampling of CSF. Such ICP monitoring devices are resource intensive. They also carry a small but significant risk of infection and hemorrhage and, in cases of intraparenchymal monitors, are prone to drift over time. Other options that require less maintenance and have lower infection risks but that do not allow for therapeutic drainage of CSF are the subdural bolt, intraparenchymal fiber-optic ICP monitor, and the epidural ICP monitor.

ICP may not be the only important intracranial variable that should be measured. Studies of TBI patients with parenchymal oxygen or microdialysis probes have shown that brain tissue hypoxia and metabolic distress occur independently of ICP or CPP.[51,52] Ischemia occurs in some patients at apparently adequate CPP levels.[50,53,54] Critics of ICP monitors are quick to point out that clinical outcome-based studies are mixed regarding the impact of ICP monitoring. Some studies evaluating protocol-driven care of severe TBI, including ICP monitoring, have shown benefit; others suggest that ICP monitoring may be associated with increased mortality, greater therapeutic intensity, and longer length of stay in the ICU.[22,55,56] In spite of the shortcomings of ICP-directed therapy, none of the other variables has been shown similar. To date, there are no RCTs that provide convincing evidence that using tissue oxygen, microdialysis, or any other modality improves outcome. All of this highlights the need for more research focused on individualized treatment protocols that may be based on multiple modality monitoring.

Because the current CPGs recommend using ICP monitoring principally, then an important treatment goal is to maintain the ICP less than 20 mm Hg and the CPP between 50 mm Hg and 70 mm Hg. If ICP remains poorly controlled after intubation with controlled ventilation and head-of-bed elevation, then mannitol should be given in a dose of 0.5 g/kg to 1 g/kg through either a peripheral or central vein. This therapy usually takes approximately 15 to 30 minutes to have an effect on ICP. Repeat boluses every 6 hours can be given. Some experts recommend using a serum osmolarity goal of 310 mOsm/L to 320 mOsm/L to achieve optimal effect. Renal function and fluid balance should be monitored while using mannitol because this is a diuretic. Osmotic diuresis occurs as does a lowering of the serum sodium level. Fluid balance can be restored using saline solutions. Studies suggest that mannitol not only lowers ICP but also improves CBF to hypoperfused areas of the brain in patients with high ICP.[57]

An increasingly popular therapy is hypertonic saline. This therapy has the advantage of increasing serum sodium and, thus, serum osmolarity without causing diuresis. It is especially useful when faced with a TBI patient who has compromised intravascular volume, such as from hemorrhagic shock. For hyperacute ICP and herniation treatment, 23% hypertonic saline is administered through a central venous line. Up to 50% reduction in ICP can occur. The onset of effect is within minutes and the effect lasts for a few hours. For prolonged therapy, a continuous IV infusion of 2% or 3% hypertonic saline is used starting at 75 mL/h and titrating as needed. The objective should be achieving an ICP goal or a desired serum osmolarity. If concentrated sodium solutions are used, sodium chloride and sodium acetate should be used as a 50/50 mix to minimize hyperchloremic metabolic acidosis. When compared with mannitol, no significant differences have been found with respect to the extent of reduction of ICP or duration of action.[37]

If initial ICP-lowering interventions are unsuccessful, pharmacologic coma or surgical decompression should be considered. The proposed effect of pharmacologic coma on ICP is via reduction of cerebral metabolic rate of oxygen, often by induction of pentobarbital coma. A few studies suggest that barbiturates are effective at reducing ICP but their effect on long-term outcomes is not clear.[58] A retrospective study of severe TBI patients with refractory intracranial hypertension treated with pentobarbital coma showed 40% survival rates with 68% of those patients achieving good functional outcomes.[59]

If the decision to use pharmacologic coma is made, pentobarbital can be administered at a loading dose of 5 mg/kg IV, followed by an infusion of 1 mg/kg/h to 3 mg/kg/h. The loading dose is 2 mg/kg IV followed by an infusion up to 200 μg/min. Continuous EEG monitoring is recommended to attain a goal of burst suppression. Decisions to initiate pharmacologic coma should not be taken lightly or in patients lacking hemodynamic stability. Pentobarbital coma carries well-known side effects, including hypotension, hypocalcemia, hepatic and renal dysfunction, and increased susceptibility for sepsis.

Propofol is another option to produce coma and has the advantage of a much shorter half-life. Propofol use often results in hypotension requiring vasopressor support and, if used for a prolonged period, may cause the rare but deadly propofol nfusion syndrome. An advantage of propofol over pentobarbital is its short half-life, allowing for wake-ups to perform neurologic examinations. Despite its widespread use, there has been some concern after a study suggested that propofol was unable to reduce ischemic burden from TBI in spite of achieving EEG burst suppression.[60]

For the past few decades, decompressive craniectomy has been used for control of refractory ICP. A recent landmark RCT—Decompressive Craniectomy (DECRA)—compared bilateral decompressive craniectomy with standard medical therapy and failed, however, to show superior 6-month neurologic outcomes after surgery.[61] Critics of this study state that the results are not generalizable because the ICP in the standard-care group was not severely elevated enough and many patients who underwent surgery did not have refractory high ICP. Consequently, this study does not invalidate the practice of resorting to decompressive craniectomy after a longer period of refractory ICP. Moreover, the study did not evaluate patients with unilateral craniectomy or those with focal space-occupying lesions, such as hematomas.

TBI patients are seriously ill; thus, meeting CPP goals may be difficult using IV fluids alone. If so, vasoactive pharmacologic agents, such as norepinephrine and phenylephrine, may be required. These 2 agents are preferred because they are considered to have the least effect on cerebral vasomotor tone. Invasive hemodynamic monitoring with a central venous pressure catheter to ascertain intravascular fluid state should be done concomitantly. It should be remembered that barbiturates and propofol are myocardial depressants and, thus, aggressive cardiovascular management probably is necessary in the event of pharmacologic coma. High CPP goals (>70 mm Hg) should be avoided due to an increased risk of developing acute respiratory distress syndrome.

VENOUS THROMBOEMBOLISM PROPHYLAXIS

Severe TBI patients are at increased risk for venous thromboembolism. Antiembolic stockings and pneumatic compression devices should be used. The risk of worsened intracranial hemorrhage with chemoprophylactic therapy for thromboembolic disease is controversial and should be approached on a case-by-case basis. Although retrospective analyses suggest that early chemoprophylactic therapy is safe in this population, there has not been an RCT.[62] Therefore, the CPGs do not give recommendations on agent preference, dosing, or timing of chemoprophylaxis. If patients are deemed unsuited for chemoprophylaxis or develop a thrombosis, an inferior vena cava filter may be placed. Although hopefully reducing the risk of embolism from the lower extremities, these filters themselves can be a nidus for clot and are by no means a guarantee against pulmonary embolism. Thus, they should be used as a temporary measure only. Screening duplex ultrasound studies of the legs should be done whenever there is clinical suspicion to DVT development.

SEIZURES

Prophylactic use of antiepileptic is not recommended for preventing late posttraumatic seizures. Antiepileptics are indicated on admission and for the first week, however, to decrease the incidence of early posttraumatic seizures. The incidence of early posttraumatic seizures (first week) is reported between 10% and 30% for severe TBI patients.[63,64] Seizures may aggravate secondary brain injury or increase ICP. As discussed previously, a low index of suspicion should be used when deciding to obtain EEG monitoring in brain-injured patients due to the high risk of both convulsive and nonconvulsive seizures.

STEROIDS

Steroid use is contraindicated in TBI. These drugs have not been shown to decrease ICP or improve clinical outcome. They have been shown to increase risk of infection, hyperglycemic state, and metabolic derangement.

NUTRITION

Initially, an orogastric tube should be inserted to decompress the stomach and reduce the aspiration risk. Typically, the nasal route is avoided because it can perforate through a skull base fracture or obstruct sinus drainage.

TBI patients have increased metabolic demands, so feeding should begin as soon as tolerated. Nutritional target goals should be met by day 7 per the CPG. Early enteral or parenteral feeding with the aim of providing at least 140% of the basal metabolic caloric needs each day. Although enteral feeding is generally preferred over the parenteral route, there are data to suggest that parenteral feeding in this population is safe with the exception of mildly worsened hyperglycemia.[65] Studies have shown that TBI patients treated with barbiturate coma often develop severe ileus, which rarely improves with postpyloric feeding. Thus, in this population, switching to parenteral nutrition should be strongly considered.[66]

POSITIONING

In patients with increased ICP, frequent turning and repositioning may not be possible because small position changing movements may lead to increased ICP. It is important to keep the head of the bed elevated at least 30° with the patient's neck in neutral alignment. This position also decreases the risk of aspiration and thus ventilator-associated pneumonia. When faced with a TBI patient with impaired oxygenation and ventilation, using a kinetic therapy bed or even a prone position may need to be considered. Measures should be in place to prevent skin breakdown.

BRAIN OXYGEN MONITORING

Continuous brain oxygen monitoring is accomplished by inserting a small probe through the skull into the parenchyma or by insertion of a jugular bulb catheter. Neither technique is optimal. The parenchymal monitor only samples a small discrete region of brain. The jugular bulb monitor is a measure of global brain oxygenation and, thus, is insensitive to focal areas of pathology. Both monitors within their limits, however, do provide some information of adequacy of perfusion. These data are complementary to ICP and CPP because it has been shown that brain tissue oxygenation varies independently of cerebral hemodynamics and ICP.[67] Because no RCT evidence exists to support or refute the clinical use of brain oxygen monitors, CPGs do not recommend the routine use of brain oxygen monitors in TBI patients but do define oxygen thresholds with a level III recommendation. Treatment thresholds for these devices are less than 15 mm Hg for partial pressure of brain parenchyma oxygen and less than 50% for jugular bulb oxygen saturation. An RCT of these devices (the BOOST [the BOOST or Brain Tissue Oxygen Monitoring in Traumatic Brain Injury project] project) will evaluate the value of these techniques. Currently, abnormally low brain oxygen levels are associated with poor outcome but it is not known whether treating low levels is efficaacious.[68,69]

CEREBRAL MICRODIALYSIS

Cerebral microdialysis is a technique that uses a catheter with a fine double-lumen probe lined with a semipermeable membrane that is placed in the interstitial space to sample local brain chemistry. It is placed inside a lesion, perilesion, or normal brain. It is most often placed in perilesion brain tissue, which is most vulnerable to secondary injury. The objective is to detect neurochemical changes associated with secondary brain injury. Cerebral microdialysis measures interstitial glucose, lactate, glycerol, and glutamate, among others. Studies by Belli[70] and Vespa[71] have shown that microchemical changes precede the development of intracranial hypertension. Disadvantages to cerebral microdialysis include wide variability over time, invasive nature, and cost. Advantages, however, include individualized, real-time assessment of local cerebral metabolism. Like brain oxygen monitoring, this is a potentially promising technique, which presently lacks evidence to endorse a CPG recommendation for its use. Further research is needed on this topic, including RCT.

FEVER AND HYPOTHERMIA

Fever is common in TBI patients and is associated with worse outcome and accelerated neuronal damage. Additionally, it has been shown that intracranial temperature and core temperature are not equal with intracranial temperature, often significantly exceeding core temperature.[72] Thus, it is advised to treat fever aggressively with a goal of normothermia. Acetaminophen, cooling blankets, or cooling jackets are common effective techniques to cool patients. In addition, there should be a low index of suspicion for infection and atelectasis for which appropriate evaluation and, if appropriate, treatment should be instituted.

Hypothermia has been used as a treatment of high ICP as well as a prophylactic treatment to arrest ongoing secondary brain injury. The CPGs do not support, however, routine prophylaxis with hypothermia. This is because as a treatment of high ICP, hypothermia studies have yielded mixed results. One large study of 392 patients did not show any benefit whereas another demonstrated modest improvement. Overall, hypothermia may be helpful in reducing death and unfavorable outcomes for TBI patients, but conclusive evidence for significant benefit remains elusive.[73] Because some studies suggest benefit among certain patient populations, this therapy is considered an option but should be reserved for those practitioners familiar with narrow indications.

HYPERGLYCEMIA

Hyperglycemia is associated with worse outcome in TBI, leading to the conclusion by many that strict glucose control could improve outcome.[74,75] This assumption has been recently questioned based on a cerebral microdialysis study that linked strict glucose control to reduced cerebral glucose availability, correlating with worse outcome.[76] It is not clear whether treatment of hyperglycemia improves or exacerbates outcomes in TBI. Because of this limited understanding, a prudent approach is to avoid extremes of blood glucose levels by targeting levels to 140 mg/dL to180 mg/dL.

DYSAUTONOMIA

Episodic dysautonomia after TBI is known as sympathetic storms, autonomic dysreflexia, and paroxysmal autonomic instability with dystonia. Occurring in 8% to 33% of patients with severe TBI, these are defined as paroxysmal episodes of tachycardia plus 2 of the following: fever, tachypnea, agitation, diaphoresis, or dystonia. Episodes are usually stimulus induced and often associated with marked hypertension and/or increased ICP. TBI patients with these storms have longer, more complicated hospital courses, but the effect on long-term outcomes is not yet fully understood.[77] Several different classes of medications, including γ-aminobutyric acid agonists, α-adrenergic agonists, β-adrenergic antagonists, and dopamine agonists, have been used successfully to treat these episodes. A recent retrospective review of β-blocker use in TBI suggested that there is a significant reduction in mortality, which the investigators attribute to control of the hyperadrenergic state.[78]

SUMMARY

Moderate to severe TBI is a serious condition. When managed by appropriate specialized neurocritical care teams using CPGs as treatment guides, most patients survive, with many achieving reasonable neurologic and functional outcomes. These CPGs are, however, continually evolving. As the underlying neurophysiologic and neurochemical bases of TBI are elucidated, clinical treatment will improve. Thus, patients can expect even better outcomes as this process advances.

REFERENCES

1. Patel H. Trends in head injury outcome from 1989 to 2003 and the effect of neurosurgical care: an observational study. Lancet 2005;366:1538.
2. Suarez J. Length of stay and mortality in neurocritically ill patients: impact of a specialized neurocritical care team. Crit Care Med 2004;32:2311.
3. Thillai M. Neurosurgical units working beyond safe capacity. BMJ 2000;320:399.
4. Varelas P. The impact of a neurointensivist-led team on a semiclosed neurosciences intensive care unit. Crit Care Med 2004;32:2191.
5. Chesnut R. The role of secondary brain injury in determining outcome from severe head injury. J Trauma 1993;34:216.
6. McHugh G. Prognostic value of secondary insults in traumatic brain injury: results from the IMPACT study. J Neurotrauma 2007;24:287.
7. Vespa P. Metabolic crisis without brain ischemia is common after traumatic brain injury: a combined microdialysis and positron emission tomography study. J Cereb Blood Flow Metab 2005;25:763.
8. Morganti-Kossmann M. Inflammatory response in acute traumatic brain injury: a double-edged sword. Curr Opin Crit Care 2002;8:101.
9. Oertel M. Posttraumatic vasospasm: the epidemiology, severity, and time course of an underestimated phenomenon: a prospective study performed in 299 patients. J Neurosurg 2005;103:812.
10. Manz HJ. Pathophysiology and pathology of elevated intracranial pressure. Pathobiol Annu 1979;9:359–81.
11. Wijdicks E. The practice of emergency and criical care neurology. New York: Oxford University Press; 2010.
12. Doczi T. Volume regulation of the brain tissue–a survey. Acta Neurochir (Wien) 1993;121(1–2):1–8.
13. McComb JG. Recent research into the nature of cerebrospinal fluid formation and absorption. J Neurosurg 1983;59(3):369–83.
14. Gjerris F. Pathophysiology of cerebrospinal fluid circulation. Oxford (United Kingdom): Blackwell Science; 2000.
15. Lyons MK, Meyer FB. Cerebrospinal fluid physiology and the management of increased intracranial pressure. Mayo Clin Proc 1990;65(5): 684–707.
16. Arienta C. Management of head-injured patients in the emergency department: a practice protocol. Surg Neurol 1997;48:213–9.
17. Balestreri M, Balestreri M, Czosnyka M, et al. Predictive value of Glasgow Coma Scale after brain trauma: change in trend over the past ten years. J Neurol Neurosurg Psychiatry 2004;75:161.
18. Stocchetti N. Inaccurate early assessment of neurological severity in head injury. J Neurotrauma 2004;21:1131.
19. Stead L, Stead LG, Wijdicks EF, et al. Validation of a new coma scale, the FOUR score, in the emergency department. Neurocrit Care 2009;10:50.
20. Wijdicks E. Validation of a new coma scale: the FOUR score. Ann Neurol 2005;58:585.
21. Eken C. Comparison of the Full Outline of Unresponsiveness Score Coma Scale and the Glasgow Coma Scale in an emergency setting population. Eur J Emerg Med 2009;16:29.
22. Shafi S. Intracranial pressure monitoring in brain-injured patients is associated with worsening of survival. J Trauma 2008;64:335–40.
23. Stocchetti N. Hypoxemia and arterial hypotension at the accident scene in head injury. J Trauma 1996;40:764.

24. Manley G. Hypotension, hypoxia, and head injury: frequency, duration, and consequences. Arch Surg 2001;136:1118.

25. Andrews P. Predicting recovery in patients suffering from traumatic brain injury by using admission variables and physiological data: a comparison between decision tree analysis and logistic regression. J Neurosurg 2002;97:326.

26. Stone M. The effect of rigid cervical collars on internal jugular vein dimensions. Acad Emerg Med 2010;17(1):100–2.

27. Raphael J. Effects of the cervical collar on cerebrospinal fluid pressure. Anaesthesia 1994;49(5):437–9.

28. Bernard S. Prehospital rapid sequence intubation improves functional outcome for patients with severe traumatic brain injury: a randomized controlled trial. Ann Surg 2010;252:959.

29. Davis D. The effect of paramedic rapid sequence intubation on outcome in patients with severe traumatic brain injury. J Trauma 2003;54:444.

30. Shribman A. Cardiovascular and catecholamine responses to laryngoscopy with and without tracheal intubation. Br J Anaesth 1987;59:295.

31. Stoelting R. Hemodynamic responses to tracheal intubation with laryngoscope versus lightwand intubating device (Trachlight) in adults with normal airway. Anesthesiology 1977;47:381.

32. Moulton C. Relation between Glasgow coma score and cough reflex. Lancet 1994;343:1261.

33. Butler J. Towards evidence based emergency medicine: best BETs from Manchester Royal Infirmary. Lignocaine premedication before rapid sequence induction in head injuries. Emerg Med J 2002;19:554.

34. Robinson N. In patients with head injury undergoing rapid sequence intubation, does pretreatment with intravenous lignocaine/lidocaine lead to an improved neurological outcome? A review of the literature. Emerg Med J 2001;18:453.

35. Muizelaar J. Adverse effects of prolonged hyperventilation in patients with severe head injury: a randomized clinical trial. J Neurosurg 1991;75:731.

36. Diringer M. No reduction in cerebral metabolism as a result of early moderate hyperventilation following severe traumatic brain injury. J Neurosurg 2000;92:7.

37. Sakellaridis N. Comparison of mannitol and hypertonic saline in the treatment of severe brain injuries. J Neurosurg 2011;114(2):545–8.

38. Zhang X. Impact of positive end-expiratory pressure on cerebral injury patients with hypoxemia. Am J Emerg Med 2011;29(7):699–703.

39. Clifton G. Fluid thresholds and outcome from severe brain injury. Crit Care Med 2002;30(4):739–45.

40. Cooper D. Prehospital hypertonic saline resuscitation of patients with hypotension and severe traumatic brain injury: a randomized controlled trial. JAMA 2004;291:1350.

41. Bulger E. Out-of-hospital hypertonic resuscitation following severe traumatic brain injury: a randomized controlled trial. JAMA 2010;304:1445.

42. Finfer S. A comparison of albumin and saline for fluid resuscitation in the intensive care unit. N Engl J Med 2004;350:2247–56.

43. Investigators SS. Saline or albumin for fluid resuscitation in patients with traumatic brain injury. N Engl J Med 2007;357:874.

44. Ley E. Elevated admission systolic blood pressure after blunt trauma predicts delayed pneumonia and mortality. J Trauma 2011;71(6):1689–93.

45. Vespa P. Nonconvulsive seizures after traumatic brain injury are associated with hippocampal atrophy. Neurology 2010;75(9):792–8.

46. Kubal W. Updated imaging of traumatic brain injury. Radiol Clin North Am 2012;50(1):15–41.

47. Juul N. Intracranial hypertension and cerebral perfusion pressure: influence on neurological deterioration and outcome in severehead injury. The Executive Committee of the International Selfotel Trial. J Neurosurg 2000;92:1–6.

48. Bouma G. Cerebral blood flow, cerebral blood volume, and cerebrovascular reactivity after severe head injury. J Neurotrauma 1992;9(1):S333.

49. Bouma G. Blood pressure and intracranial pressure-volume dynamics in severe head injury: relationship with cerebral blood flow. J Neurosurg 1992;77:15.

50. Bratton S. Guidelines for the management of severe traumatic brain injury. J Neurotrauma 2007;24:S1–106.

51. Chang J. Physiologic and functional outcome correlates of brain tissue hypoxia in traumatic brain injury. Crit Care Med 2009;37:283–90.

52. Vespa P. Pericontusional brain tissue exhibits persistent elevation of lactate/pyruvate ratio independent of cerebral perfusion pressure. Crit Care Med 2007;35:1153–60.

53. Czosnyka M. Cerebral autoregulation following head injury. J Neurosurg 2001;95:756–63.

54. Coles J. Incidence and mechanisms of cerebral ischemia in early clinical head injury. J Cereb Blood Flow Metab 2004;24:202–11.

55. Bulger E. Management of severe head injury: institutional variations in care and effect on outcome. Crit Care Med 2002;30:1870–6.

56. Cremer O. Effect of intracranial pressure monitoring and targeted intensive care on functional outcome after severe head injury. Crit Care Med 2005;33:2207–13.

57. Scalfani M. Effect of osmotic agents on regional cerebral blood flow in traumatic brain injury. J Crit Care 2012;27(5):526.e7–12.

58. Eisenberg H. High-dose barbiturate control of elevated intracranial pressure in patients with severe head injury. J Neurosurg 1988;69:15–23.

59. Marshall G. Pentobarbital coma for refractory intracranial hypertension after severe traumatic brain injury: mortality predictions and one-year outcomes in 55 patients. J Trauma 2010;69(2):275–83.

60. Johnston A. Effects of propofol on cerebral oxygenation and metabolism after head injury. Br J Anaesth 2003;91(6):781–6.

61. Cooper D. Decompressive craniectomy in diffuse traumatic brain injury. N Engl J Med 2011;364:1493.

62. Koehler D. Is early venous thromboembolism prophylaxis safe in trauma patients with intracranial hemorrhage? J Trauma 2011;70(2):324–9.

63. Temkin N. Risk factors for posttraumatic seizures in adults. Epilepsia 2003;44(10):18.

64. Frey L. Epidemiology of posttraumatic epilepsy: a critical review. Epilepsia 2003;44(10):11.

65. Meirelles CJ. Enteral or parenteral nutrition in traumatic brain injury: a prospective randomised trial. Nutr Hosp 2011;26(5):1120–4.

66. Bochicchio G. Tolerance and efficacy of enteral nutrition in traumatic brain-injured patients induced into barbiturate coma. JPEN J Parenter Enteral Nutr 2006;30(6):503–6.

67. Eriksson E. Cerebral perfusion pressure and intracranial pressure are not surrogates for brain tissue oxygenation in traumatic brain injury. Clin Neurophysiol 2012;123(6):1255–60.

68. Cruz J. On-line monitoring of global cerebral hypoxia in acute brain injury: relationship to intracranial hypertension. J Neurosurg 1993;79:228–33.

69. Sheinberg M. Continuous monitoring of jugular venous oxygen saturation in head-injured patients. J Neurosurg 1992;76:212–7.

70. Belli A, Sen J, Petzold A, et al. Metabolic failure precedes intracranial pressure rises in traumatic brain injury: a microdialysis study. Acta Neurochem (Wien) 2008;150:461–9.

71. Stein NR, McArthur DL, Etchepare M, et al. Early cerebral metabolic crisis after TBI influences outcome despite adequate hemodynamic resuscitation. Neurocrit Care 2011;32:1639–51.

72. Rossi S. Brain temperature, body core temperature, and intracranial pressure in acute cerebral damage. J Neurol Neurosurg Psychiatry 2001; 71(4):448–54.

73. Sydenham E. Hypothermia for traumatic head injury. Cochrane Database Syst Rev 2009;(2): CD001048.

74. Rovlias A. The influence of hyperglycemia on neurological outcome in patients with severe head injury. Neurosurgery 2000;46:335.

75. Jeremitsky E. The impact of hyperglycemia on patients with severe brain injury. J Trauma 2005; 58:47.

76. Oddo M. Impact of tight glycemic control on cerebral glucose metabolism after severe brain injury: a microdialysis study. Crit Care Med 2008;36: 3233.

77. Fernandez-Ortega J. Paroxysmal Sympathetic Hyperactivity after Traumatic Brain Injury: clinical and prognostic implications. J Neurotrauma 2012; 29(7):1364–70.

78. Cotton BA, Snodgrass KB, Fleming SB, et al. Beta-blocker exposure is associated with improved survival after severe traumatic brain injury. J Trauma 2007;62(1):26–33 [discussion: 5].

Managing Subarachnoid Hemorrhage in the Neurocritical Care Unit

Justin M. Caplan, MD[a], Geoffrey P. Colby, MD, PhD[b],
Alexander L. Coon, MD[c], Judy Huang, MD[d],
Rafael J. Tamargo, MD[e],*

KEYWORDS

- Aneurysm • Subarachnoid hemorrhage • Vasospasm • Delayed cerebral ischemia
- Neurocritical care

KEY POINTS

- The management of patients with aneurysmal subarachnoid hemorrhage is challenging and requires a multidisciplinary team approach, and is best done at high-volume centers.
- There is a paucity of randomized, blinded, placebo-controlled, prospective trials to aid in the management of aneurysmal subarachnoid hemorrhage.
- The critical care management of aneurysmal subarachnoid hemorrhage varies between patients with microsurgical clipping and those with endovascular occlusion, and the critical care practitioner should be aware of these differences.
- Much of the morbidity from aneurysmal subarachnoid hemorrhage occurs in a delayed manner following the initial hemorrhage. It is the role of the neurocritical care unit to understand and manage these complications.

INTRODUCTION

Aneurysmal subarachnoid hemorrhage (aSAH) can be a devastating condition that leads to significant morbidity and mortality. Over the past several decades, there has been an overall decrease in the incidence of strokes in high-income countries, but without a concomitant decrease in the incidence of SAH.[1] Unlike other causes of SAH (ie, trauma), aSAH represents a unique physiology, which sets up a cascade of events that leads to further pathologic processes involving multiple organ systems. If a patient survives the initial hemorrhage, it is these pathologic processes that are the source of the significant morbidity and mortality following aSAH. As such, a thorough understanding of these processes and their management are a necessity for any practitioner caring for patients with aSAH. Furthermore, given the complexity of the management of these patients, this care is best done in a dedicated neurocritical care unit (NCCU).

In 2011 and 2012, 2 sets of guidelines were published on the management of aSAH.[2,3] These guidelines by the Neurocritical Care Society and

Disclosures: None.
[a] Department of Neurosurgery, Johns Hopkins University School of Medicine, 1800 Orleans Street, Room 6007, Baltimore, MD 21287, USA; [b] Department of Neurosurgery, Johns Hopkins University School of Medicine, 1800 Orleans Street, Room 6115C, Baltimore, MD 21287, USA; [c] Department of Neurosurgery, Johns Hopkins University School of Medicine, 1800 Orleans Street, Room 6115E, Baltimore, MD 21287, USA; [d] Department of Neurosurgery, Johns Hopkins University School of Medicine, 1800 Orleans Street, Room 6115F, Baltimore, MD 21287, USA; [e] Division of Cerebrovascular Neurosurgery, Department of Neurosurgery, Johns Hopkins University School of Medicine, 1800 Orleans Street, Room 6115G, Baltimore, MD 21287, USA
* Corresponding author.
E-mail address: rtamarg@jhmi.edu

the American Heart Association/American Stroke Association (AHA/ASA), and their supporting articles, provide comprehensive reviews of the literature combined with expert consensus opinions. These articles note that there is a paucity of prospective, randomized, placebo-controlled trials in the literature showing that an intervention improves outcome, which might aid in guiding the management of aSAH. In fact, the use of nimodipine (Nimotop) is the only such intervention supported by level 1A class evidence.[3] As such, much of the management of this disease is left to the interpretation of the literature by an experienced clinician. The goal of this article is to review the pertinent literature in a condensed format, in combination with our own experiences in managing these patients, in an attempt to provide a practical aid to those managing this challenging disease in the NCCU.

In addition to reviewing the evidence behind the current management of aSAH in the NCCU, this article is also meant to serve as a practical reference to those who are involved in the day-to-day management of these patients (ie, residents and fellows). To this end a table is included to aid with admission orders, and which can be used as a quick reference on daily NCCU rounds. In their NCCU, we often use a "systems-based" method of rounding, and have organized the table and article in this manner (**Table 1**).

CARE SETTING

The care of patients with aSAH requires a multidisciplinary approach. Team members include neurosurgeons, neurointensivists, neurologists, neuroradiologists, and interventional neuroradiologists. Patients also require specialized critical care nursing with specialized training in neurosciences. We believe that these patients are best served in dedicated NCCUs that treat a high volume of such patients. This scenario is also supported in the literature, which shows that outcomes are improved at high-volume centers.[4] It is also important that patients be transferred expeditiously to the high-volume centers, as rebleeding before transfer or during transfer is reported.[5]

NEUROLOGIC
Hydrocephalus

Hydrocephalus is a known complication of aSAH, first described experimentally in 1928 by Bagley.[6] The incidence of acute hydrocephalus varies widely, and many studies report a range from 15% to 53%.[7–13] The incidence of patients with

SAH who go on to require permanent shunting also varies widely in the literature. Shunt rates from 2.3% to 36% have been reported.[7–16] This large variation is likely multifactorial, including varying indications for shunting across institutions and surgeons, effects of clot/blood removal from the subarachnoid space at the time of surgery, and fenestration of the lamina terminalis.

Hydrocephalus following aSAH can be of both the obstructive and the communicating variant. In obstructive hydrocephalus, there may be intraventricular extension of the subarachnoid blood or an intraparenchymal hematoma. In the communicating variant the ventricular system may be free of blood, but the arachnoid granulations may become obstructed by the subarachnoid blood, limiting reabsorption of cerebrospinal fluid (CSF). Recognition of the cause of the patient's hydrocephalus is important, as it can affect the means by which the hydrocephalus is treated (lumbar drain, external ventriculostomy drainage, endoscopic third ventriculostomy, shunt, and so forth).

There are many factors involved in managing hydrocephalus following subarachnoid hemorrhage that are important to the neurointensivist, including ventriculostomy or lumbar drain weaning, risk of aneurysmal rebleeding in the setting of CSF drainage, and indications and timing of permanent CSF diversion (ie, shunting).

The timing of ventriculostomy weaning and removal is not agreed upon. The role of rapid versus gradual weaning from external ventricular drainage (EVD) was examined in a prospective randomized trial by Klopfenstein and colleagues.[17] In this study 81 patients with aSAH with EVDs were randomized to either rapid (24 hours) or gradual (96 hours) wean. This study found no difference in rates of shunt implantation between groups. The gradual-wean group did have longer stays in the intensive care unit (ICU) and hospital. However, we have found that persistence in ventriculostomy weaning is very effective in preventing the need for shunting. Serial EVD clamp trials are effective as long as the amount of CSF draining through the ventriculostomy decreases daily. Although this may lead to a more prolonged EVD wean and ICU/hospital stay, it reduces the number of shunts placed.

After initial ventriculostomy or lumbar drain placement, the risk of aneurysm rebleeding is often quoted as a concern against aggressive CSF drainage in the setting of an unsecured aneurysm. Some data suggest, however, that this is safe. Hellingman and colleagues[18] retrospectively reviewed 34 patients who underwent EVD placement against matched controls with untreated hydrocephalus and a control without ventricular enlargement.

Rebleeding occurred in 21% of patients with treated hydrocephalus as well as untreated hydrocephalus, and 18% of those without hydrocephalus. In the lumbar puncture (LP) group, rebleeding occurred in 5% of patients, in 14% of patients with hydrocephalus without LP, and in none of the controls without hydrocephalus. It was concluded that there was no statistically significant difference between rebleeding in those patients treated with either EVD or LP versus those who were not. McIver and colleagues[19] retrospectively reviewed 304 patients with aneurysmal subarachnoid hemorrhage. Of these patients, 45 had ventriculostomies placed. Rebleeding occurred in 5.4% of patients not undergoing ventriculostomy placement and in 4.4% of those who did undergo ventriculostomy placement. The ability to safely drain CSF following aSAH is important, as there are data to suggest it may lead to a reduction in vasospasm.[20]

Temporary CSF diversion may typically be achieved with ventriculostomy, serial LPs, or lumbar catheter placement. Knowledge of the cause of the hydrocephalus is important, as this may influence a particular approach. We routinely use ventriculostomy as a means to achieve CSF diversion. This approach is well tolerated and, in addition to CSF drainage, allows for accurate measurement of intracranial pressure, which may be important, particularly in high-grade patients with a poor neurologic examination.

Shunt dependence following aSAH varies. Factors predicting the development of shunt-dependent hydrocephalus include age, acute hydrocephalus, ventilation on admission, posterior circulation, and giant aneurysms.[14] Fenestration of the lamina terminalis is a microsurgical maneuver, the utility of which is debated. In our experience, routine fenestration of the lamina terminalis is associated with an 80% decrease in the incidence of shunt-dependent hydrocephalus.[8] We routinely perform this straightforward microsurgical technique in all cases of aSAH where access to the lamina terminalis is easily obtainable (ie, fronto-spheno-temporal [pterional] craniotomies). However, the issue of fenestrating the lamina terminalis is debated, as some literature suggests it does not reduce the incidence of shunt-dependent hydrocephalus.[15] The AHA guidelines do not recommend this maneuver, and classify the evidence as level IIIB.[3]

Seizures

Seizures after aSAH hemorrhage are common. One retrospective review found a prevalence of 15.2% in 547 patients.[21] Seizure frequency in subarachnoid hemorrhage after surgery was 9.4% in the 307 patients studied prospectively by Ohman.[22] Furthermore, in this study a history of hypertension was found to be a significant risk factor for the development of epilepsy after aSAH and surgery. Epilepsy developed in 7% of 247 patients alive with follow-up 12 months after aSAH.[23] Subdural hematoma and cerebral infarction were predictors of epilepsy.

The risk of seizures in patients undergoing clip occlusion or coil embolization of ruptured aneurysms was assessed in the International Subarachnoid Aneurysm Trial (ISAT).[24] There was an overall incidence of seizures in 10.9% of the patients. Among those patients randomized to endovascular intervention, 8.3% had seizures, whereas 13.6% of patients randomized to open surgery had seizures, a difference that was found to be significant. Furthermore, on long-term follow-up after discharge, the risk of seizures was also significantly greater in the neurosurgical group. The study also identified the following risk factors for developing seizures: younger age, Fisher grade greater than 1 on computed tomography (CT), delayed ischemic neurologic deficit due to vasospasm, thromboembolic complication, and middle cerebral artery (MCA) location of the aneurysm.

Lanzino and colleagues[25] reviewed 56 articles from 1980 to 2010 on the topic of the incidence and treatment of seizures after aneurysmal subarachnoid hemorrhage. Seizures occurred at the time of SAH in 4% to 26% of patients. Only a small proportion of patients had a seizure after admission but before aneurysm treatment. This review also addressed the role of anticonvulsants after SAH. The study notes that there are no randomized controlled trials addressing the safety and efficacy of antiepileptics in SAH. The AHA/ASA guidelines are similarly vague, stating that "the use of prophylactic anticonvulsants may be considered in the immediate post-hemorrhagic period."[3] There are data to suggest that the use of phenytoin (Dilantin, Phenytek) for seizure prophylaxis is associated with poor functional outcome.[26]

The duration of prophylactic anticonvulsant use is also not well agreed upon. A short course of phenytoin (3 days), however, may be equivalent to a longer (7-day) course, but with fewer side effects in preventing seizures.[27] While the routine use of antiepileptic drugs (AEDs) in SAH is common, it is not trivial. A study pooling the data of 3552 patients from 4 prospective, randomized, double-blind, placebo-controlled trials from 1991 to 1997 looked at the outcomes in patients with subarachnoid hemorrhage treated with AEDs.[28] In this study, 65.1% of patients received antiepileptic drugs. Patients who received treatment with AEDs had a worse outcome based on the Glasgow Outcome

Table 1
Admission orders and rounding template for patients with aSAH in the NCCU

System	Orders	Notes
General	Admit to NCCU, neurosurgery, attending of record	
Neurologic	Noncontrast head CT	
	Conventional 4-vessel cerebral-angiogram	
	Aneurysm precautions	Dark, quiet room, limited interruptions
	Levetiracetam 1 g q12 h	Seizure prophylaxis
	q6 h Na/K checks	To monitor for CSW/SIADH
	Na goal: 135–145	May be adjusted depending on patient's clinical status and evidence of cerebral edema
	Ventriculostomy-if symptomatic hydrocephalus	Pop-off set to 15–20 mm Hg in setting of unsecured aneurysm. After aneurysm occlusion, pop-off may be lowered depending on clinical scenario
	Dexamethasone (Decadron) 4 mg q6 h × 24 h	
	Daily TCDs	
	Nimodipine 60 mg q4 h × 21 d	
Cardiac	SBP goal <160	Nicardipine (Cardene) continuous infusion if needed. SBP goal may be liberalized if vasospasm/DCI
	MAP goal >70	
	Baseline ECG	
	Baseline echocardiogram	
Pulmonary	Incentive spirometry	
	Chest radiograph	On admission and then daily if intubated
	Ventilator settings if patient requires mechanical ventilation	

Renal	IV fluids: 0.9% normal saline at 150 mL/h Goal euvolemia	May use 2% or 3% hypertonic saline based on sodium goal Volume status goal may change as clinical scenario changes (ie, goal hypervolemia in setting of vasospasm/DCI)
GI	NPO on admission Pantoprazole (Protonix) 40 mg q24 h	Resume enteral feeds when clinically stable GI ulcer prophylaxis
ID	Follow temperature curves	Initiate cooling measures if persistently febrile despite antipyretics
	Periprocedural antibiotics	Cefazolin 1–2 g × 1 for EVD or lumbar drain placement Cefazolin 1–2 g q8 × 3 doses for craniotomy (may use clindamycin 600 mg if cefazolin allergy)
	Fever workup if T_{max} >38.4°C	Urine analysis, blood and urine cultures, CXR, ± CSF studies/culture
Endocrine	Glucose checks q4 h while NPO Insulin sliding scale	Glucose goal ≤150 mg/dL
Hematology	Hemoglobin goal ≥10 g/dL	
DVT prophylaxis	Compression stockings Sequential compression devices Unfractionated heparin 5000 units SC q8–12 h	Start 24 h after stable head CT or after craniotomy
Check labs	BMP, CBC, coags, type and screen, UA/urine culture, urine pregnancy test (if applicable)	
Consent	Consent for angiogram, intraoperative angiogram, ventriculostomy, craniotomy	Done at time of admission to NCCU

Abbreviations: aSAH, aneurysmal subarachnoid hemorrhage; BMP, basic metabolic panel; CBC, complete blood count; coags, coagulation panel; CSF, cerebrospinal fluid; CSW, cerebral salt wasting; CT, computed tomography; CXR, chest radiography; DCI, delayed cerebral ischemia; DVT, deep venous thrombosis; ECG, electrocardiography; EVD, external ventricular drainage; GI, gastrointestinal; ID, infectious disease; IV, intravenous; MAP, mean arterial pressure; NCCU, neurocritical care unit; NPO, nothing by mouth; q, every; SBP, systolic blood pressure; SC, subcutaneous; SIADH, syndrome of inappropriate antidiuretic hormone secretion; TCD, transcranial Doppler ultrasonography; UA, urinalysis.

Scale, and were more likely to have vasospasm, neurologic deterioration, cerebral infarction, and elevated temperatures during hospitalization. We routinely use levetiracetam (Keppra), 500 to 1000 mg every 12 hours, for seizure prophylaxis. This medication has a favorable side-effect profile in comparison with phenytoin. The duration of therapy is tailored to the individual patient, and takes into account the extent and location of SAH/intraparenchymal hemorrhage and the presence or absence of seizures.

Rebleeding

Rebleeding rates after aSAH vary in the literature. Starke and Connolly,[29] on behalf of the participants of the International Multidisciplinary Consensus Conference on the Critical Care Management of Subarachnoid Hemorrhage, recently published a review of the literature on this topic. Early studies (through 1990) showed that rebleeding rates for untreated aneurysms were 4% within the first 24 hours, 1% to 2% per day for the next 14 days, 50% for the first 6 months, and 3% per year following this. In the ISAT trial, approximately 2.1% of patients rebled before treatment.[30] In the International Cooperative Study on the Timing of Aneurysm Surgery, rebleeding occurred in 6% of patients with planned surgery for days 0 to 3 and 22% in patients with planned surgery for days 15 to 32.[31] In this study, after the initial effects of the hemorrhage and vasospasm, rebleeding was the next largest cause of poor results.[32] This finding has led to the standard of care that aneurysms should be occluded as soon as possible following rupture.

Many risk factors can help to predict rebleeding. Naidech and colleagues[33] looked at 574 patients enrolled in the Columbia University SAH Outcomes project. Rebleeding occurred in 6.9% of patients, 73% of which occurred in the first 3 days. In their multilogistic regression model, independent predictors of rebleeding were Hunt-Hess grade on admission and maximal aneurysm diameter. Of note, rebleeding was associated with a decrease in survival with functional independence. Timing of rebleeding was also related to Hunt-Hess grade. Patients with higher grades (IV and V) rebled earlier than those with lower grades. Rebleeding time did not correlate with aneurysm size. Patients with rebleeding have worse outcomes compared with those who do not, including higher rates of brain death and poor outcomes.[34]

Risk of rebleeding following treatment of ruptured intracranial aneurysms was studied in the Cerebral Aneurysm Rerupture After Treatment (CARAT) study,[35] which looked at 1001 patients across 9 centers treated with either coil embolization or surgical clipping. In this study there were 19 reruptures following treatment, 58% of which led to death. Degree of aneurysm occlusion was associated with the risk of rerupture. There was no statistically significant difference between rebleeding risk following coil embolization in comparison with surgical clipping.

Given the important finding that rebleeding is associated with worse outcomes, many have sought to identify interventions that can reduce this risk. As mentioned earlier, early aneurysm occlusion is one such intervention that has been an important development in the management of these patients. Another intervention that has been studied is the use of antifibrinolytic therapy, which has been evaluated mainly with the antifibrinolytics tranexamic acid (Lysteda, Cyklokapron) and ε-aminocaproic acid (EACA) (Amicar). The use of tranexamic acid (TXA) and EACA has been studied extensively. The goal of this therapy is to prevent clot dissipation by means of inhibiting fibrinolysis. However, despite the theoretical benefits, clinical outcomes have been varied.

In 2003 a Cochrane review looked at the use of antifibrinolytic therapy in aSAH, and concluded there was no benefit for poor outcome or death.[36] There was a reduction in rebleeding but this was countered by the increased risk of cerebral ischemia, therefore the review rejected the routine use of antifibrinolytic therapy in aSAH.

Given worse outcomes from delayed ischemia in patients treated with antifibrinolytics, more recent studies have evaluated the potential benefit of a short course of antifibrinolytic therapy. A prospective, randomized controlled trial published in 2002 looked at the use of early TXA (1 g) at the time of SAH diagnosis and 1 g every 6 hours until the aneurysm was occluded.[37] However, treatment with TXA did not exceed 72 hours. A total of 505 patients were randomized (254 to TXA, and 251 to control). Rebleeding decreased from 10.8% in controls to 2.4% in the treatment group. A prospective observational study looked at the use of EACA at the time of SAH diagnosis, but continued only for a maximum of 72 hours.[38] The study compared 73 patients treated with EACA and 175 patients not treated with EACA. This protocol resulted in a significant decrease in bleeding among those patients treated with EACA (2.7%) versus non-EACA treated patients (11.4%). Of importance, as had been previously seen in trials with prolonged use of antifibrinolytic therapy, there were no differences in ischemic complications between those treated and those not treated. There was, however, an increase in the incidence of deep venous thrombosis (DVT) in the treatment group. There was no statistically significant difference in outcome between cohorts.

Given these data, the AHA/ASA SAH guidelines offer a Class IIA recommendation that it is reasonable to give antifibrinolytic therapy for less than 72 hours in patients with an unavoidable delay in aneurysm occlusion, a significant risk of rebleeding, and no medical contraindication.[3] We currently do not routinely use antifibrinolytic therapy. However, we do aim to treat all ruptured aneurysms within 24 hours of admission, thereby reducing the risk of rerupture.

Vasospasm and Delayed Cerebral Ischemia

Nomenclature

aSAH is associated with significant morbidity and mortality. Much of the morbidity is secondary to cerebral ischemia, which can occur in a delayed manner (ie, several days after the ictus). If severe enough, the ischemia can lead to brain tissue infarction. Although this has often been correlated with angiographic vessel narrowing ("vasospasm"), vasospasm can occur without ischemia/infarction, and ischemia/infarction can occur without vasospasm.[39] Vasospasm has been a well-known sequela of SAH since early descriptions by Robertson[40] in 1949 and Ecker and Riemenschneider[41] in 1951. Owing to the large variability in nomenclature, an international ad hoc panel of experts was assembled to propose a universal definition of delayed cerebral ischemia (DCI) to standardize outcome measures.[42] The investigators correctly observe that the diagnosis of DCI is one of exclusion. We make the diagnosis of DCI when there is a deterioration in the neurologic examination, etiology such as hydrocephalus, cerebral salt wasting (CSW), infection, and hemorrhage have been ruled out, and the deterioration improves with triple-H therapy within 6 to 12 hours; or, if there is no improvement, an angiogram is obtained to show radiographic vessel narrowing. It is important to recognize failure to respond to therapy, as lack of early improvement leads to a high risk of poor outcomes and thus may be an indication for conventional angiography.[43]

It is important to distinguish vasospasm (a radiographic finding) from clinical deterioration secondary to DCI, which can be a multifactorial process that includes vessel narrowing (ie, vasospasm).[42,44] A prospective study of 508 patients with subarachnoid hemorrhage also supports the notion that DCI is a more meaningful definition than arterial narrowing alone.[45] Given the significant morbidity and mortality associated with vasospasm and DCI, over the past several decades a significant effort has been made to establish monitoring and interventions that can improve outcomes from this process. A comprehensive review of all of these trials and measures is beyond the scope of this article; however, an outline follows of what we believe to be the most important, including transcranial Doppler ultrasonography (TCD), calcium-channel blockers, triple-H therapy, endovascular therapy, endothelin receptor antagonists, and statins.

Monitoring for vasospasm and DCI

Monitoring for the development of vasospasm and DCI remains an important role of the NCCU. In addition to serial neurologic examinations and imaging studies (ie, CT, CT perfusion, and conventional angiography), TCD is an important method for evaluating the cerebral vasculature. Despite the widespread use of TCD, however, its accuracy in predicting DCI and vasospasm is limited.[46,47] In a review of 441 patients with aSAH, almost 40% of patients with DCI did not have TCD velocities above the vasospasm threshold of 120 cm/s.[46] We use TCD data as an adjuvant to the clinical examination and other diagnostic modalities (such as CT perfusion scanning), and will follow trends in TCD velocities, but elevation in these numbers alone without clinical evidence of DCI does not lead them to make interventions.

Calcium-channel blockers

There are few multi-institutional, randomized, placebo-controlled, double-blind trials in the neurosurgical literature on improvement of outcomes that are available to guide management. The use of nimodipine following aSAH, however, represents one such trial.[48] The use of nimodipine following aSAH was pioneered by Allen and colleagues[48] at Johns Hopkins University School of Medicine. In this trial, 125 neurologically intact patients with aSAH were randomized to either nimodipine or placebo for 21 days. Only 1 patient of 56 treated with nimodipine versus 8 of 60 in the placebo group developed a persistent deficit from cerebral arterial spasm ($P = .03$).

Recently, a meta-analysis was completed looking at the use of calcium antagonists for aSAH.[49,50] The review included 16 trials with 3361 patients. Three of these trials included magnesium sulfate. Oral nimodipine provided a relative risk of 0.67 (95% confidence interval [CI] 0.55–0.81) for poor outcome. There was no statistically significant reduction for other calcium-channel antagonists alone or with intravenous nimodipine. Calcium-channel antagonists overall reduced the occurrence of secondary ischemia with a relative risk of 0.66 (95% CI 0.59–0.75). Based on this evidence, the investigators recommend oral nimodipine, 60 mg every 4 hours for 21 days[50]; this is also our practice.

As already mentioned, it has been hypothesized that magnesium sulfate may also reduce the risk of DCI and poor outcome after aSAH. The MASH-2 (Magnesium for Aneurysmal Subarachnoid Hemorrhage) trial was a phase 3 randomized, placebo-controlled, multicenter trial aimed at addressing this question.[51] Patients were randomized to magnesium sulfate, 64 mmol/d, or placebo. There were 606 patients in the magnesium group and 597 in the placebo group. Poor outcome was found in 26.2% of patients receiving magnesium and in 25.3% of patients receiving placebo (relative risk 1.03, 95% CI 0.85–1.25). Based on this evidence and an updated review of meta-analysis data, the investigators do not recommend intravenous magnesium sulfate after aSAH. We do not use magnesium sulfate in managing these patients.

Triple-H therapy

The treatment of vasospasm following subarachnoid hemorrhage has classically been the so-called triple-H therapy, consisting of hypertension, hypervolemia, and hemodilution. This therapy evolved from 1972 to 1982, initially as monotherapies and subsequently as a combination of all 3.[52–55] The relative importance of each component of triple-H therapy has recently come under review. The literature seems to support that of each component; hypertension is the most important in increasing cerebral blood flow (CBF) and/or oxygenation, whereas hypervolemia does not increase CBF.[56–58] Further studies are needed to best identify the role triple-H therapy should play in managing vasospasm/DCI, as it is not a benign therapy and is associated with many complications, including pulmonary edema, hyponatremia, and myocardial infarction.[59] Furthermore, accurate hemodynamic management of these patients often requires invasive catheter lines. We routinely use the PiCCO (Pulsion Medical Systems SE, Feldkirchen, Germany) catheter system in preference to traditional Swan-Ganz catheters in managing these patients.

In patients with unsecured, unruptured aneurysms, hypertensive, hypervolemia therapy seems to be safe and does not lead to rupture.[60] When hypotension is a concern, if nimodipine administration results in unwanted lowering of blood pressure, we will routinely change the dosage from 60 mg every 4 hours to 30 mg every 2 hours. This change often will mitigate the antihypertensive effects of this calcium-channel blocker while maintaining the total daily dose.

During triple-H therapy, we aim for a mean arterial pressure goal that is 20% above the patient's baseline. If this fails to produce a favorable response in the patient, it will then be increased by another 10% of the new baseline. Extrapolating from the ischemic stroke guidelines, this elevation will be continued up to a systolic blood pressure of 220 mm Hg or diastolic blood pressure of 120 mm Hg.[61]

Endovascular management of vasospasm

Balloon catheter for angioplasty for vasospasm in aSAH was introduced in 1984.[62] In their review of the literature, Hoh and Ogilvy[63] found a 62% rate of clinical improvement following balloon angioplasty, although this was associated with a 5% major complication rate and 1.1% rate of vessel rupture. The decision to proceed with angioplasty rather than intra-arterial vasodilators is beyond the scope of this article. For a recent review of the literature, see Kimball and colleagues.[64] We proceed with angiography in patients with suspected DCI/vasospasm who do not improve clinically within 6 to 12 hours of initiation of triple-H therapy. If vasospasm is found radiographically, it is treated with either angioplasty or intra-arterial vasodilators.

Inflammation and endothelin receptor antagonists and statins

As discussed earlier, DCI is a major source of morbidity following subarachnoid hemorrhage. Vasospasm is thought to play at least some role in this process. Laboratory evidence supports the hypothesis that vasospasm is at least partially mediated by inflammatory processes.[65–68] Given this theory, considerable efforts have been made to evaluate promising therapies aimed at the inflammatory nature of vasospasm/DCI.

Endothelin, a vasoconstrictor, is thought to be a potential mediator of vasospasm, produced by a variety of cell types, including leukocytes in the CSF.[69,70] As such, there have been efforts to show that endothelin antagonists (such as clazosentan) can improve vasospasm, and therefore improve outcomes in aSAH. The CONSCIOUS trials (Clazosentan to Overcome Neurologic Ischemia and Infarction Occurring after Subarachnoid Hemorrhage) have sought to answer this question. CONSCIOUS-1 was a randomized, double-blind, placebo-controlled phase 2b dose-finding trial, which found that clazosentan significantly decreased moderate and severe angiographic vasospasm in a dose-dependent manner.[71] Encouragingly the investigators also found that there was some evidence suggesting a decrease in morbidity and mortality related to vasospasm. However, the study, was not powered to detect differences in clinical outcome.

The CONSCIOUS-2 trial was a randomized, double-blind, placebo-controlled phase 3 trial to assess the efficacy in reducing all-cause mortality, vasospasm-related new infarcts, delayed ischemic neurologic deficit secondary to vasospasm, and rescue therapy for vasospasm in patients with aSAH undergoing surgical clipping.[72] The study failed to show any significant benefit in clazosentan use. The CONSCIOUS-3 trial aimed to assess the same question in aSAH patients undergoing endovascular coiling.[73] This study was ended prematurely given the results of the CONSCIOUS-2 trial. The study did show a significant reduction of vasospasm-related morbidity and all-cause mortality at the high dose, but there was no statistically significant improvement in patient outcome. A recent review of the literature further supports these findings, and do not support the use of endothelin receptor antagonists for patients with aSAH.[74]

Given the proposed inflammatory nature of vasospasm and DCI, the use of statins has also been proposed and studied as a possible means to improve outcomes. Two recent meta-analyses, however, have failed to suggest that there is a significant enough benefit to warrant its routine use.[75,76] We do not routinely use endothelin antagonists in patients with aSAH. Furthermore, we do not routinely start patients on statins when admitted with aSAH, but will continue them if the patient had been using the medication before the hemorrhage.

CARDIAC

Troponin elevation following subarachnoid hemorrhage is a well-known phenomenon. Elevation in troponin I was found to be associated with an increased risk of left ventricular dysfunction, pulmonary edema, DCI, and death or poor functional outcomes in a cohort of 253 patients at the time of discharge.[77] Cardiac dysfunction following aSAH (also known as stunned myocardium, and the more recently proposed neurogenic stress cardiomyopathy) presents a challenge to the management of these patients.[78] It manifests as an increase in troponins, multiterritorial regional wall-motion abnormalities on echocardiogram, electrocardiogram abnormalities, a chest radiograph with pulmonary edema, and a normal coronary angiogram.[78] These findings are important, as their presence may hinder the treatment of vasospasm and DCI. Tako-tsubo cardiomyopathy is a subset of cardiomyopathy that can be seen following aSAH, particularly in postmenopausal women.[79,80] It is important to be aware of the diagnosis of cardiomyopathy following subarachnoid hemorrhage, as this has implications

in the augmentative therapy needed in DCI (ie, inotropic pressors may be more appropriate than vasoconstrictors). Cardiomyopathy, whether pre-existing or secondary to aSAH, can be detrimental in the setting of vasospasm when hemodynamic augmentation (triple-H therapy) is required. We previously reported on the successful use of an intra-aortic balloon counterpulsation pump in such a setting.[81]

Although the causality has not been well established, it has been shown that bradycardia, tachycardia, and nonspecific ST-wave and T-wave abnormalities have been associated with mortality following aSAH.[82]

PULMONARY

Pulmonary complications have been reported in 22% of patients with aSAH, with pneumonia and congestive heart failure being the most common.[83] In their study of 305 patients, Friedman and colleagues[83] found that the incidence of symptomatic vasospasm was higher in patients with pulmonary complications. This finding is important, as it may relate to the fact that optimal treatment of vasospasm/DCI can be limited by the presence of pulmonary complications. Mechanisms by which pulmonary function is impaired following subarachnoid hemorrhage include pneumonia, pulmonary edema, atelectasis, acute lung injury, and acute respiratory distress syndrome.[84–86]

RENAL
Fluid Balance

An understanding of the fluid balance of patients with aSAH is important,[87] as is sodium balance, which is closely linked to fluid physiology. Standard calculations of fluid-balance measurements do not accurately predict actual circulating blood volumes as measured by pulse dye densitometry.[88] Given these findings, in a prospective controlled study Hoff and colleagues[89] used pulse dye densitometry to measure blood volumes daily in 102 patients in the first 10 days following SAH. In the intervention group, fluid management was based on blood-volume measurements, compared with the control group in which fluid management was based on fluid balance. The investigators found that severe hypovolemia (defined as blood volume <50 mL/kg) was seen more often in patients being managed by fluid calculation alone.

Swan-Ganz catheterization is one means of invasive measurement of hemodynamic parameters. However, there are numerous complications associated with this method.[90] One more recent method of monitoring volume status is by means of transpulmonary thermodilution monitoring with the PiCCO system.[91] The effectiveness of the PiCCO system, compared with conventional pulmonary artery catheter–derived measurements, was compared in 16 patients with subarachnoid hemorrhage.[92] Cardiac output by the PiCCO system showed high correlation and low error compared with conventional catheter-based measurements. Once the accuracy of the PiCCO system was validated in the 16 patients, 100 subsequent patients were then randomized to either PiCCO or traditional catheters and the outcomes compared. Patients receiving early goal-directed therapy by PiCCO had decreased occurrences of vasospasm and cardiopulmonary complications compared with those managed by standard management based on use of central venous or pulmonary artery catheters. In the NCCU, we prefer the use of the PiCCO system to Swan-Ganz catheterization when more precise hemodynamic monitoring is needed beyond a central venous line.

Fluid-balance goals should constantly be assessed in patients with aSAH. The role of prophylactic hypervolemia has been studied. Eighty-two patients were randomized to either hypervolemia or euvolemia in a prospective randomized trial following aneurysm clipping.[58] There was no benefit in CBF in the patients randomized to hypervolemia. Similarly, in their study of 32 patients randomized to triple-H therapy or euvolemia, Egge and colleagues[93] did not find any benefit to prophylactic triple-H therapy. Given these data and the complications associated with hypervolemia, we aim for a goal of euvolemia unless otherwise indicated (ie, vasospasm/DCI). To this end, 0.9% normal saline is routinely used as maintenance fluids. In the setting of CSW or syndrome of inappropriate antidiuretic hormone secretion (SIADH), however, hypertonic saline may be required.

Sodium Goals

Derangements in maintenance levels of blood sodium are common in aSAH. Sodium levels are important, as outcomes have been associated with abnormal valves.[94] Two common causes of hyponatremia in patients with aSAH are CSW and SIADH. In CSW there is a renal loss of sodium, resulting in diuresis and hypovolemia, whereas in SIADH there is a retention of free water, leading to euvolemia or hypervolemia.[95] It is important to distinguish the 2 disorders clinically, as treatment will vary depending on the origin of the hyponatremia. We have previously reported favorable experience using 3% sodium chloride/acetate for hyponatremia in 29 patients with symptomatic

vasospasm.[96] Most patients with hyponatremia after aSAH have CSW and not SIADH.

Corticosteroids have been used to treat hyponatremia in aSAH. In one randomized, placebo-controlled trial, hydrocortisone (Cortef) was effectively used to prevent hyponatremia, although there was no overall difference in patient outcome.[97] Fludrocortisone (Florinef) has also been shown to be effective in preventing natriuresis in randomized studies.[98,99] A recent study showed that early use of fludrocortisone was effective in preventing symptomatic vasospasm, but had no effect on overall outcomes.[100] We use fludrocortisone when the diagnosis of CSW has been made by presence of excessive diuresis accompanied by declining levels of blood sodium; we do not routinely use corticosteroids in a prophylactic manner.

INFECTIOUS DISEASE
Fever

Fever following subarachnoid hemorrhage is common. Predictors include poor Hunt-Hess grade and the presence of intraventricular hemorrhage.[101] Of importance, refractory fever following SAH is associated with increased mortality and worse outcomes.[101,102] Despite this, the role of fever reduction in improving outcomes is not well known. The side effects of treating fever either by pharmacologic means (ie, potential antiplatelet effects of nonsteroidal anti-inflammatories) or by cooling devices such as cooling blankets and intravascular devices (ie, shivering) must be weighed against the potential benefit in reducing the patient's temperature. In the NCCU, we treat fevers (>38.4°C) first with acetaminophen, and simultaneously send a diagnostic workup for the etiology of the fever and treatment of identifiable causes. If this is ineffective, methods of cooling such as surface cooling devices are used. Initial fever workup consists of urine analysis, urine culture, blood cultures, and chest radiography. CSF studies are sent on patients with ventriculostomies or lumbar catheters. If the patient has had an intracranial procedure but does not have a CSF drain in place, consideration is given to LP to obtain CSF in the appropriate clinical setting. Thorough investigation to identify and treat infectious causes of fever is prudent, as both pneumonia and bloodstream infections are independently associated with death or severe disability at 3 months.[103] Of importance is that delayed fever may also be present in the setting of vasospasm.[104]

Periprocedural Antibiotics

Periprocedural antibiotics are given for invasive procedures involving the central nervous system.

We use cefazolin (Ancef, Kefzol) unless the patient has an allergy or contraindication, in which case clindamycin (Cleocin) is substituted. One dose is given immediately before placement of ventriculostomy or lumbar drain. For patients undergoing craniotomy, antibiotics are continued for an additional 24 hours after surgery while in the NCCU.

ENDOCRINE
Glucose Control

Persistently elevated glucose (>200 mg/dL for 2 or more consecutive days), has been shown to result in patients being 7 times more likely of having a poor outcome at 10 months after treatment for aSAH than those patients who did not have persistently elevated glucose.[105] Furthermore, elevated glucose levels at admission are also associated with an increased risk of poor outcome.[106] Prolonged elevated glucose (ie, over a week) is also associated with worse outcomes.[107] However, treatment of hyperglycemia can lead to increased incidence of hypoglycemia, which has been shown, in both the SAH literature and the general medical literature, to be associated with worse outcomes.[108,109] As such, we place patients on an insulin sliding scale to target a glucose goal of 150 mg/dL or less at the time of admission. Continuous insulin infusions are only used when hyperglycemia is refractory to intermittent subcutaneous insulin dosing regimens.

HEMATOLOGY
Anemia

The ideal hemoglobin goal in patients with aSAH is not certain. Early animal data suggested that a hematocrit near 30% was optimal for protecting the brain in a canine model of ischemia.[110] Subsequently, several human studies have shown that anemia and lower hemoglobin values are associated with worse outcomes in patients with aSAH, and that higher hemoglobin is associated with improved outcomes.[111–114] A recent prospective, randomized trial randomized 44 patients to a hemoglobin goal of at least either 10 or 11.5 g/dL to evaluate the safety of this practice.[115] Although those in the higher hemoglobin group received more transfusions, this was found to be safe with similar safety and outcome end points. This finding is an important one for the SAH population, as studies from the critical care literature have suggested that a higher hemoglobin goal is not necessarily better and may actually result in worse outcomes.[116] We aim for a hemoglobin goal of at least 10 g/dL, and transfuse accordingly.

Deep Venous Thrombosis

The incidence of DVT in patients with SAH varies. Ray and colleagues[117] report an incidence of 18% in 250 patients with aSAH over a 4-year period, and Mack and colleagues[118] report an incidence of 3.4% in 178 patients who had screening lower extremity Doppler ultrasonography. A recent meta-analysis looking at venous thromboembolism (VTE) prevention, with pooled data from 30 studies with a total of 7779 patients, showed that low molecular weight heparin and intermittent compression devices were effective in decreasing the rate of VTE.[119]

Typically all patients at our center receive compression stockings and sequential compression devices at the time of admission. We will typically hold medical thromboprophylaxis until definitive treatment of the aneurysm. At this point, 5000 units unfractionated heparin given subcutaneously every 8 to 12 hours is begun, starting 24 hours after treatment. We do not routinely use low molecular weight heparin, although this may be considered for patients at high risk for DVT.[120] Rates of intracranial hemorrhage vary depending on the method of prophylaxis used. Lowest rates were seen if no heparin was used (0.04 per 1000 patients), and was 0.35 per 1000 patients if unfractionated heparin was used. Rates were highest in the group receiving low molecular weight heparin (1.52 per 1000 patients).[119]

NCCU MANAGEMENT OF ENDOVASCULAR VERSUS SURGICALLY TREATED PATIENTS

It should be noted that patients treated endovascularly rather than with surgical clipping of aneurysms following aSAH present unique challenges, which vary with treatment modality. Some aneurysms are best treated with endovascular therapy (ie, mid-basilar aneurysms), whereas others are best treated with microsurgical clipping (ie, MCA aneurysms). However, the decision of whether to treat a particular aneurysm with microsurgical clipping versus endovascular occlusion is complex and beyond the scope of this article. We have previously reviewed this literature, and in general favor surgical clipping over endovascular therapy in aSAH patients.[121] Regardless of which treatment modality is ultimately used, it is important that those caring for these patients in the NCCU recognize the differences in their management. Patients who have had coil embolization or stent-assisted coil embolization, may require antiplatelet therapy, which creates a challenge if the patient requires subsequent invasive interventions (ventriculostomy, lumbar drain, craniotomy, and so

forth). For example, rates of hemorrhagic complications associated with ventriculostomy placement in aSAH patients undergoing stent-assisted
coiling, and thus on dual antiplatelet therapy, are
higher than those undergoing coiling without
a stent.[122] Patients who have undergone craniotomies are susceptible to postoperative complications (eg, wound infections, postoperative
hematoma) that patients treated by endovascular
means are not. It is important for the practitioner
caring for these patients to be aware of these
differences.

SUMMARY

aSAH can be a devastating disease. Those patients who survive the initial hemorrhage are best
cared for in specialized NCCUs with personnel
well trained in the management of this disease.
Despite the progress made over the last decades,
there still remains a paucity of high-quality evidence with which to guide the management of
these patients. This article aims to provide those
caring for these patients with a brief review of
some of the literature combined with our own experiences. **Table 1** provides an outline for admission orders and a daily rounding template based
on this experience, to help those who take on the
challenge of managing this disease.

REFERENCES

1. Feigin VL, Lawes CM, Bennett DA, et al. Worldwide stroke incidence and early case fatality reported in 56 population-based studies: a systematic review. Lancet Neurol 2009;8(4):355–69.
2. Diringer MN, Bleck TP, Claude Hemphill J, et al. Critical care management of patients following aneurysmal subarachnoid hemorrhage: recommendations from the Neurocritical Care Society's Multidisciplinary Consensus Conference. Neurocrit Care 2011;15:211–40.
3. Connolly ES, Rabinstein AA, Carhuapoma JR, et al. Guidelines for the management of aneurysmal subarachnoid hemorrhage: a guideline for healthcare professionals from the American Heart Association/American Stroke Association. Stroke 2012;43:1711–37.
4. Cross DT, Tirschwell DL, Clark MA, et al. Mortality rates after subarachnoid hemorrhage: variations according to hospital case volume in 18 states. J Neurosurg 2003;99(5):810–7.
5. Ohkuma H, Tsurutani H, Suzuki S. Incidence and significance of early aneurysmal rebleeding before neurosurgical or neurological management. Stroke 2001;32(5):1176–80.
6. Bagley C. Blood in the cerebrospinal fluid resultant functional and organic alterations in the central nervous system A. Experimental data. Arch Surg 1928;17(1):18.
7. Dorai Z, Hynan LS, Kopitnik TA, et al. Factors related to hydrocephalus after aneurysmal subarachnoid hemorrhage. Neurosurgery 2003;52(4):763–71.
8. Komotar RJ, Olivi A, Rigamonti D, et al. Microsurgical fenestration of the lamina terminalis reduces the incidence of shunt-dependent hydrocephalus after aneurysmal subarachnoid hemorrhage. Neurosurgery 2002;51(6):1403–12 [discussion: 1412–3].
9. Komotar RJ, Hahn DK, Kim GH, et al. The impact of microsurgical fenestration of the lamina terminalis on shunt-dependent hydrocephalus and vasospasm after aneurysmal subarachnoid hemorrhage. Neurosurgery 2008;62(1):123–32 [discussion: 132–4].
10. van Gijn J, Hijdra A, Wijdicks EF, et al. Acute hydrocephalus after aneurysmal subarachnoid hemorrhage. J Neurosurg 1985;63(3):355–62.
11. de Oliveira JG, Beck J, Setzer M, et al. Risk of shunt-dependent hydrocephalus after occlusion of ruptured intracranial aneurysms by surgical clipping or endovascular coiling: a single-institution series and meta-analysis. Neurosurgery 2007;61(5):924–33 [discussion: 933–4].
12. Dehdashti AR, Rilliet B, Rufenacht DA, et al. Shunt-dependent hydrocephalus after rupture of intracranial aneurysms: a prospective study of the influence of treatment modality. J Neurosurg 2004;101(3):402–7.
13. Rincon F, Gordon E, Starke RM, et al. Predictors of long-term shunt-dependent hydrocephalus after aneurysmal subarachnoid hemorrhage. Clinical article. J Neurosurg 2010;113(4):774–80.
14. O'Kelly CJ, Kulkarni AV, Austin PC, et al. Shunt-dependent hydrocephalus after aneurysmal subarachnoid hemorrhage: incidence, predictors, and revision rates. Clinical article. J Neurosurg 2009;111(5):1029–35.
15. Komotar RJ, Hahn DK, Kim GH, et al. Efficacy of lamina terminalis fenestration in reducing shunt-dependent hydrocephalus following aneurysmal subarachnoid hemorrhage: a systematic review. Clinical article. J Neurosurg 2009;111(1):147–54.
16. Little AS, Zabramski JM, Peterson M, et al. Ventriculoperitoneal shunting after aneurysmal subarachnoid hemorrhage: analysis of the indications, complications, and outcome with a focus on patients with borderline ventriculomegaly. Neurosurgery 2008;62(3):618–27 [discussion: 618–27].
17. Klopfenstein JD, Kim LJ, Feiz-Erfan I, et al. Comparison of rapid and gradual weaning from external ventricular drainage in patients with aneurysmal subarachnoid hemorrhage: a prospective randomized trial. J Neurosurg 2004;100(2):225–9.

18. Hellingman CA, van den Bergh WM, Beijer IS, et al. Risk of rebleeding after treatment of acute hydrocephalus in patients with aneurysmal subarachnoid hemorrhage. Stroke 2007;38(1):96–9.

19. McIver JI, Friedman JA, Wijdicks EF, et al. Preoperative ventriculostomy and rebleeding after aneurysmal subarachnoid hemorrhage. J Neurosurg 2002;97(5):1042–4.

20. Klimo P, Kestle JR, MacDonald JD, et al. Marked reduction of cerebral vasospasm with lumbar drainage of cerebrospinal fluid after subarachnoid hemorrhage. J Neurosurg 2004;100(2):215–24.

21. Choi KS, Chun HJ, Yi HJ, et al. Seizures and epilepsy following aneurysmal subarachnoid hemorrhage: incidence and risk factors. J Korean Neurosurg Soc 2009;46(2):93–8.

22. Ohman J. Hypertension as a risk factor for epilepsy after aneurysmal subarachnoid hemorrhage and surgery. Neurosurgery 1990;27(4):578–81.

23. Claassen J, Peery S, Kreiter KT, et al. Predictors and clinical impact of epilepsy after subarachnoid hemorrhage. Neurology 2003;60(2):208–14.

24. Hart Y, Sneade M, Birks J, et al. Epilepsy after subarachnoid hemorrhage: the frequency of seizures after clip occlusion or coil embolization of a ruptured cerebral aneurysm: results from the International Subarachnoid Aneurysm Trial. J Neurosurg 2011; 115(6):1159–68.

25. Lanzino G, D'Urso PI, Suarez J, Participants in the International Multi-Disciplinary Consensus Conference on the Critical Care Management of Subarachnoid Hemorrhage. Seizures and anticonvulsants after aneurysmal subarachnoid hemorrhage. Neurocrit Care 2011;15(2):247–56.

26. Naidech AM, Kreiter KT, Janjua N, et al. Phenytoin exposure is associated with functional and cognitive disability after subarachnoid hemorrhage. Stroke 2005;36(3):583–7.

27. Chumnanvej S, Dunn IF, Kim DH. Three-day phenytoin prophylaxis is adequate after subarachnoid hemorrhage. Neurosurgery 2007;60(1): 99–102 [discussion: 102–3].

28. Rosengart AJ, Huo JD, Tolentino J, et al. Outcome in patients with subarachnoid hemorrhage treated with antiepileptic drugs. J Neurosurg 2007;107(2): 253–60.

29. Starke RM, Connolly ES, Participants in the International Multi-Disciplinary Consensus Conference on the Critical Care Management of Subarachnoid Hemorrhage. Rebleeding after aneurysmal subarachnoid hemorrhage. Neurocrit Care 2011; 15(2):241–6.

30. Molyneux AJ, Kerr RS, Yu LM, et al. International subarachnoid aneurysm trial (ISAT) of neurosurgical clipping versus endovascular coiling in 2143 patients with ruptured intracranial aneurysms: a randomised comparison of effects on survival, dependency, seizures, rebleeding, subgroups, and aneurysm occlusion. Lancet 2005;366(9488): 809–17.

31. Kassell NF, Torner JC, Jane JA, et al. The International Cooperative Study on the Timing of Aneurysm Surgery. Part 2: surgical results. J Neurosurg 1990;73(1):37–47.

32. Kassell NF, Torner JC, Haley EC, et al. The International Cooperative Study on the Timing of Aneurysm Surgery. Part 1: overall management results. J Neurosurg 1990;73(1):18–36.

33. Naidech AM, Janjua N, Kreiter KT, et al. Predictors and impact of aneurysm rebleeding after subarachnoid hemorrhage. Arch Neurol 2005;62(3): 410–6.

34. Lord AS, Fernandez L, Schmidt JM, et al. Effect of rebleeding on the course and incidence of vasospasm after subarachnoid hemorrhage. Neurology 2011;78(1):31–7.

35. Johnston SC, Dowd CF, Higashida RT, et al. Predictors of rehemorrhage after treatment of ruptured intracranial aneurysms: the Cerebral Aneurysm Rerupture After Treatment (CARAT) study. Stroke 2008;39(1):120–5.

36. Roos YB, Rinkel GJ, Vermeulen M, et al. Antifibrinolytic therapy for aneurysmal subarachnoid haemorrhage. Cochrane Database Syst Rev 2003;(2):CD001245.

37. Hillman J, Fridriksson S, Nilsson O, et al. Immediate administration of tranexamic acid and reduced incidence of early rebleeding after aneurysmal subarachnoid hemorrhage: a prospective randomized study. J Neurosurg 2002;97(4):771–8.

38. Starke RM, Kim GH, Fernandez A, et al. Impact of a protocol for acute antifibrinolytic therapy on aneurysm rebleeding after subarachnoid hemorrhage. Stroke 2008;39(9):2617–21.

39. Brown RJ, Kumar A, Dhar R, et al. The relationship between delayed infarcts and angiographic vasospasm after aneurysmal subarachnoid hemorrhage. Neurosurgery 2013. [Epub ahead of print].

40. Robertson EG. Cerebral lesions due to intracranial aneurysms. Brain 1949;72(Pt. 2):150–85.

41. Ecker A, Riemenschneider PA. Arteriographic demonstration of spasm of the intracranial arteries, with special reference to saccular arterial aneurysms. J Neurosurg 1951;8(6):660–7.

42. Vergouwen MD, Vermeulen M, van Gijn J, et al. Definition of delayed cerebral ischemia after aneurysmal subarachnoid hemorrhage as an outcome event in clinical trials and observational studies: proposal of a multidisciplinary research group. Stroke 2010;41(10):2391–5.

43. Frontera JA, Fernandez A, Schmidt JM, et al. Clinical response to hypertensive hypervolemic therapy and outcome after subarachnoid hemorrhage. Neurosurgery 2010;66(1):35–41 [discussion: 41].

44. Vergouwen MD, Participants in the International Multi-Disciplinary Consensus Conference on the Critical Care Management of Subarachnoid Hemorrhage. Vasospasm versus delayed cerebral ischemia as an outcome event in clinical trials and observational studies. Neurocrit Care 2011; 15(2):308–11.

45. Frontera JA, Fernandez A, Schmidt JM, et al. Defining vasospasm after subarachnoid hemorrhage: what is the most clinically relevant definition? Stroke 2009;40(6):1963–8.

46. Carrera E, Schmidt JM, Oddo M, et al. Transcranial Doppler for predicting delayed cerebral ischemia after subarachnoid hemorrhage. Neurosurgery 2009;65(2):316–23 [discussion: 323–4].

47. Lysakowski C, Walder B, Costanza MC, et al. Transcranial Doppler versus angiography in patients with vasospasm due to a ruptured cerebral aneurysm: a systematic review. Stroke 2001; 32(10):2292–8.

48. Allen GS, Ahn HS, Preziosi TJ, et al. Cerebral arterial spasm—a controlled trial of nimodipine in patients with subarachnoid hemorrhage. N Engl J Med 1983;308(11):619–24.

49. Dorhout Mees SM, Rinkel GJ, Feigin VL, et al. Calcium antagonists for aneurysmal subarachnoid haemorrhage. Cochrane Database Syst Rev 2007;(3):CD000277.

50. Dorhout Mees SM, Rinkel GJ, Feigin VL, et al. Calcium antagonists for aneurysmal subarachnoid hemorrhage. Stroke 2008;39:514–5.

51. Dorhout Mees SM, Algra A, Vandertop WP, et al. Magnesium for aneurysmal subarachnoid haemorrhage (MASH-2): a randomised placebo-controlled trial. Lancet 2012;380(9836):44–9.

52. Wise G, Sutter R, Burkholder J. The treatment of brain ischemia with vasopressor drugs. Stroke 1972;3(2):135–40.

53. Hunt WE, Kosnik EJ. Timing and perioperative care in intracranial aneurysm surgery. Clin Neurosurg 1974;21:79–89.

54. Wood JH, Fleischer AS. Observations during hypervolemic hemodilution of patients with acute focal cerebral ischemia. JAMA 1982;248(22): 2999–3004.

55. Kassell NF, Peerless SJ, Durward QJ, et al. Treatment of ischemic deficits from vasospasm with intravascular volume expansion and induced arterial hypertension. Neurosurgery 1982;11(3):337–43.

56. Dankbaar JW, Slooter AJ, Rinkel GJ, et al. Effect of different components of triple-H therapy on cerebral perfusion in patients with aneurysmal subarachnoid haemorrhage: a systematic review. Crit Care 2010;14(1):R23.

57. Raabe A, Beck J, Keller M, et al. Relative importance of hypertension compared with hypervolemia for increasing cerebral oxygenation in patients with cerebral vasospasm after subarachnoid hemorrhage. J Neurosurg 2005;103(6):974–81.

58. Lennihan L, Mayer SA, Fink ME, et al. Effect of hypervolemic therapy on cerebral blood flow after subarachnoid hemorrhage: a randomized controlled trial. Stroke 2000;31(2):383–91.

59. Sen J, Belli A, Albon H, et al. Triple-H therapy in the management of aneurysmal subarachnoid haemorrhage. Lancet Neurol 2003;2(10):614–21.

60. Hoh BL, Carter BS, Ogilvy CS. Risk of hemorrhage from unsecured, unruptured aneurysms during and after hypertensive hypervolemic therapy. Neurosurgery 2002;50(6):1207–11 [discussion: 1211–2].

61. Adams HP, del Zoppo G, Alberts MJ, et al. Guidelines for the early management of adults with ischemic stroke: a guideline from the American Heart Association/American Stroke Association Stroke Council, Clinical Cardiology Council, Cardiovascular Radiology and Intervention Council, and the Atherosclerotic Peripheral Vascular Disease and Quality of Care Outcomes in Research Interdisciplinary Working Groups: the American Academy of Neurology affirms the value of this guideline as an educational tool for neurologists. Stroke 2007;38(5):1655–711.

62. Zubkov YN, Nikiforov BM, Shustin VA. Balloon catheter technique for dilatation of constricted cerebral arteries after aneurysmal SAH. Acta Neurochir 1984;70(1–2):65–79.

63. Hoh BL, Ogilvy CS. Endovascular treatment of cerebral vasospasm: transluminal balloon angioplasty, intra-arterial papaverine, and intra-arterial nicardipine. Neurosurg Clin N Am 2005;16(3): 501–16, vi.

64. Kimball MM, Velat GJ, Hoh BL, Participants in the International Multi-Disciplinary Consensus Conference on the Critical Care Management of Subarachnoid Hemorrhage. Critical care guidelines on the endovascular management of cerebral vasospasm. Neurocrit Care 2011;15:336–41.

65. Froehler MT, Kooshkabadi A, Miller-Lotan R, et al. Vasospasm after subarachnoid hemorrhage in haptoglobin 2-2 mice can be prevented with a glutathione peroxidase mimetic. J Clin Neurosci 2010;17(9):1169–72.

66. Pradilla G, Chaichana KL, Hoang S, et al. Inflammation and cerebral vasospasm after subarachnoid hemorrhage. Neurosurg Clin N Am 2010; 21(2):365–79.

67. Chaichana KL, Pradilla G, Huang J, et al. Role of inflammation (leukocyte-endothelial cell interactions) in vasospasm after subarachnoid hemorrhage. World Neurosurg 2010;73(1):22–41.

68. Gallia GL, Tamargo RJ. Leukocyte-endothelial cell interactions in chronic vasospasm after subarachnoid hemorrhage. Neurol Res 2006;28(7):750–8.

69. Fassbender K, Hodapp B, Rossol S, et al. Endothelin-1 in subarachnoid hemorrhage: an acute-phase reactant produced by cerebrospinal fluid leukocytes. Stroke 2000;31(12):2971–5.

70. Ardelt A. From bench-to-bedside in catastrophic cerebrovascular disease: development of drugs targeting the endothelin axis in subarachnoid hemorrhage-related vasospasm. Neurol Res 2012;34:195–210.

71. MacDonald RL, Kassell NF, Mayer S, et al. Clazosentan to overcome neurological ischemia and infarction occurring after subarachnoid hemorrhage (CONSCIOUS-1): randomized, double-blind, placebo-controlled phase 2 dose-finding trial. Stroke 2008;39(11):3015–21.

72. MacDonald RL, Higashida RT, Keller E, et al. Clazosentan, an endothelin receptor antagonist, in patients with aneurysmal subarachnoid haemorrhage undergoing surgical clipping: a randomised, double-blind, placebo-controlled phase 3 trial (CONSCIOUS-2). Lancet Neurol 2011;10(7):618–25.

73. MacDonald RL, Higashida RT, Keller E, et al. Randomized trial of clazosentan in patients with aneurysmal subarachnoid hemorrhage undergoing endovascular coiling. Stroke 2012;43(6):1463–9.

74. Vergouwen MD, Algra A, Rinkel GJ. Endothelin receptor antagonists for aneurysmal subarachnoid hemorrhage: a systematic review and meta-analysis update. Stroke 2012;43(10):2671–6.

75. Kramer AH, Fletcher JJ. Statins in the management of patients with aneurysmal subarachnoid hemorrhage: a systematic review and meta-analysis. Neurocrit Care 2010;12(2):285–96.

76. Vergouwen MD, de Haan RJ, Vermeulen M, et al. Effect of statin treatment on vasospasm, delayed cerebral ischemia, and functional outcome in patients with aneurysmal subarachnoid hemorrhage: a systematic review and meta-analysis update. Stroke 2010;41(1):e47–52.

77. Naidech AM, Kreiter KT, Janjua N, et al. Cardiac troponin elevation, cardiovascular morbidity, and outcome after subarachnoid hemorrhage. Circulation 2005;112(18):2851–6.

78. Lee VH, Oh JK, Mulvagh SL, et al. Mechanisms in neurogenic stress cardiomyopathy after aneurysmal subarachnoid hemorrhage. Neurocrit Care 2006;5(3):243–9.

79. Lee VH, Connolly HM, Fulgham JR, et al. Takotsubo cardiomyopathy in aneurysmal subarachnoid hemorrhage: an underappreciated ventricular dysfunction. J Neurosurg 2006;105(2):264–70.

80. Ako J, Honda Y, Fitzgerald PJ. Tako-tsubo-like left ventricular dysfunction. Circulation 2003;108(23): e158 [author reply: e158].

81. Lazaridis C, Pradilla G, Nyquist PA, et al. Intra-aortic balloon pump counterpulsation in the setting of subarachnoid hemorrhage, cerebral vasospasm, and

neurogenic stress cardiomyopathy. Case report and review of the literature. Neurocrit Care 2010; 13(1):101–8.

82. Coghlan LA, Hindman BJ, Bayman EO, et al. Independent associations between electrocardiographic abnormalities and outcomes in patients with aneurysmal subarachnoid hemorrhage: findings from the intraoperative hypothermia aneurysm surgery trial. Stroke 2009;40(2):412–8.

83. Friedman JA, Pichelmann MA, Piepgras DG, et al. Pulmonary complications of aneurysmal subarachnoid hemorrhage. Neurosurgery 2003;52(5): 1025–31 [discussion: 1031–2].

84. Vespa PM, Bleck TP. Neurogenic pulmonary edema and other mechanisms of impaired oxygenation after aneurysmal subarachnoid hemorrhage. Neurocrit Care 2004;1(2):157–70.

85. Kahn JM, Caldwell EC, Deem S, et al. Acute lung injury in patients with subarachnoid hemorrhage: incidence, risk factors, and outcome. Crit Care Med 2006;34(1):196–202.

86. Bruder N, Rabinstein A, Participants in the International Multi-Disciplinary Consensus Conference on the Critical Care Management of Subarachnoid Hemorrhage. Cardiovascular and pulmonary complications of aneurysmal subarachnoid hemorrhage. Neurocrit Care 2011;15(2):257–69.

87. Gress DR, Participants in the International Multi-Disciplinary Consensus Conference on the Critical Care Management of Subarachnoid Hemorrhage. Monitoring of volume status after subarachnoid hemorrhage. Neurocrit Care 2011;15(2):270–4.

88. Hoff RG, van Dijk GW, Algra A, et al. Fluid balance and blood volume measurement after aneurysmal subarachnoid hemorrhage. Neurocrit Care 2008; 8(3):391–7.

89. Hoff R, Rinkel G, Verweij B, et al. Blood volume measurement to guide fluid therapy after aneurysmal subarachnoid hemorrhage: a prospective controlled study. Stroke 2009;40(7):2575–7.

90. Rosenwasser RH, Jallo JI, Getch CC, et al. Complications of Swan-Ganz catheterization for hemodynamic monitoring in patients with subarachnoid hemorrhage. Neurosurgery 1995;37(5):872–5 [discussion: 875–6].

91. Mutoh T, Kazumata K, Ajiki M, et al. Goal-directed fluid management by bedside transpulmonary hemodynamic monitoring after subarachnoid hemorrhage. Stroke 2007;38(12):3218–24.

92. Mutoh T, Kazumata K, Ishikawa T, et al. Performance of bedside transpulmonary thermodilution monitoring for goal-directed hemodynamic management after subarachnoid hemorrhage. Stroke 2009;40(7):2368–74.

93. Egge A, Waterloo K, Sjøholm H, et al. Prophylactic hyperdynamic postoperative fluid therapy after aneurysmal subarachnoid hemorrhage: a clinical,

prospective, randomized, controlled study. Neurosurgery 2001;49(3):593–605 [discussion: 605–6].

94. Qureshi AI, Suri MF, Sung GY, et al. Prognostic significance of hypernatremia and hyponatremia among patients with aneurysmal subarachnoid hemorrhage. Neurosurgery 2002;50(4):749–55 [discussion: 755–6].

95. Harrigan MR. Cerebral salt wasting syndrome. Crit Care Clin 2001;17(1):125–38.

96. Suarez JI, Qureshi AI, Parekh PD, et al. Administration of hypertonic (3%) sodium chloride/acetate in hyponatremic patients with symptomatic vasospasm following subarachnoid hemorrhage. J Neurosurg Anesthesiol 1999;11(3):178–84.

97. Katayama Y, Haraoka J, Hirabayashi H, et al. A randomized controlled trial of hydrocortisone against hyponatremia in patients with aneurysmal subarachnoid hemorrhage. Stroke 2007;38(8):2373–5.

98. Hasan D, Lindsay KW, Wijdicks EF, et al. Effect of fludrocortisone acetate in patients with subarachnoid hemorrhage. Stroke 1989;20(9):1156–61.

99. Mori T, Katayama Y, Kawamata T, et al. Improved efficiency of hypervolemic therapy with inhibition of natriuresis by fludrocortisone in patients with aneurysmal subarachnoid hemorrhage. J Neurosurg 1999;91(6):947–52.

100. Nakagawa I, Hironaka Y, Nishimura F, et al. Early inhibition of natriuresis suppresses symptomatic cerebral vasospasm in patients with aneurysmal subarachnoid hemorrhage. Cerebrovasc Dis 2013;35(2):131–7.

101. Fernandez A, Schmidt JM, Claassen J, et al. Fever after subarachnoid hemorrhage: risk factors and impact on outcome. Neurology 2007;68(13):1013–9.

102. Naidech AM, Bendok BR, Bernstein RA, et al. Fever burden and functional recovery after subarachnoid hemorrhage. Neurosurgery 2008;63(2):212–7 [discussion: 217–8].

103. Frontera JA, Fernandez A, Schmidt JM, et al. Impact of nosocomial infectious complications after subarachnoid hemorrhage. Neurosurgery 2008;62(1):80–7 [discussion: 87].

104. Rousseaux P, Scherpereel B, Bernard MH, et al. Fever and cerebral vasospasm in ruptured intracranial aneurysms. Surg Neurol 1980;14(6):459–65.

105. McGirt MJ, Woodworth GF, Ali M, et al. Persistent perioperative hyperglycemia as an independent predictor of poor outcome after aneurysmal subarachnoid hemorrhage. J Neurosurg 2007;107(6):1080–5.

106. Kruyt ND, Biessels GJ, de Haan RJ, et al. Hyperglycemia and clinical outcome in aneurysmal subarachnoid hemorrhage: a meta-analysis. Stroke 2009;40(6):e424–30.

107. Frontera JA, Fernandez A, Claassen J, et al. Hyperglycemia after SAH: predictors, associated complications, and impact on outcome. Stroke 2006;37(1):199–203.

108. Naidech AM, Levasseur K, Liebling S, et al. Moderate hypoglycemia is associated with vasospasm, cerebral infarction, and 3-month disability after subarachnoid hemorrhage. Neurocrit Care 2010;12(2):181–7.

109. NICE-SUGAR Study Investigators, Finfer S, Chittock DR, et al. Intensive versus conventional glucose control in critically ill patients. N Engl J Med 2009;360(13):1283–97.

110. Lee SH, Heros RC, Mullan JC, et al. Optimum degree of hemodilution for brain protection in a canine model of focal cerebral ischemia. J Neurosurg 1994;80(3):469–75.

111. Kramer AH, Zygun DA, Bleck TP, et al. Relationship between hemoglobin concentrations and outcomes across subgroups of patients with aneurysmal subarachnoid hemorrhage. Neurocrit Care 2009;10(2):157–65.

112. Kramer AH, Gurka MJ, Nathan B, et al. Complications associated with anemia and blood transfusion in patients with aneurysmal subarachnoid hemorrhage. Crit Care Med 2008;36(7):2070–5.

113. Naidech AM, Drescher J, Ault ML, et al. Higher hemoglobin is associated with less cerebral infarction, poor outcome, and death after subarachnoid hemorrhage. Neurosurgery 2006;59(4):775–9 [discussion: 779–80].

114. Naidech AM, Jovanovic B, Wartenberg KE, et al. Higher hemoglobin is associated with improved outcome after subarachnoid hemorrhage. Crit Care Med 2007;35(10):2383–9.

115. Naidech AM, Shaibani A, Garg RK, et al. Prospective, randomized trial of higher goal hemoglobin after subarachnoid hemorrhage. Neurocrit Care 2010;13(3):313–20.

116. Hébert PC, Wells G, Blajchman MA, et al. A multicenter, randomized, controlled clinical trial of transfusion requirements in critical care. Transfusion Requirements in Critical Care Investigators, Canadian Critical Care Trials Group. N Engl J Med 1999;340(6):409–17.

117. Ray WZ, Strom RG, Blackburn SL, et al. Incidence of deep venous thrombosis after subarachnoid hemorrhage. J Neurosurg 2009;110(5):1010–4.

118. Mack WJ, Ducruet AF, Hickman ZL, et al. Doppler ultrasonography screening of poor-grade subarachnoid hemorrhage patients increases the diagnosis of deep venous thrombosis. Neurol Res 2008;30(9):889–92.

119. Collen JF, Jackson JL, Shorr AF, et al. Prevention of venous thromboembolism in neurosurgery: a meta-analysis. Chest 2008;134(2):237–49.

120. Vespa P, Participants in the International Multi-Disciplinary Consensus Conference on the Critical Care Management of Subarachnoid Hemorrhage. Deep venous thrombosis prophylaxis. Neurocrit Care 2011;15(2):295–7.

121. Raja PV, Huang J, Germanwala AV, et al. Microsurgical clipping and endovascular coiling of intracranial aneurysms: a critical review of the literature. Neurosurgery 2008;62(6):1187–202 [discussion: 1202–3].

122. Kung DK, Policeni BA, Capuano AW, et al. Risk of ventriculostomy-related hemorrhage in patients with acutely ruptured aneurysms treated using stent-assisted coiling. J Neurosurg 2011;114(4): 1021–7.

Management of Acute Spinal Cord Injury in the Neurocritical Care Unit

Linton T. Evans, MD[a],*, Stuart Scott Lollis, MD[a], Perry A. Ball, MD[a,b]

KEYWORDS

• Spinal cord injury • Neurogenic shock • Mechanical ventilation • Thromboembolism

KEY POINTS

- Traumatic spinal cord injury (SCI) is frequently accompanied by multiple injuries and widespread derangements requiring aggressive monitoring and management in the intensive care unit.
- Neuroprotective therapies are designed to minimize further neurologic deterioration. Several pharmacologic agents and hypothermia are currently under investigation.
- Cardiovascular complications including hypotension and arrhythmias are not uncommon, and represent an important source of morbidity following acute SCI.
- SCI may lead to absent or inefficient respiratory mechanics, atelectasis, pneumonia, and pulmonary dysfunction requiring intubation and mechanical ventilation.
- Prophylaxis and surveillance of deep venous thrombosis is paramount in individuals with SCI, and should be instituted within 72 hours of injury.

INTRODUCTION

Acute spinal cord injury (SCI) is often devastating, and imposes significant emotional and economic costs to the individual and society. The morbidity and sequelae are severe and frequently fatal. Mortality at the time of injury is 48% to 79%, with another 4.4% to 16% of deaths occurring before hospital discharge. Traumatic SCI occurs with an annual incidence of approximately 15 to 40 cases per million in the United States. Estimates of prevalence are 236,000 to 327,000.[1–3] SCI disproportionately affects young adults. The mean age at injury is 41 years, although two-thirds of individuals are younger than 30. Motor vehicle accidents account for 40% to 50% of SCI followed by falls (20%), violence (14%), and recreational and work-related activities.[4,5] The epidemiology and mechanism of SCI have important implications on preventive measures, the type of injury sustained, and subsequent management in the critical care unit.

Evaluation and management of acute SCI is complicated by broad pathophysiologic derangements that require timely identification and intervention. Respiratory insufficiency or other pulmonary dysfunction, systemic hypotension, cardiac arrhythmias, and delayed neurologic decline are well-described phenomena following SCI. Additional systemic injuries are commonplace, with 20% to 57% of those with SCI having other significant injuries typically involving the head or chest. Isolated SCIs are reported to occur in only 20% of individuals.[6] The management of these

[a] Section of Neurosurgery, Dartmouth-Hitchcock Medical Center, One Medical Center Drive, Lebanon, NH 03756, USA; [b] Department of Anesthesiology, Dartmouth-Hitchcock Medical Center, One Medical Center Drive, Lebanon, NH 03756, USA
* Corresponding author.
E-mail address: Linton.T.Evans@Hitchcock.org

Neurosurg Clin N Am 24 (2013) 339–347
http://dx.doi.org/10.1016/j.nec.2013.02.007
1042-3680/13/$ – see front matter © 2013 Elsevier Inc. All rights reserved.

patients in the intensive care unit is frequently directed by treatment of concurrent injuries. The majority of traumatic SCIs (55%) involve the cervical spine.[7] The last 3 decades have witnessed an increase in the proportion of cervical spine injuries. Specifically this has been injury to C1 to C4, nearly tripling the number of individuals requiring intubation and ventilator dependence from 1.4% in 1970 to 4.6% in 2004.[3] During this same period there has been a concomitant decrease in the number of complete SCIs from more than 60% to 45%.[8] This decline is multifactorial and reflects improvements in prehospital resuscitation and retrieval, immobilization, and motor vehicle restraint and safety devices. Advances in monitoring and medical management also hold an important role in limiting secondary injury from hypoxia or hypotension. Several studies have demonstrated improved morbidity and mortality with monitoring and aggressive management of SCI in the critical care setting.[9] The median length of hospital admission following SCI is 67 days, with 11 of those days spent in the acute care setting at a cost of $95,203.[10] This review discusses the potential complications and medical management of acute SCI in the neurocritical care unit.

MANAGEMENT OF NEUROLOGIC INJURY

Treatment of acute SCI in the intensive care unit focuses on prevention of secondary injury and neuroprotection. Following an initial insult or trauma producing spinal cord compression, contusion, laceration, or shear, a cascade of pathologic events develops. These abnormalities include loss of normal blood flow in the spine, ischemia, vasospasm, thrombosis, hemorrhage, impaired autoregulation of the microcirculation, and systemic hypotension from neurogenic shock; electrolyte disturbances; neurotransmitter accumulation and excitotoxicity; lipid peroxidation; arachidonic acid production and inflammation; free radical production; edema; apoptosis; and necrosis.[2,11,12] Delayed neurologic deterioration is well described, with a reported incidence of 1.8% to 10%, and may be seen from hours to days following the onset of injury.[13] Intensive monitoring and rapid correction of hypotension or hypoxia is essential (see later discussion). Pharmacologic strategies to blunt secondary injury have also been used, perhaps the most well described being methylprednisolone.

Glucocorticoids offer neuroprotection by increasing cell membrane integrity, augmenting spinal cord perfusion, inhibiting endogenous endorphin release, and decreasing inflammation and free radical production, as well as by limiting vasogenic edema through stabilization of the blood–spinal cord barrier. The largest clinical trials investigating the efficacy of methylprednisolone are the 3 multicenter randomized NASCIS (National Acute Spinal Cord Injury Study) trials. The first of these studies (NASCIS I) compared motor and sensory scores in individuals with SCI following administration of either a 100-mg or 1000-mg bolus of methylprednisolone followed by a daily dose for 10 days. There was no placebo, and comparison of the outcomes at 6 weeks and 6 months showed no difference.[14] With the NASCIS II study, the dose of methylprednisolone was increased and individuals with SCI were randomized to 3 different treatments: (1) methylprednisolone (30 mg/kg bolus followed by 5.4 mg/kg/h for 23 hours); (2) the opioid antagonist naloxone (5.4 mg/kg bolus followed by 4.0 mg/kg/h for 23 hours); and (3) placebo. Through post hoc analysis the investigators reported improved motor and sensory scores at 6 months if methylprednisolone was administered within 8 hours of injury. This benefit was observed for both complete and incomplete injuries, but was not present in patients receiving steroids more than 8 hours following injury, naloxone, or placebo.[15,16] A third trial (NASCIS III) randomized patients to receive methylprednisolone for 24 or 48 hours or the antioxidant tirilazad mesylate for 48 hours after a bolus of methylprednisolone. Tirilazad mesylate impairs lipid peroxidation but does not contain the steroid moiety to interact with and activate glucocorticoid receptors, and is thus thought to avoid the adverse effects of methylprednisolone. Neurologic outcomes were similar for all treatment groups if initiated within 3 hours of injury. When comparing individuals treated between 3 and 8 hours following injury, motor scores and functional measures were improved at 6 weeks and 6 months in participants treated with methylprednisolone for 48 hours. The neurologic outcomes were equivocal for subjects who received 24 hours of methylprednisolone and 48 hours of tirilazad mesylate. No difference in functional outcome scores was seen in the 3 groups at 1 year.[17,18]

Several limitations to the NASCIS trials exist. The studies excluded pediatric SCI, penetrating injury, or cauda equina injuries, and do not specifically address these entities. Administration of methylprednisolone was associated with increased incidence of pulmonary embolism and pneumonia, wound infection, sepsis, and gastrointestinal complications in NASCIS II and III. Other reports have also noted increased length of admission and altered immune function.[12,19] Several methodological flaws have also been identified, including a post hoc versus prospectively defined time course (ie,

8 hours), inclusion of patients with minimal deficits and lesions below T12, use of right-sided motor scores only, lack of functional measures, and no standardization with respect to surgical or medical treatment.[12,20] For these reasons, the use of methylprednisolone in SCI is controversial. The Cochrane database offers the NASCIS experience as a recommendation for the use of methylprednisolone within 8 hours of injury.[21] Guidelines published by the American Association of Neurological Surgeons (AANS) and the Congress of Neurological Surgeons (CNS) recently modified the recommendations against the use of methylprednisolone in the management of spinal cord injury.[22]

Other pharmacologic agents have also been studied in the setting of acute SCI.[20] In laboratory studies, GM-1 ganglioside has been associated with increased neural plasticity following injury, diminished excitotoxicity, and reduced apoptosis. A prospective study randomizing 37 individuals with SCI to placebo or GM-1 ganglioside demonstrated improved Frankel and ASIA (American Spinal Injury Association) scores at 1-year follow-up in participants who received 100 mg of GM-1 for 30 days.[23] This study served as the impetus for a large multicenter randomized trial examining the effects of low-dose GM-1, high-dose GM-1, and placebo. All subjects received methylprednisolone as described in the NASCIS II study. In this large study of 797 patients, there was no significant difference in neurologic outcome between the treatment groups, limiting the use of GM-1.[24] Opioid antagonists such as naloxone, glutamate antagonists, nimodipine, other anti-inflammatories, and erythropoietin have all garnered interest following optimistic findings in laboratory models.

In addition to pharmacologic methods of neuroprotection, there is increasing interest in therapeutic hypothermia. In laboratory models, moderate hypothermia has led to alterations in apoptosis as well as reduced mitochondrial dysfunction, metabolic demand, cell membrane injury, and inflammation. In rodents, prompt cooling following induced SCI offered improved motor outcomes, and the use of hypothermia is reported to decrease SCI following aortic cross-clamping.[25] Fourteen patients with complete SCI underwent moderate hypothermia (33°C) for 48 hours in a study by Levi and colleagues[26] in 2009. At median follow-up of 12 months, 6 individuals (43%) had neurologic improvement.[27] The most frequent complications were pulmonary (pneumonia or atelectasis), but occurred at a rate similar to that of controls. Another study had similar results following endovascular cooling in 35 individuals with complete cervical SCI. The duration of hypothermic therapy was 48 hours, and 15 (43%) had

improvement based on the International Standards for Neurological Classification of Spinal Cord Injury scale.[28] Following completion of phase I trials, large multicenter studies are currently being conducted (see clinicaltrials.gov).

CARDIOVASCULAR COMPLICATIONS

Severe SCI is frequently associated with hemodynamic instability. Disruption of sympathetic fibers through injury to the cervical or high-thoracic (>T6) spinal cord produces hypotension and cardiac arrhythmias. Fifty percent to 90% of individuals with acute cervical SCI require aggressive fluid resuscitation or initiation of vasopressors to maintain a mean arterial pressure greater than 80 mm Hg.[29] Typically the degree of cardiac instability is related to the severity of the SCI. At autopsy, individuals with cervical SCI developing significant hypotension, arrhythmia, or autonomic dysreflexia had increased degeneration compared with those without cardiac instability.[30] In addition, these individuals had fewer preserved axons within the lateral funiculus. Descending sympathetic fibers originating in the hypothalamus or brainstem are located within the intermediolateral and dorsolateral aspects of the lateral funiculus.[31] Injury leads to loss of sympathetic outflow and unopposed parasympathetic tone with decreased cardiac contractility, heart rate, and vasoconstrictor tone.

The hypotension and neurogenic shock following acute SCI is a distributive process resulting from loss of vasoconstrictor tone in peripheral arterioles and pooling of blood within the peripheral vasculature. Initial attempts at correction should include volume resuscitation with intravenous fluids. Administration of fluids transiently increases venous return. However, with disruption of sympathetic innervation to the heart and predominance of parasympathetic tone, cardiac output remains low because of impaired cardiac contractility and decreased heart rate. If after 1 to 2 L of intravenous fluids the blood pressure has not improved, vasopressor therapy may be indicated. Vasoactive agents with α-adrenergic and β-adrenergic effects, such as dopamine and norepinephrine, increase vasoconstrictor tone and chronotropic support to the heart. Vasopressors with exclusive α-adrenergic function have no chronotropic effect and are of limited use in neurogenic shock. Furthermore, phenylephrine frequently produces a reflex bradycardia. Throughout these interventions frequent monitoring of blood pressure, heart rate, urine output, and resolution of acidosis are vital. Echocardiography offers the ability to efficiently assess cardiac output and filling. In select situations, invasive monitoring with a pulmonary artery catheter assists in treatment by measuring cardiac output and peripheral vascular resistance, although this has largely been replaced by the echocardiogram.[32]

In a study by Levi and colleagues,[33] 82% of individuals with incomplete cervical SCI required vasopressor therapy for an average of 5.7 days following injury to maintain a mean arterial pressure (MAP) of greater than 90 mm Hg. Another study correlated level and severity of spinal injury with the need for vasopressors: complete cervical SCI 90%, incomplete cervical SCI 52%, complete thoracic SCI 33%, and incomplete thoracic 25%.[34] Management of hypotension following SCI is commonplace in the neurocritical care unit. Throughout the resuscitation efforts it is important to continually reassess and ensure that other events such as hemorrhage, tension pneumothorax, or cardiac tamponade are not etiologic.

Although avoidance of systemic hypotension and adequate tissue perfusion are well accepted, blood pressure targets are not as clearly defined. In addition, it is difficult to accurately assess spinal cord perfusion. There are several uncontrolled studies describing improved neurologic outcomes with a MAP greater than 85 to 90 mm Hg. Vale and colleagues[34] used a MAP of 85 mm Hg to direct aggressive fluid resuscitation and vasopressors for 7 days following injury. The small series reported improved outcomes, but the MAP in this study was selected arbitrarily. The AANS/CNS guidelines recommend maintenance of a MAP of between 85 and 90 mm Hg for the first 7 days as an option for treatment.[22]

Loss of sympathetic innervation with unopposed vagal tone produces frequent and often severe cardiac arrhythmias such as bradycardia and, less often, supraventricular tachycardia or ventricular tachycardia. Estimates of cardiac arrest following cervical SCI are as high as 15%. The arrhythmias typically develop within 3 to 5 days following injury and become less pronounced at day 14. The severity of cardiac instability is influenced by the degree of spinal injury as well as other factors such as hypoxia, endotracheal suctioning, and physical stimulation. Treatment includes continuous monitoring and, when symptomatic bradycardia develops, oxygen, atropine, inotropes, and aminophylline. These pharmacologic measures are usually effective, but if bradycardia persists patients may require a cardiac pacemaker. The number of individuals with cervical SCI requiring cardiac pacing ranges from 9% to 17%.[35]

Orthostatic hypotension and autonomic dysreflexia are known to occur following SCI. Typically these are seen in the subacute or chronic phase of injury,[36] but may complicate admission to the neurocritical care unit. Orthostatic hypotension is defined as a decrease in systolic blood pressure of greater than 20 mm Hg or diastolic blood pressure greater than 10 mm Hg when transitioning from a supine to upright position. The prevalence of orthostatic hypotension is approximately 80% and 50% for quadriplegics and paraplegics, respectively.[37] Nearly 50% of individuals with cervical SCI will experience symptoms of orthostatic hypotension, and require treatment. This orthostasis results from venous pooling of blood resulting from the loss of vasoconstrictor tone and arterial baroreceptors caudal to the injury level, an ineffective increase in heart rate from unopposed vagal tone, and loss of muscular tone in the lower extremities, impairing venous return to the heart. Treatment measures include volume expansion through fluids, increased salt intake, or fludrocortisone; pressure devices such as abdominal binders; devices supplying electrical stimulation to and contraction of the lower extremity musculature; midodrine, a potent α-agonist; or ephedrine. The most well-described pharmacologic agents are fludrocortisone and midodrine.[38]

Individuals with severe SCI rostral to T6 are subject to autonomic dysreflexia. During these periods noxious or seemingly benign stimulation below the level of injury, such as bowel or bladder distention, leads to rapid and dramatic elevation in blood pressure and heart rate. By definition this is characterized by an elevation in blood pressure greater than 20%, tachycardia, or bradycardia, and is associated with other symptoms of overactive autonomic stimulation such as piloerection, diaphoresis, or flushing. Dysreflexia is seen in up to 90% of individuals with complete tetraplegia but in less than 30% of those with incomplete tetraplegia. Autonomic dysreflexia is typically a chronic complication following SCI. In a study of 58 patients with cervical SCI, however, approximately 3% of subjects exhibited dysreflexic episodes acutely. Prompt recognition and treatment is important in avoiding complications of hypertensive crisis such as intracranial or retinal hemorrhages, seizure, or death.[38,39]

Treatment of autonomic dysreflexia begins with identification of the offending stimulus. A distended bladder or bowel should be relieved and all other noxious stimuli removed. Pharmacologic interventions designed to shorten the disturbance include nitrates, prostaglandin E2, hydralazine, labetalol, or captopril. Prevention of dysreflexic episodes involves avoidance of noxious stimuli. In addition, the use of prazosin or terazosin is described in the literature.[40–42] Nifedipine had once been used for this purpose but has since been abandoned following reports of deaths associated with this medication.

RESPIRATORY INSUFFICIENCY AND PULMONARY DYSFUNCTION

SCI has profound effects on the mechanics of ventilation and respiratory physiology. Inspiration occurs through contraction of the diaphragm and internal intercostal muscles, leading to expansion of the chest cavity. At strenuous levels of respiration, the accessory muscles defined by the pectoralis major, scalene, and sternocleidomastoid are recruited. Expiration is largely a passive process, but is augmented by contraction of the abdominal wall. The diaphragm is innervated by the C3-C5 segments forming the phrenic nerve. Innervation of the accessory muscles is variable, involving several spinal segments: thoracic nerves (intercostal), C1-C2 (sternocleidomastoid), and C4-C8 (scalene). SCI above the C3 level leads to loss of diaphragmatic function and immediate respiratory insufficiency. Typically the injury is fatal unless mechanical ventilation is initiated. Although function of the diaphragm is spared with injury below the C3 level, ventilation remains significantly compromised. Acutely following injury there is flaccid paralysis of the accessory muscles innervated by the lower cervical and thoracic segments. The accessory muscles normally stabilize the chest wall, and in their absence contraction of the diaphragm causes the chest wall to contract rather than expand, with paradoxic motion and decreased volumes.[32] The loss of ventilatory function is profound, with a decrease in maximal inspiratory force of 70%.[43,44]

The mechanics of the diaphragm are similarly affected by paralysis of the abdominal musculature. Integrated action of the intact intercostal and abdominal musculature functions as a fulcrum against which the diaphragm contracts. Loss of this mechanical advantage leads to increased diaphragmatic work. In addition, with flaccid paralysis of the abdominal muscles, the abdominal contents and viscera are displaced inferiorly away from the diaphragm. The diaphragm subsequently flattens, diminishing the radius of curvature and placing the diaphragm at a mechanical disadvantage. This effect is further exaggerated when a quadriplegic patient is positioned in the upright position; paradoxically, ventilation is improved when supine. Similarly, the loss of abdominal-wall contraction during expiration decreases the maximal expiratory force, leading to a decreased ability to cough and clear secretions. With resolution of spinal shock, the intercostal muscles develop a spastic paralysis and the chest wall regains its rigidity, no longer collapsing with inspiration. This process leads to improved ventilation. At 5 months following injury, the forced vital capacity and maximal inspiratory force approach 60% of preinjury levels.[32,43,44]

Other factors contributing to respiratory insufficiency and pulmonary dysfunction following SCI include loss of compliance and bronchial hyperresponsiveness. Spastic paresis of the intercostal muscles stiffens the thoracic cage, decreasing compliance. In addition, persistent low lung volumes and altered surfactant have been reported to contribute to reduced lung compliance in cervical SCI.[45,46] Increased bronchial responsiveness and reversible airflow limitation have also been reported in individuals with quadriplegia. This finding reflects unopposed vagal or cholinergic tone to the bronchioles mediating bronchoconstriction, and is reversed with anticholinergic agents. The loss of postganglionic sympathetic innervation and impaired smooth muscle relaxation from low lung volumes has a minor effect.[47]

Intubation and Mechanical Ventilation

The inefficient and compromised ventilation that occurs following SCI is initially tolerated and is compensated by an increase in respiratory rate. Arterial blood gas is often within normal limits, or notable only for mild hypoxia. The rapid and shallow breathing is difficult to maintain, owing to increased work. The proportion of each breath participating in gas exchange decreases because of the fixed dead space of the trachea and bronchi. Low lung volumes promote atelectasis, further contributing to respiratory insufficiency and fatigue. Approximately one-third of patients with injuries to the cervical spine require intubation within the first 24 hours of injury.[48] Ninety percent of those developing respiratory failure do so within the first 3 days. Frequent monitoring for signs of impending respiratory insufficiency are crucial in the acute period following SCI. The decision of when to intubate is often difficult, but should be considered with increasing respiratory rate, rising partial pressure of CO_2, and progressive decline in vital capacity.

Ideally intubation is performed under a controlled setting rather than in an emergent situation. Two large series have demonstrated the safety of endotracheal intubation in cervical SCI with manual in-line traction.[32,49,50] Paralytics facilitate control of the airway during intubation. Although succinylcholine is ideal in most instances because of its rapid onset and short half-life, it should be avoided in SCI after more than 4 days because of the risk of potentially life-threatening hyperkalemia.[32]

Over the following weeks there is progressive improvement in pulmonary function. With resolution of spinal cord inflammation and spinal shock, there is a functional descent in the level of neuro-logic injury and transition from flaccid to spastic paralysis of the intercostal muscles, restoring support to the chest wall in individuals with injury below C4. Respiratory failure is more common in complete than in incomplete injuries, and the duration of mechanical ventilation varies based on the level of injury. The average number of days on mechanical ventilation is 65 for C1-C4 injuries, 22 for C4-C8 injuries, and 12 for thoracic injuries. Typically ventilator support is not weaned until about 12 days following injury. The appropriate timing is variable, but indicators that weaning may be tolerated include an increase in the forced vital capacity, inspired oxygen content of less than 50%, and minute ventilation less than 10 L. Pressure support modes of ventilation allow for a progressive decrease in the amount of mechanical support. T-piece trials and continuous positive airway pressure are other effective methods of weaning.[32]

Tracheostomy

The timing of tracheostomy is variable, but typically will be considered after 14 days of mechanical ventilation. There are several advantages to tracheostomy, and it often facilitates transfer to lower levels of care. A tracheostomy is less irritating to the posterior pharyngeal mucosa than an endotracheal tube, and is generally better tolerated and more comfortable to the patient. For individuals with a marginal respiratory status, tracheostomy has less dead space ventilation and offers the ability to alternate between mechanical and spontaneous ventilation for periods of time. There is limited evidence from the trauma literature that tracheostomy is associated with lower rates of pneumonia.[51,52] When an anterior stabilization has been performed, the tracheostomy site is often near the incision, necessitating that the tracheostomy be delayed to allow for adequate tissue healing.

Pneumonia

Following SCI several respiratory disturbances contribute to the development of pneumonia, the most significant of which is mechanical ventilation. The incidence of ventilator-associated pneumonia increases by 1% to 3% per day of mechanical ventilation, and represents an important cause of morbidity and mortality (27%) in SCI.[53] If diagnosed within 4 days of intubation, the most common pathogens are Streptococcus pneumonia or Haemophilus influenzae, whereas gram-negative bacilli and Staphylococcus aureus dominate at later time points, affecting antibiotic selection.

Prompt diagnosis and initiation of treatment is important. Guidelines assembled by the American College of Chest Physicians to aid in the diagnosis of nosocomial pneumonia include: (1) temperature higher than 38°C or lower than 36°C; (2) leukocytosis or leukopenia; (3) purulent secretions; (4) hypoxemia. Alternatively, if chest radiographs or imaging exhibit an infiltrate or air bronchograms, the selection of antibiotics is based on culture data from tracheal aspirates, either quantitative or qualitative.[54] After initiating broad-spectrum antimicrobials, the antibiotic therapy should be tailored to the offending pathogens once identified. If infection from Pseudomonas is suspected, aggressive treatment with 2 agents, a β-lactam and aminoglycoside, should be administered. The mortality from Pseudomonas pneumonia is reported to be as high as 47%.[32]

THROMBOEMBOLIC COMPLICATIONS

The incidence of venous thromboembolism following SCI is as high as 81%, with the most significant risk occurring between 72 hours and 2 weeks following injury.[38,55,56] A meta-analysis reviewing the factors associated with venous thromboembolism in trauma patients demonstrated that the risk was increased 2-fold in patients with spine fractures and 3-fold in those with injury to the cord.[57] Initiation of thromboprophylaxis following injury is essential, as is efficient diagnosis if venous thromboembolism is suspected. The options for prophylaxis are mechanical devices such as external pneumatic compression devices or stockings, and the anticoagulants unfractionated heparin, low molecular weight heparin, and warfarin. Mechanical compression devices are low risk and widely used, but alone are not sufficient. Anticoagulation is effective, with a well-documented decrease in the incidence of thromboembolism associated with its use. A potential disadvantage, however, is the increased risk of hemorrhage, particularly in the setting of intracranial or spinal hematoma. The incidence of venous thromboembolism is relatively low within the first 72 hours of SCI, and the current consensus is to start prophylactic anticoagulation within 72 hours of injury for a duration of 8 weeks. Standard mini-dose heparin administered twice daily is not sufficient in patients with SCI, and the first-line recommendation is to use low molecular weight heparin.[58,59] An inferior vena cava filter should be considered if thromboprophylaxis has failed, if anticoagulation is contraindicated because of active hemorrhage, or if a patient with a high cervical injury has a tenuous cardiopulmonary reserve.[59]

Multiple methods exist for the diagnosis of venous thrombosis or pulmonary embolism. The use of compression B-mode ultrasonography is efficient and safe, largely replacing the use of contrast venography. Similarly, the pulmonary angiogram remains the standard for the diagnosis of a pulmonary embolism, but its use has been restricted owing to concerns for complications and cost. Less invasive techniques to evaluate for a pulmonary embolism are ventilation-perfusion (V/Q) scans and spiral computed tomography (CT). Spiral CT now dominates as the diagnostic test of choice for clots in the segmental and sub-segmental pulmonary artery branches.[32] The reported sensitivity and specificity are 94% and 96%, respectively; in patients with suspected pulmonary embolism randomized to a spiral CT or V/Q scan, the diagnosis was made more frequently in those undergoing CT.[60] Finally, the hemodynamic strain often associated with a large pulmonary embolism may be appreciated on a transthoracic echocardiogram.

If not contraindicated, treatment with parenteral anticoagulation such as warfarin should be initiated immediately following diagnosis of a deep venous thrombosis (DVT) or pulmonary embolism. In the setting of a DVT, therapeutic anticoagulation for 6 weeks to 6 months helps reduce the risk of recurrent DVT, post-thrombotic syndrome, and pulmonary embolism. When a patient is found to have a pulmonary embolism, it is recommended that therapeutic unfractionated heparin or low molecular weight heparin be administered for 5 days and an International Normalized Ratio of 2 to 3 is achieved for 2 consecutive days on warfarin. The duration of anticoagulation is typically 6 months.[38]

REFERENCES

1. van den Berg ME, Castellote JM, de Pedro-Cuesta J, et al. Survival after spinal cord injury: a systematic review. J Neurotrauma 2010;27(8):1517–28.
2. Sekhon LH, Fehlings MG. Epidemiology, demographics, and pathophysiology of acute spinal cord injury. Spine 2001;26(Suppl 24):S2–12.
3. Devivo MJ. Epidemiology of traumatic spinal cord injury: trends and future implications. Spinal Cord 2012;50(5):365–72.
4. Vitale MG, Goss JM, Matsumoto H, et al. Epidemiology of pediatric spinal cord injury in the United States: years 1997 and 2000. J Pediatr Orthop 2006;26(6):745–9.
5. Jackson AB, Dijkers M, Devivo MJ, et al. A demographic profile of new traumatic spinal cord injuries: change and stability over 30 years. Arch Phys Med Rehabil 2004;85(11):1740–8.
6. Burney RE, Maio RF, Maynard F, et al. Incidence, characteristics, and outcome of spinal cord injury at trauma centers in North America. Arch Surg 1993;128(5):596–9.
7. Hasler RM, Exadaktylos AK, Bouamra O, et al. Epidemiology and predictors of cervical spine injury in adult major trauma patients: a multicenter cohort study. J Trauma Acute Care Surg 2012;72(4):975–81.
8. Tator CH, Duncan EG, Edmonds VE, et al. Changes in epidemiology of acute spinal cord injury from 1947 to 1981. Surg Neurol 1993;40(3):207–15.
9. Management of acute spinal cord injuries in an intensive care unit or other monitored setting. Neurosurgery 2002;50(Suppl 3):S51–7.
10. National Spinal Cord Injury Statistical Center, Birmingham, AL. Annual report for the model spinal cord injury care systems, Birmingham, October, 2011. (Citation is from the 2011 Annual statistical report of the National Spinal Cord Injury Statisical Center).
11. McDonald JW, Sadowsky C. Spinal-cord injury. Lancet 2002;359(9304):417–25.
12. Pharmacological therapy after acute cervical spinal cord injury. Neurosurgery 2002;50(Suppl 3):S63–72.
13. Harrop JS, Sharan AD, Vaccaro AR, et al. The cause of neurologic deterioration after acute cervical spinal cord injury. Spine 2001;26(4):340–6.
14. Bracken MB, Collins WF, Freeman DF, et al. Efficacy of methylprednisolone in acute spinal cord injury. JAMA 1984;251(1):45–52.
15. Bracken MB, Shepard MJ, Collins WF, et al. A randomized, controlled trial of methylprednisolone or naloxone in the treatment of acute spinal-cord injury. Results of the Second National Acute Spinal Cord Injury Study. N Engl J Med 1990;322(20):1405–11.
16. Bracken MB, Shepard MJ, Collins WF Jr, et al. Methylprednisolone or naloxone treatment after acute spinal cord injury: 1-year follow-up data. Results of the second National Acute Spinal Cord Injury Study. J Neurosurg 1992;76(1):23–31.
17. Bracken MB, Shepard MJ, Holford TR, et al. Administration of methylprednisolone for 24 or 48 hours or tirilazad mesylate for 48 hours in the treatment of acute spinal cord injury. Results of the Third National Acute Spinal Cord Injury Randomized Controlled Trial. National Acute Spinal Cord Injury Study. JAMA 1997;277(20):1597–604.
18. Bracken MB, Shepard MJ, Holford TR, et al. Methylprednisolone or tirilazad mesylate administration after acute spinal cord injury: 1-year follow up. Results of the third National Acute Spinal Cord Injury randomized controlled trial. J Neurosurg 1998;89(5):699–706.
19. Galandiuk S, Raque G, Appel S, et al. The two-edged sword of large-dose steroids for spinal

cord trauma. Ann Surg 1993;218(4):419–25 [discussion: 419–25].

20. Kwon BK, Tetzlaff W, Grauer JN, et al. Pathophysiology and pharmacologic treatment of acute spinal cord injury. Spine J 2004;4(4):451–64.

21. Bracken MB. Steroids for acute spinal cord injury. Cochrane Database Syst Rev 2012;(1):CD001046.

22. Hurlbert RH, Hadley MN, et al. Guidelines for the management of acute cervical spine and spinal cord injuries. Clin Neurosurg 2013;72: 93–105.

23. Geisler FH, Dorsey FC, Coleman WP. Recovery of motor function after spinal-cord injury—a randomized, placebo-controlled trial with GM-1 ganglioside. N Engl J Med 1991;324(26):1829–38.

24. Geisler FH, Coleman WP, Grieco G, et al. The Sygen multicenter acute spinal cord injury study. Spine 2001;26(Suppl 24):S87–98.

25. Castillo-Abrego G. Hypothermia in spinal cord injury. Crit Care 2012;16(Suppl 2):A12.

26. Levi AD, Green BA, Wang MY, et al. Clinical application of modest hypothermia after spinal cord injury. J Neurotrauma 2009;26(3):407–15.

27. Levi AD, Casella G, Green BA, et al. Clinical outcomes using modest intravascular hypothermia after acute cervical spinal cord injury. Neurosurgery 2010;66(4):670–7.

28. Dididze M, Green BA, Dalton Dietrich W, et al. Systemic hypothermia in acute cervical spinal cord injury: a case-controlled study. Spinal Cord 2012; 50(12):1–6.

29. Zahra M, Samdani A, Piggott K, et al. Acute changes in systemic hemodynamics and serum vasopressin after complete cervical spinal cord injury in piglets. Neurocrit Care 2010;13(1):132–40.

30. Furlan JC, Fehlings MG, Shannon P, et al. Descending vasomotor pathways in humans: correlation between axonal preservation and cardiovascular dysfunction after spinal cord injury. J Neurotrauma 2003;20(12):1351–63.

31. Nathan PW, Smith MC. The location of descending fibres to sympathetic preganglionic vasomotor and sudomotor neurons in man. J Neurol Neurosurg Psychiatr 1987;50(10):1253–62.

32. Ball PA. Critical care of spinal cord injury. Spine 2001;26(Suppl 24):S27–30.

33. Levi L, Wolf A, Belzberg H. Hemodynamic parameters in patients with acute cervical cord trauma: description, intervention, and prediction of outcome. Neurosurgery 1993;33(6):1007–16 [discussion: 1016–7].

34. Vale FL, Burns J, Jackson AB, et al. Combined medical and surgical treatment after acute spinal cord injury: results of a prospective pilot study to assess the merits of aggressive medical resuscitation and blood pressure management. J Neurosurg 1997;87(2):239–46.

35. Rangappa P, Jeyadoss J, Flabouris A, et al. Cardiac pacing in patients with a cervical spinal cord injury. Spinal Cord 2010;48(12):867–71.

36. Helkowski WM, Ditunno JF Jr, Boninger M. Autonomic dysreflexia: incidence in persons with neurologically complete and incomplete tetraplegia. J Spinal Cord Med 2003;26(3):244–7.

37. Illman A, Stiller K, Williams M. The prevalence of orthostatic hypotension during physiotherapy treatment in patients with an acute spinal cord injury. Spinal Cord 2000;38(12):741–7.

38. Furlan JC, Fehlings MG. Cardiovascular complications after acute spinal cord injury: pathophysiology, diagnosis, and management. Neurosurg Focus 2008;25(5):E13.

39. Krassioukov AV, Furlan JC, Fehlings MG. Autonomic dysreflexia in acute spinal cord injury: an under-recognized clinical entity. J Neurotrauma 2003;20(8):707–16.

40. Karlsson AK. Autonomic dysreflexia. Spinal Cord 1999;37(6):383–91.

41. Chancellor MB, Erhard MJ, Hirsch IH, et al. Prospective evaluation of terazosin for the treatment of autonomic dysreflexia. J Urol 1994; 151(1):111–3.

42. Vaidyanathan S, Soni BM, Sett P, et al. Pathophysiology of autonomic dysreflexia: long-term treatment with terazosin in adult and paediatric spinal cord injury patients manifesting recurrent dysreflexic episodes. Spinal Cord 1998;36(11): 761–70.

43. Ledsome JR, Sharp JM. Pulmonary function in acute cervical cord injury. Am Rev Respir Dis 1981;124(1):41–4.

44. McMichan JC, Michel L, Westbrook PR. Pulmonary dysfunction following traumatic quadriplegia. Recognition, prevention, and treatment. JAMA 1980;243(6):528–31.

45. Scanlon PD, Loring SH, Pichurko BM, et al. Respiratory mechanics in acute quadriplegia. Lung and chest wall compliance and dimensional changes during respiratory maneuvers. Am Rev Respir Dis 1989;139(3):615–20.

46. Brown R, DiMarco AF, Hoit JD, et al. Respiratory dysfunction and management in spinal cord injury. Respir Care 2006;51(8):853–68 [discussion: 869–70].

47. Almenoff PL, Alexander LR, Spungen AM, et al. Bronchodilatory effects of ipratropium bromide in patients with tetraplegia. Paraplegia 1995;33(5): 274–7.

48. Gardner BP, Watt JW, Krishnan KR. The artificial ventilation of acute spinal cord damaged patients: a retrospective study of forty-four patients. Paraplegia 1986;24(4):208–20.

49. Grande CM, Barton CR, Stene JK. Appropriate techniques for airway management of emergency

patients with suspected spinal cord injury. Anesth Analg 1988;67(7):714–5.

50. Shatney CH, Brunner RD, Nguyen TQ. The safety of orotracheal intubation in patients with unstable cervical spine fracture or high spinal cord injury. Am J Surg 1995;170(6):676–9 [discussion: 679–80].

51. Rodriguez JL, Steinberg SM, Luchetti FA, et al. Early tracheostomy for primary airway management in the surgical critical care setting. Surgery 1990;108(4):655–9.

52. Kane TD, Rodriguez JL, Luchette FA. Early versus late tracheostomy in the trauma patient. Respir Care Clin N Am 1997;3(1):1–20.

53. Fagon JY, Chastre J, Hance AJ, et al. Nosocomial pneumonia in ventilated patients: a cohort study evaluating attributable mortality and hospital stay. Am J Med 1993;94(3):281–8.

54. Grossman RF, Fein A. Evidence-based assessment of diagnostic tests for ventilator-associated pneumonia. Executive summary. Chest 2000;117(4 Suppl 2):177S–81S.

55. Furlan JC, Fehlings MG. Role of screening tests for deep venous thrombosis in asymptomatic adults with acute spinal cord injury: an evidence-based analysis. Spine 2007;32(17):1908–16.

56. Geerts WH, Code KI, Jay RM, et al. A prospective study of venous thromboembolism after major trauma. N Engl J Med 1994;331(24):1601–6.

57. Green D, Rossi EC, Yao JS, et al. Deep vein thrombosis in spinal cord injury: effect of prophylaxis with calf compression, aspirin, and dipyridamole. Paraplegia 1982;20(4):227–34.

58. Merli GJ, Herbison GJ, Ditunno JF, et al. Deep vein thrombosis: prophylaxis in acute spinal cord injured patients. Arch Phys Med Rehabil 1988;69(9):661–4.

59. Deep venous thrombosis and thromboembolism in patients with cervical spinal cord injuries. Neurosurgery 2002;50(Suppl 3):S73–80.

60. van Rossum AB, Pattynama PM, Ton ER, et al. Pulmonary embolism: validation of spiral CT angiography in 149 patients. Radiology 1996;201(2):467–70.

Intracerebral Hemorrhage
New Challenges and Steps Forward

Jose Javier Provencio, MD[a,b,*],
Ivan Rocha Ferreira Da Silva, MD[a],
Edward Michael Manno, MD[a]

KEYWORDS

- Intracerebral hemorrhage • Acute brain injury • Anticoagulation

KEY POINTS

- Intracerebral hemorrhage (ICH) takes a toll on patients and society. Advances in the treatment of ICH have not kept pace with those of stroke and acute myocardial infarction.
- The cause of ICH and complications afterward are related to blood pressure control, making this the central strategy for prevention and treatment.
- Limited surgery for some ICH may be beneficial. Studies are ongoing.
- Anticoagulation associated ICH is best treated by early correction of coagulopathy.

INTRODUCTION

Intracerebral hemorrhage (ICH) is a devastating disease that all too frequently leaves patients dead or severely disabled. Attempts over the last decade to improve the outcome of these patients have met with only marginal success. As the population ages and the use of anticoagulation for the treatment of atrial fibrillation increases, the incidence of ICH is expected to rise.[1] This will have a major impact on health resources because the number of patients who remain permanently debilitated after ICH is high.

Any hemorrhage that primarily affects the substance of the brain or the ventricular spaces (compared with the subarachnoid spaces) is considered ICH. There is considerable overlap between ICH and subarachnoid hemorrhage in regard to the causes of the ictus and many patients have bleeding in more than one compartment. Most intraventricular hemorrhage (IVH) is a consequence of ICH where the hemorrhage ruptures into the ventricular space. There seems to be an independent entity of isolated IVH that differs from ICH but likely constitutes a small proportion of patients with IVH.[2] In addition, there are a considerable number of patients who have ICH as a consequence of secondary hemorrhage subsequent to ischemic stroke.

This article deals specifically with nontraumatic isolated ICH with or without IVH. The frequency, causes, treatments, and outcomes of patients with ICH are discussed. In addition, some of the more recent scientific inquiries into the causes of ICH are explored.

EPIDEMIOLOGY, PROGNOSIS, AND IMPACT

The annual incidence rate for ICH is approximately 28 hemorrhages per 100,000 people.[3] It is the second most common form of stroke accounting for 10% to 15% of new strokes per year.[1] Thirty-day mortality is estimated to be 30% to 50%, although these numbers are likely skewed by the reluctance

[a] Cerebrovascular Center, S80, Cleveland Clinic, 9500 Euclid Avenue Cleveland, OH 44195, USA;
[b] Neuroinflammation Research Center, Neuroscience, NC30, Cleveland Clinic, 9500 Euclid Avenue Cleveland, OH 44195, USA
* Corresponding author. Neuroinflammation Research Center, Neuroscience, NC30, Cleveland Clinic, 9500 Euclid Avenue Cleveland, OH 44195.
E-mail address: provenj@ccf.org

Neurosurg Clin N Am 24 (2013) 349–359
http://dx.doi.org/10.1016/j.nec.2013.03.002
1042-3680/13/$ – see front matter © 2013 Elsevier Inc. All rights reserved.

of physicians and family to aggressively manage patients with ICH.[4] This self-fulfilling prophecy has limited the evaluation of the actual mortality of the disease.[5] There is concern that therapeutic nihilism may lead to abnormally high mortality projections, which lead physicians and families to limit care in patients with the potential for recovery. It has been observed that hospitals with a higher proportion of patients with "do not resuscitate" orders have higher mortality for ICH.[4,6]

The most common risk factors for ICH are chronic hypertension and evidence of previous microhemorrhages on magnetic resonance imaging (MRI).[7] The most rapidly increasing population of patients with ICH is patients on oral anticoagulation therapy (OAT), discussed later.

The incidence and prevalence of ICH varies among different ethnic and racial groups largely because of racial variation in the incidence and management of hypertension.[8] Across the board, chronic hypertension is responsible for approximately 50% of ICH. The classic vessel damage associated with chronic hypertension–associated hemorrhages occurs in small penetrating arteries that come off of larger parent vessels, such as the lenticulostriate arteries emanating from the middle cerebral artery and perforators that arise from the basilar artery. These small arteries feed deep central areas of the brain.

The next most common cause of ICH is cerebral amyloid angiopathy, which accounts for about 20% of cases.[1] The angiopathy typically occurs in older patients and is unrelated to systemic amyloidosis.[9,10] Although there has traditionally been a view that lobar hemorrhages are more likely to be associated with amyloid angiopathy, it is more accurate to say that amyloid angiopathy hemorrhages are more likely to be lobar than deep.[10]

ICHs often have small subclinical hemorrhages that can now be visualized by MRI sequences that exploit the susceptibility artifact that is generated by hemosiderin deposits in the brain. These small hemorrhages, termed "microhemorrhages," also have been associated with stroke and vascular dementia suggesting that they are a general marker of microvascular disease of the brain (**Fig. 1**).[11–16] How chronic hypertension and anticoagulation contribute to microhemorrhages is not clear.

Prediction of outcome after ICH is essential for informed discussions with patient families. It is clear that the size of the hemorrhage, location, and age of the patient are strong predictors of mortality.[1] The ICH score uses these risk factors to quantify the chance of survival.[17] Points are assigned for age greater than 80, Glasgow Coma Score, hemorrhage volume greater than 30 mL

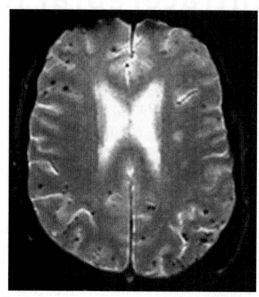

Fig. 1. Magnetic resonance imaging of multiple cerebral microbleeds detected on spin echo gradient imaging. These microbleeds most likely represent amyloid angiopathy but may also be a marker for small vessel disease. (*Data from* Walker DA, Broderick DF, Kotsenas AL, et al. Routine use of gradient-echo MRI to screen for cerebral amyloid angiopathy in elderly patients. Am J Roentgenol 2004;182:1547–50.)

by computed tomography (CT) scan, infratentorial location, and intraventricular extension of blood. The grading scale predicts mortality from a score of 0 at 0% mortality to a score of 5 with a mortality of 100%.[17] A similar score was developed to predict independent functional survival, which also includes an assessment of prehospital cognitive status.[18] Both scores have been validated and seem to be useful in clinical practice. Neither scale took into account the effect of therapeutic nihilism that may have resulted in the reporting of increased mortality.

The impact of ICH on society is great. Stroke of all kinds is particularly costly because of the prolonged disability of patients who survive. It is estimated that ICH costs $125,000 per ICH per year resulting in $6 billion cost per year in the United States.[19] In a similar assessment, the lifetime cost of ICH in Spain was found to be €46,193 (euros) per patient suggesting that the costs in the United States may be higher than other developed countries.[20]

INTENSIVE CARE UNIT MANAGEMENT

Most patients with ICH are critically ill on admission, so appropriate critical care management seems likely to make an important contribution to outcome. Important issues that arise in patients with ICH include poor control of their airway protective reflexes, hypoventilation, and increased intracranial pressure (reviewed in[21]). In a few patients with severe damage to critical areas of the brain, specific cardiac and pulmonary complications, such as takasubo cardiomyopathy and neurogenic pulmonary edema, may occur.[22,23] These entities are more common in patients with subarachnoid hemorrhage and traumatic brain injury. In addition, pressure on the hypothalamic-pituitary axis can lead to several electrolyte abnormalities, such as diabetes insipidus and cerebral salt wasting.

Specific understanding of systemic complications that occur in ICH may lead to improved outcomes. A retrospective review of outcome data from the Project IMPACT database of intensive care units showed that admission to a dedicated intensive care unit with neurologic specialization was an independent predictor of decreased mortality.[24] In addition, a before-and-after study of management of patients with ICH showed that the addition of physicians trained in neurointensive care decreased mortality.[25]

The mainstay of ICH management for the last 30 years has been the control of systolic blood pressure to prevent hematoma expansion.[7] Until recently, this was done without convincing evidence that control of blood pressure made a difference. There is concern that untreated systolic blood pressure leads to hemorrhage expansion. However, concerns were also raised that aggressive control of blood pressure could lead to ischemia in the perihematomal area. Previous evidence by positron emission tomography scanning of patients with ICH showed that moderately decreasing blood pressure does not significantly decrease perihematomal perfusion.[26] In fact, positron emission tomography scans evaluating cerebral metabolism suggest that any decreased blood flow to the perihematomal area is caused by matched perfusion-metabolism demand, which precludes the worry about ischemia.[27]

Recently, two studies have supported the suspicion that blood pressure control is valuable. The Intensive Blood Pressure Reduction in Acute Cerebral Hemorrhage Trial randomized 404 patients to aggressive blood pressure control (systolic blood pressure <140 mm Hg) or standard therapy (systolic blood pressure <180 mm Hg).[28] CT scan comparing a baseline CT imaging with 24- and 72-hour scans showed significantly less hemorrhage and cerebral edema in the aggressive blood pressure management group. The study was not powered to evaluate clinical outcome but a larger study to address this is planned.

A second, large randomized trial called the Antihypertensive Treatment of Acute Cerebral Hemorrhage is also planned to specifically assess acute blood pressure control and clinical outcome. The phase 1 dose-escalation arm of the study randomized 60 patients to different dosing regimens of antihypertensives. Patients with lower blood pressure were less likely to have hematoma expansion, perihematomal edema, and poor 3-month outcome.[29] It is hoped that the results of the larger trial will address the question of the benefit of acute blood pressure management.

TREATMENT BASED ON PATHOPHYSIOLOGY

The brain injury that occurs after a spontaneous ICH evolves over time but the initial injury is likely caused by mechanical disruption of brain tissue and the subsequent mass effect of the blood compressing vital brain structures. Hematoma size is a powerful predictor of mortality and hematoma expansion correlates with increase mortality.[30] Hematoma growth occurs in approximately 38% of patients with most occurring within the first hour and the remaining over the subsequent 20 hours.[31] Hematoma expansion may be predicted by the patient's presenting blood pressure but has been difficult to quantify. Patients with contrast extravasation inside of the hematoma area seen on contrasted CT of the brain (called the spot sign) have been clearly documented to predict hematoma expansion (**Fig. 2**).[32]

Secondary injury after ICH is still not well understood. Neurotransmitters (mostly glutamate),[33] inflammatory cytokines,[34] matrix metalloproteinases,[35] heme,[36] iron,[37,38] and thrombin[39] injure the brain at different times in the evolution of the hematoma. It is likely that there is temporal evolution of susceptibility of the brain to injury. The development of toxic mediators may take a similar course making the identification of a particular offending agent at a particular time difficult.[40]

Secondary injury after ICH may be related to the development of perihematomal edema. Perihematomal edema is a zone of viable tissue around the core of the hemorrhage that is vulnerable to secondary insults similar to the ischemic penumbra in ischemic stroke. Perihematomal edema is believed to develop in three phases.[41] Within the first few hours after the hemorrhage, the hematoma develops and retracts as the red cell mass and coagulation factors organize into a compact mass leaving serum molecules from the hematoma into the surrounding tissue. These proteins seem to be toxic to neurons. During the ensuing 2 to 3 days, these toxic elements lead to

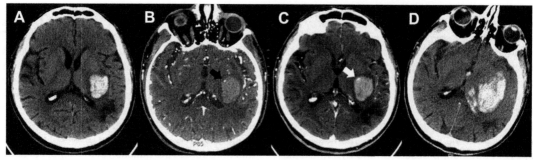

Fig. 2. (A) Computed topographic imaging of a left putaminal hemorrhage. (B, C) CT angiography demonstrating contrast extravasation (spot sign) black arrow in image B and white arrow in image C. (D) Subsequent hematoma expansion detected on CT. (*From* Wada R, Aviv RI, Fox AJ, et al. CT angiography "spot sign" predicts hematoma expansion in acute intracerebral hemorrhage. Stroke 2007;38(4):1257–62; with permission.)

endothelial activation and extravasation of inflammatory mediators. In the final step, as the clot dissolves, red blood cells are lysed and hemoglobin breakdown products mediate toxicity.

Thrombin, a trypsin-like serum protease that plays a pivotal role in the coagulation cascade, is present in high concentrations in the brain after an ICH and may be neurotoxic.[39,42] Studies done in animals show that injection of thrombin inhibitors in the hematoma site results in less edema formation suggesting that thrombin plays a direct role in production of perihematomal edema.[43,44]

From these data, there seems to be competition between hematoma expansion prevention (in part by thrombin) and thrombin-mediated neuronal damage. One report found that patients with higher relative volumes of perihematomal edema have better prognosis.[45] This study could reflect a more intact coagulation system with correspondent clot retraction and less hematoma expansion highlighting the possible balance of expanding clot and neuronal toxicity.

Possibly the most detrimental preventable complication of ICH is hematoma expansion after the original hemorrhage. Recent studies show that hematoma expansion is common and independently affects mortality.[46] There has not been much research into the specific cellular or molecular changes that lead to rehemorrhage but clinical evidence suggests that systolic hypertension contributes. Several studies have tested procoagulants in patients on anticoagulation but only one randomized study investigated procoagulants in patients not on anticoagulation therapy.[47,48] The FAST trial analyzed the effect of administering recombinant activated factor VIIa acutely in patients with spontaneous ICH who were not receiving anticoagulation.[49] A lower incidence of hematoma expansion was observed in the treatment group without significant change in the overall prognosis.

The disappointing results could be a reflection of increased thrombin concentrations inside of the hematoma or the increased rate of secondary thrombotic complications.

Several trials have investigated preventing secondary brain injury by affecting molecular and cellular mechanisms. To date, no clinical studies have shown significant benefit. A neuroprotective free radical scavenger NXY-059 was tested in patients with ICH to evaluate safety and tolerability. The purpose of the study was to test the feasibility of administering medications to symptomatic patients before CT evaluation.[50,51] Although the study was not powered for efficacy, there was no trend toward improvement in the study group.

The most promising current medical therapy being investigated is an iron-chelating drug called deferoximine. The development of reactive oxidant species formation during iron metabolism has been well established; however, the development of these agents was thought to be too early in the course of the disease to be good targets for treatment.[52,53] Ferric iron, stored in hemoglobin, is converted to ferrous iron, a reactive oxidant species, when red blood cells are lysed. Lysis may be delayed for several hours or days making the approach of chelating iron before its conversion a hopeful treatment target.

Animal studies have been promising and a safety and tolerability study was significantly promising to support a phase 3 trial.[52,54] It is possible that if chelating iron is not feasible, other ways of interacting with the late radicalization of iron may still represent meaningful treatment targets.

SURGERY FOR ICH

It has long been recognized that surgery for cerebellar hemorrhages with significant mass effect on the brainstem can be life saving.[55] There is still controversy about whether there is a role for external ventricular drainage alone in patients with hydrocephalus from impingement of the fourth ventricle without decompressive craniectomy, or whether both therapies should be initiated together.

Surgery for supratentorial ICH has been attempted for years without evidence of improvement in patient outcome. Previous small, randomized studies with one exception showed no benefit compared with aggressive medical therapy. Interestingly, the one study that did show benefit in the surgery arm used a minimally invasive technique to decompress hemorrhages that came close to the surface.[56]

An attempt to definitively address the possible benefit of surgery for ICH was undertaken with the Surgical Trial in Intracerebral Hemorrhage (STICH) trial.[57] The design of this multinational trial was to randomize patients based on the theory of equipoise randomizing patients when the admitting surgeon was unsure if surgery would be beneficial. This left two groups (patients the surgeon believed would definitely benefit from surgery and patients in whom the surgeon at the local facility believed would not benefit from surgery) out of the study. There were thus large differences in how severe and what types of hemorrhages were included between centers.

The study randomized 1000 patients. Six-month mortality, modified Rankin Scale scores, and Barthal Index scores were no different between the surgery and medical management groups. Subgroup analysis did show that hemorrhages that were closer to the surface had better outcomes with surgery (similar to the previous study by Auer and coworkers[56]).

The failure of open surgery to improve outcomes in deep hemorrhages and the suggestion that less invasive surgery may be beneficial has led to three ongoing trials. The STICH trial investigators have devised a follow-up study to investigate open surgery for peripheral hemorrhages. In addition, a single center trial using a minimally invasive approach with external ventricular devices placed into the clot with lytic agents shows promising results.[58] This new approach using external ventricular catheters to administer recombinant tissue plasminogen activator into the clot with removal of lysed blood is being tested in The Minimally Invasive Surgery Plus T-PA for Intracerebral Hemorrhage Evacuation trial.[59] This trial exploits the CT scan volumetric evaluation of the hemorrhage to determine the approach of the external ventricular catheters and the administration of the lytic medicine. The result of these studies is expected in 1 to 3 years.

ICH ASSOCIATED WITH ORAL ANTICOAGULATION

ICH in patients on OAT (OAT-ICH) is an increasing problem, mostly because of the aging population and the increased use of anticoagulants for patients at high risk for thrombosis.[60] It is speculated that approximately 5.6 million patients in the United States will have atrial fibrillation by 2050 and many of them will likely be taking oral anticoagulants.[61] Moreover, ICHs are eight times more frequent in patients on oral anticoagulants,[62] with an annual estimated incidence of 0.25% to 1.1%.[63]

The mechanism through which anticoagulation promotes ICH has not been completely elucidated, but animal data using a mouse model demonstrated that hematoma size was directly related to the intensity of anticoagulation.[64,65] Although anticoagulation may not increase the risk of ICH, it is hypothesized that a greater bleeding tendency increases the size of spontaneous ICHs that otherwise might be asymptomatic.

Not surprisingly, anticoagulated patients have a higher risk of hematoma expansion. This has been observed in up to 56% of patients[66] occurring as far as 7 days postictus (despite correction of the underlying coagulopathy).[67,68]

Patients on oral anticoagulation also have increased incidence of volume expansion into the ventricular system.[69,70] Some studies have observed an association of higher mortality with the presence of IVH, especially in patients in which all the ventricles were involved.[70] In general, patients with OAT-ICH have an overall worse prognosis than patients with spontaneous ICH[67,71,72] with mortality rates almost doubling those reported in noncoagulopathic patients.[71,73]

Risk factors for OAT-ICH are advanced age; hypertension; history of cerebrovascular disease; the intensity of anticoagulation (mainly if international normalized ratio [INR] >4)[74,75]; and the concomitant use of aspirin.[76] Recently, the presence of microhemorrhages on brain MRI gradient echo weighted scans,[77] leukoaraiosis,[78] and genetic factors (CYP2C9, VKORC1, and apolipoprotein E genotype variants)[79–84] are believed to contribute to an increased risk of OAT-ICH. Although most OAT-ICH occurs in patients with INR less than 3,[60] higher INR values (>3.5) are directly correlated with OAT-ICH occurrence[85–87] and the size of the hematoma on arrival to the hospital.[88]

A radiographic finding observed in roughly 60% of patients with OAT-ICH is a distinct fluid level in the hematoma. This is believed to occur because of the inability of the blood to coagulate creating a level of serum over red blood cells as the patient is laying flat for the scan.[89,90] At the same time, the

Table 1
Suggestions for reversal of anticoagulants commonly used in clinical practice

Agent	Coagulation Monitoring	Reversal Strategies	Comments[a]
Heparinoids			
Heparin	Activated partial thromboplastin time or anti-Xa heparin assay (in patients in whom activated partial thromboplastin time is unreliable)	Protamine sulfate	Typical dosing: 1 mg of protamine/100 IU of heparin infused during the previous 6 h maximum dose of 50 mg. Smaller doses may be appropriate for infusions that are stopped >2 h (heparin half-life approximately 90 min)
Low-molecular-weight heparins	Anti-Xa heparin assay	Protamine sulfate	No consensus on appropriate dosing. Protamine is less effective to reverse the effects of low-molecular-weight heparin than heparin sulfate.
Vitamin K antagonists			
Warfarin	Prothrombin time INR	PCC, fresh frozen plasma, vitamin K, recombinant activated factor VII	For reversal of therapeutic INR: 10 mg intravenous vitamin K plus 50 IU/kg PCC For patients with INR >4: 10 mg of vitamin K plus 10–20 mcg/kg although higher doses of PCC plus the addition of recombinant activated factor VII or fresh frozen plasma to replete factor VII depletion (not necessary if a four-factor PCC is used)
Direct thrombin inhibitors			
Dabigatran	Possibly echarin clotting time, thrombin time, thromboelastography	Hemodialysis, possible reversal with PCC	PCC can be tried but there are no data to support efficacy or specific dosing. Currently, only hemodyalysis has been shown to reverse the effect.
Factor Xa inhibitors			
Rivaroxaban	Possibly thromboelastography	Possibly PCC	Some existing data support PCC use (usually 50 IU/kg)

Abbreviations: INR, international normalized ratio; PCC, prothrombin complex concentrates.
[a] The described doses have not been validated. The comments are suggestions based on common practice at the authors' institution and are not the only possible therapies.

hematoma shape is usually not significantly different than what is observed in spontaneous ICH. Similarly, the standard ABC/2 volumetric measuring method offers reasonable approximation of hematoma volume in OAT-ICH.[91] Interestingly, OAT-ICH has a predilection for the cerebellum. The reason for this is unclear.[72,92,93]

OAT-ICH is a neurologic emergency, because patients with elevated INR are at high risk of hematoma expansion during the first 24 to 48 hours. Even small hematomas can transform into neurologic catastrophes in a matter of minutes. Currently, there are no randomized trials assessing clinical outcomes of different anticoagulation reversal strategies in patients with OAT-ICH. Most of the evidence and guidelines derive from several small studies or case series, most of which are retrospective analyses.

There is no absolute consensus on how to reverse the effects of anticoagulation. For warfarin there are well-studied choices, but for heparinoids and direct thrombin inhibitors there are fewer options. **Table 1** summarizes suggested reversal strategies for the most used anticoagulants.

There is a theoretical concern that reversing anticoagulation could lead to thrombus generation especially in patients with mechanical heart valves and procoagulant states, which was refuted by recent studies.[94–96] Finally, the four pillars of OAT-ICH treatment are (1) prompt reversal of anticoagulation; (2) hypertension control; (3) surgery (if indicated); and (4) specialized neurologic intensive care. It is important to collect a meticulous history about the kind of anticoagulant the patient is receiving, last dose, renal and liver function, and the indication for anticoagulation and occurrence of previous bleedings.

IVH COMPLICATING ICH

IVH occurs in 50% of patients with spontaneous ICH. Mortality is five times higher than in patients with isolated ICH.[97] IVH complicates the management of patients in several ways. In addition to forming a low-pressure outlet for hematoma expansion, blood in the cerebrospinal fluid spaces often leads to hydrocephalus that can cause further brain damage from increased intracranial pressure.

Traditional management of IVH is cerebrospinal fluid diversion by placing an external ventricular drain. Further treatment of the IVH component is still investigational. One study of patients with predominant IVH with small volume of ICH is currently underway. The Clot Lysis Evaluating Accelerated Resolution of Intraventricular Hemorrhage trial seeks to evaluate whether administration of small

doses of intraventricular recombinant tissue plasminogen activator can decrease IVH size and improve outcome.[98] Preliminary results show decreased intraventricular clot in the intervention group without obviously increased rates of infection and rebleeding. The final results of the study are expected in the next few years.

SUMMARY

For many years, the management of ICH was left to convention and predictions based on the pathophysiology of the hemorrhage. Unlike such diseases as subarachnoid hemorrhage and traumatic brain injury that have been subjects for serious clinical trials for many years, ICH has only in the last 10 to 15 years begun the period of systematic research to evaluate therapies. Although no great breakthroughs have yet been made, there is a great deal of optimism that effective therapies for the management and treatment of ICH will be developed in the near future. Because of the significant impact of this disease financially and the human toll on patients and caregivers, improvements in therapy are welcomed.

REFERENCES

1. Manno EM, Atkinson JL, Fulgham JR, et al. Emerging medical and surgical management strategies in the evaluation and treatment of intracerebral hemorrhage. Mayo Clin Proc 2005;80(3):420–33.
2. Gaab MR. Intracerebral hemorrhage (ICH) and intraventricular hemorrhage (IVH): improvement of bad prognosis by minimally invasive neurosurgery. World Neurosurg 2011;75(2):206–8.
3. Nilsson OG, Lindgren A, Stahl N, et al. Incidence of intracerebral and subarachnoid haemorrhage in southern Sweden. J Neurol Neurosurg Psychiatry 2000;69(5):601–7.
4. Zahuranec DB, Brown DL, Lisabeth LD, et al. Early care limitations independently predict mortality after intracerebral hemorrhage. Neurology 2007;68(20):1651–7.
5. Becker KJ, Baxter AB, Cohen WA, et al. Withdrawal of support in intracerebral hemorrhage may lead to self-fulfilling prophecies. Neurology 2001;56(6):766–72.
6. Zahuranec DB, Morgenstern LB, Sanchez BN, et al. Do-not-resuscitate orders and predictive models after intracerebral hemorrhage. Neurology 2010;75(7):626–33.
7. Morgenstern LB, Hemphill JC 3rd, Anderson C, et al. Guidelines for the management of spontaneous intracerebral hemorrhage: a guideline for healthcare professionals from the American Heart

Association/American Stroke Association. Stroke 2010;41(9):2108–29.

8. Morgenstern LB, Spears WD. A triethnic comparison of intracerebral hemorrhage mortality in Texas. Ann Neurol 1997;42(6):919–23.

9. Yamada M, Naiki H. Cerebral amyloid angiopathy. Prog Mol Biol Transl Sci 2012;107:41–78.

10. Charidimou A, Gang Q, Werring DJ. Sporadic cerebral amyloid angiopathy revisited: recent insights into pathophysiology and clinical spectrum. J Neurol Neurosurg Psychiatry 2012;83(2):124–37.

11. Flaherty ML. Anticoagulant-associated intracerebral hemorrhage. Semin Neurol 2010;30(5): 565–72.

12. Goos JD, Henneman WJ, Sluimer JD, et al. Incidence of cerebral microbleeds: a longitudinal study in a memory clinic population. Neurology 2010;74(24):1954–60.

13. Shimoyama T, Iguchi Y, Kimura K, et al. Stroke patients with cerebral microbleeds on MRI scans have arteriolosclerosis as well as systemic atherosclerosis. Hypertens Res 2012;35(10):975–9.

14. Dassan P, Brown MM, Gregoire SM, et al. Association of cerebral microbleeds in acute ischemic stroke with high serum levels of vascular endothelial growth factor. Arch Neurol 2012;69(9):1186–9.

15. Gregoire SM, Smith K, Jager HR, et al. Cerebral microbleeds and long-term cognitive outcome: longitudinal cohort study of stroke clinic patients. Cerebrovasc Dis 2012;33(5):430–5.

16. Walker DA, et al. Routine use of gradient-echo MRI to screen for cerebral amyloid angiopathy in elderly patients. AJR Am J Roentgenol 2004;182: 1547–50.

17. Hemphill JC III, Bonovich DC, Besmertis L, et al. The ICH score: a simple, reliable grading scale for intracerebral hemorrhage. Stroke 2001;32(4): 891–7.

18. Rost NS, Smith EE, Chang Y, et al. Prediction of functional outcome in patients with primary intracerebral hemorrhage: the FUNC score. Stroke 2008; 39(8):2304–9.

19. Hsieh PC, Awad IA, Getch CC, et al. Current updates in perioperative management of intracerebral hemorrhage. Neurol Clin 2006;24(4):745–64.

20. Navarrete-Navarro P, Hart WM, Lopez-Bastida J, et al. The societal costs of intracerebral hemorrhage in Spain. Eur J Neurol 2007;14(5):556–62.

21. Manno EM. Update on intracerebral hemorrhage. Continuum (Minneap Minn) 2012;18(3):598–610.

22. Rahimi AR, Katayama M, Mills J. Cerebral hemorrhage: precipitating event for a tako-tsubo-like cardiomyopathy? Clin Cardiol 2008;31(6):275–80.

23. Goncalves V, Silva-Carvalho L, Rocha I. Cerebellar haemorrhage as a cause of neurogenic pulmonary edema: case report. Cerebellum 2005; 4(4):246–9.

24. Diringer MN, Edwards DF. Admission to a neurologic/neurosurgical intensive care unit is associated with reduced mortality rate after intracerebral hemorrhage. Crit Care Med 2001;29(3):635–40.

25. Varelas PN, Conti MM, Spanaki MV, et al. The impact of a neurointensivist-led team on a semiclosed neurosciences intensive care unit. Crit Care Med 2004;32(11):2191–8.

26. Powers WJ, Zazulia AR, Videen TO, et al. Autoregulation of cerebral blood flow surrounding acute (6 to 22 hours) intracerebral hemorrhage. Neurology 2001;57(1):18–24.

27. Zazulia AR, Diringer MN, Videen TO, et al. Hypoperfusion without ischemia surrounding acute intracerebral hemorrhage. J Cereb Blood Flow Metab 2001;21(7):804–10.

28. Anderson CS, Huang Y, Arima H, et al. Effects of early intensive blood pressure-lowering treatment on the growth of hematoma and perihematomal edema in acute intracerebral hemorrhage: the Intensive Blood Pressure Reduction in Acute Cerebral Haemorrhage Trial (INTERACT). Stroke 2010; 41(2):307–12.

29. Qureshi AI, Palesch YY, Martin R, et al. Effect of systolic blood pressure reduction on hematoma expansion, perihematomal edema, and 3-month outcome among patients with intracerebral hemorrhage: results from the antihypertensive treatment of acute cerebral hemorrhage study. Arch Neurol 2010;67(5):570–6.

30. Broderick JP, Brott TG, Duldner JE, et al. Volume of intracerebral hemorrhage. A powerful and easy-to-use predictor of 30-day mortality. Stroke 1993; 24(7):987–93.

31. Brott T, Broderick J, Kothari R, et al. Early hemorrhage growth in patients with intracerebral hemorrhage. Stroke 1997;28(1):1–5.

32. Wada R, Aviv RI, Fox AJ, et al. CT angiography "spot sign" predicts hematoma expansion in acute intracerebral hemorrhage. Stroke 2007;38(4): 1257–62.

33. Castillo J, Davalos A, Alvarez-Sabin J, et al. Molecular signatures of brain injury after intracerebral hemorrhage. Neurology 2002;58(4):624–9.

34. Wang J, Dore S. Inflammation after intracerebral hemorrhage. J Cereb Blood Flow Metab 2007; 27(5):894–908.

35. Rosenberg GA, Navratil M. Metalloproteinase inhibition blocks edema in intracerebral hemorrhage in the rat. Neurology 1997;48(4):921–6.

36. Figueiredo RT, Fernandez PL, Mourao-Sa DS, et al. Characterization of heme as activator of Toll-like receptor 4. J Biol Chem 2007;282(28):20221–9.

37. Kruman I, Bruce-Keller AJ, Bredesen D, et al. Evidence that 4-hydroxynonenal mediates oxidative stress-induced neuronal apoptosis. J Neurosci 1997;17(13):5089–100.

38. Hua Y, Keep RF, Hoff JT, et al. Brain injury after intracerebral hemorrhage: the role of thrombin and iron. Stroke 2007;38(Suppl 2):759–62.

39. Xi G, Reiser G, Keep RF. The role of thrombin and thrombin receptors in ischemic, hemorrhagic and traumatic brain injury: deleterious or protective? J Neurochem 2003;84(1):3–9.

40. Xi G, Keep RF, Hoff JT. Mechanisms of brain injury after intracerebral haemorrhage. Lancet Neurol 2006;5(1):53–63.

41. Xi G, Keep RF, Hoff JT. Pathophysiology of brain edema formation. Neurosurg Clin N Am 2002; 13(3):371–83.

42. Lee KR, Colon GP, Betz AL, et al. Edema from intracerebral hemorrhage: the role of thrombin. J Neurosurg 1996;84(1):91–6.

43. Lee KR, Betz AL, Keep RF, et al. Intracerebral infusion of thrombin as a cause of brain edema. J Neurosurg 1995;83(6):1045–50.

44. Kitaoka T, Hua Y, Xi G, et al. Delayed argatroban treatment reduces edema in a rat model of intracerebral hemorrhage. Stroke 2002;33(12):3012–8.

45. Gebel JM Jr, Jauch EC, Brott TG, et al. Relative edema volume is a predictor of outcome in patients with hyperacute spontaneous intracerebral hemorrhage. Stroke 2002;33(11):2636–41.

46. Dowlatshahi D, Demchuk AM, Flaherty ML, et al. Defining hematoma expansion in intracerebral hemorrhage: relationship with patient outcomes. Neurology 2011;76(14):1238–44.

47. Makris M, Greaves M, Phillips WS, et al. Emergency oral anticoagulant reversal: the relative efficacy of infusions of fresh frozen plasma and clotting factor concentrate on correction of the coagulopathy. Thromb Haemost 1997;77(3): 477–80.

48. Huttner HB, Schellinger PD, Hartmann M, et al. Hematoma growth and outcome in treated neurocritical care patients with intracerebral hemorrhage related to oral anticoagulant therapy: comparison of acute treatment strategies using vitamin K, fresh frozen plasma, and prothrombin complex concentrates. Stroke 2006;37(6):1465–70.

49. Mayer SA, Brun NC, Begtrup K, et al. Efficacy and safety of recombinant activated factor VII for acute intracerebral hemorrhage. N Engl J Med 2008; 358(20):2127–37.

50. Shuaib A, Lees KR, Lyden P, et al. NXY-059 for the treatment of acute ischemic stroke. N Engl J Med 2007;357(6):562–71.

51. Lyden PD, Shuaib A, Lees KR, et al. Safety and tolerability of NXY-059 for acute intracerebral hemorrhage: the CHANT Trial. Stroke 2007;38(8): 2262–9.

52. Okauchi M, et al. Effects of deferoxamine on intracerebral hemorrhage-induced brain injury in aged rats. Stroke 2009;40(5):1858–63.

53. Okauchi M, et al. Deferoxamine treatment for intracerebral hemorrhage in aged rats: therapeutic time window and optimal duration. Stroke 2010;41(2): 375–82.

54. Selim M, Yeatts S, Goldstein JN, et al. Safety and tolerability of deferoxamine mesylate in patients with acute intracerebral hemorrhage. Stroke 2011; 42(11):3067–74.

55. Dammann P, Asgari S, Bassiouni H, et al. Spontaneous cerebellar hemorrhage: experience with 57 surgically treated patients and review of the literature. Neurosurg Rev 2011;34(1):77–86.

56. Auer LM, Deinsberger W, Niederkorn K, et al. Endoscopic surgery versus medical treatment for spontaneous intracerebral hematoma: a randomized study. J Neurosurg 1989;70(4):530–5.

57. Mendelow AD, Gregson BA, Fernandes HM, et al. Early surgery versus initial conservative treatment in patients with spontaneous supratentorial intracerebral haematomas in the International Surgical Trial in Intracerebral Haemorrhage (STICH): a randomised trial. Lancet 2005;365(9457):387–97.

58. Newell DW, Shah MM, Wilcox R, et al. Minimally invasive evacuation of spontaneous intracerebral hemorrhage using sonothrombolysis. J Neurosurg 2011;115(3):592–601.

59. Morgan T, Zuccarello M, Narayan R, et al. Preliminary findings of the minimally-invasive surgery plus rtPA for intracerebral hemorrhage evacuation (MISTIE) clinical trial. Acta Neurochir Suppl 2008; 105:147–51.

60. Flaherty ML, Kissela B, Woo D, et al. The increasing incidence of anticoagulant-associated intracerebral hemorrhage. Neurology 2007;68(2): 116–21.

61. Go AS, Hylek EM, Phillips KA, et al. Prevalence of diagnosed atrial fibrillation in adults: national implications for rhythm management and stroke prevention: the AnTicoagulation and Risk Factors in Atrial Fibrillation (ATRIA) Study. JAMA 2001; 285(18):2370–5.

62. Franke CL, de Jonge J, van Swieten JC, et al. Intracerebral hematomas during anticoagulant treatment. Stroke 1990;21(5):726–30.

63. Butler AC, Tait RC. Management of oral anticoagulant-induced intracranial haemorrhage. Blood Rev 1998;12(1):35–44.

64. Foerch C, Arai K, Jin G, et al. Experimental model of warfarin-associated intracerebral hemorrhage. Stroke 2008;39(12):3397–404.

65. Illanes S, Zhou W, Heiland S, et al. Kinetics of hematoma expansion in murine warfarin-associated intracerebral hemorrhage. Brain Res 2010;1320: 135–42.

66. Cucchiara B, Messe S, Sansing L, et al. Hematoma growth in oral anticoagulant related intracerebral hemorrhage. Stroke 2008;39(11):2993–6.

67. Flibotte JJ, Hagan N, O'Donnell J, et al. War-farin, hematoma expansion, and outcome of intracerebral hemorrhage. Neurology 2004;63(6):1059–64.

68. Yasaka M, et al. Predisposing factors for enlargement of intracerebral hemorrhage in patients treated with warfarin. Thromb Haemost 2003;89(2):278–83.

69. Biffi A, Battey TW, Ayres AM, et al. Warfarin-related intraventricular hemorrhage: imaging and outcome. Neurology 2011;77(20):1840–6.

70. Zubkov A, Claassen DO, Rabinstein AA. Warfarin-associated intraventricular hemorrhage. Neurol Res 2007;29(7):661–3.

71. Rosand J, Eckman MH, Knudsen KA, et al. The effect of warfarin and intensity of anticoagulation on outcome of intracerebral hemorrhage. Arch Intern Med 2004;164(8):880–4.

72. Flaherty ML, Haverbusch M, Sekar P, et al. Location and outcome of anticoagulant-associated intracerebral hemorrhage. Neurocrit Care 2006;5(3):197–201.

73. Steiner T, Rosand J, Diringer M. Intracerebral hemorrhage associated with oral anticoagulant therapy: current practices and unresolved questions. Stroke 2006;37(1):256–62.

74. Hart RG, Tonarelli SB, Pearce LA. Avoiding central nervous system bleeding during antithrombotic therapy: recent data and ideas. Stroke 2005;36(7):1588–93.

75. Schulman S, Beyth RJ, Kearon C, et al. Hemorrhagic complications of anticoagulant and thrombolytic treatment: American College of Chest Physicians Evidence-Based Clinical Practice Guidelines (8th edition). Chest 2008;133(Suppl 6):257S–98S.

76. Hart RG, Benavente O, Pearce LA. Increased risk of intracranial hemorrhage when aspirin is combined with warfarin: a meta-analysis and hypothesis. Cerebrovasc Dis 1999;9(4):215–7.

77. Lee GH, Kwon SU, Kang DW. Warfarin-induced intracerebral hemorrhage associated with microbleeds. J Clin Neurol 2008;4(3):131–3.

78. Smith EE, Rosand J, Knudsen KA, et al. Leukoaraiosis is associated with warfarin-related hemorrhage following ischemic stroke. Neurology 2002;59(2):193–7.

79. Gage BF. Pharmacogenetics-based coumarin therapy. Hematology Am Soc Hematol Educ Program 2006;467–73.

80. Higashi MK, Veenstra DL, Kondo LM, et al. Association between CYP2C9 genetic variants and anticoagulation-related outcomes during warfarin therapy. JAMA 2002;287(13):1690–8.

81. Rieder MJ, Reiner AP, Gage BF, et al. Effect of VKORC1 haplotypes on transcriptional regulation and warfarin dose. N Engl J Med 2005;352(22):2285–93.

82. Sanderson S, Emery J, Higgins J. CYP2C9 gene variants, drug dose, and bleeding risk in warfarin-treated patients: a HuGEnet systematic review and meta-analysis. Genet Med 2005;7(2):97–104.

83. Tzourio C, Arima H, Harrap S, et al. APOE genotype, ethnicity, and the risk of cerebral hemorrhage. Neurology 2008;70(16):1322–8.

84. Woo D, Sauerbeck LR, Kissela BM, et al. Genetic and environmental risk factors for intracerebral hemorrhage: preliminary results of a population-based study. Stroke 2002;33(5):1190–5.

85. A randomized trial of anticoagulants versus aspirin after cerebral ischemia of presumed arterial origin. The Stroke Prevention in Reversible Ischemia Trial (SPIRIT) Study Group. Ann Neurol 1997;42(6):857–65.

86. Fang MC, Chang Y, Hylek EM, et al. Advanced age, anticoagulation intensity, and risk for intracranial hemorrhage among patients taking warfarin for atrial fibrillation. Ann Intern Med 2004;141(10):745–52.

87. Hylek EM, Evans-Molina C, Shea C, et al. Major hemorrhage and tolerability of warfarin in the first year of therapy among elderly patients with atrial fibrillation. Circulation 2007;115(21):2689–96.

88. Radberg JA, Olsson JE, Radberg CT. Prognostic parameters in spontaneous intracerebral hematomas with special reference to anticoagulant treatment. Stroke 1991;22(5):571–6.

89. Hart RG, Boop BS, Anderson DC. Oral anticoagulants and intracranial hemorrhage. Facts and hypotheses. Stroke 1995;26(8):1471–7.

90. Pfleger MJ, Hardee EP, Contant CF, et al. Sensitivity and specificity of fluid-blood levels for coagulopathy in acute intracerebral hematomas. AJNR Am J Neuroradiol 1994;15(2):217–23.

91. Sheth KN, Cushing TA, Wendell L, et al. Comparison of hematoma shape and volume estimates in warfarin versus non-warfarin-related intracerebral hemorrhage. Neurocrit Care 2010;12(1):30–4.

92. Kase CS, Robinson RK, Stein RW, et al. Anticoagulant-related intracerebral hemorrhage. Neurology 1985;35(7):943–8.

93. Toyoda K, Okada Y, Ibayashi S, et al. Antithrombotic therapy and predilection for cerebellar hemorrhage. Cerebrovasc Dis 2007;23(2–3):109–16.

94. Ananthasubramaniam K, Beattie JN, Rosman HS, et al. How safely and for how long can warfarin therapy be withheld in prosthetic heart valve patients hospitalized with a major hemorrhage? Chest 2001;119(2):478–84.

95. Phan TG, Koh M, Wijdicks EF. Safety of discontinuation of anticoagulation in patients with intracranial hemorrhage at high thromboembolic risk. Arch Neurol 2000;57(12):1710–3.

96. Wijdicks EF, Schievink WI, Brown RD, et al. The dilemma of discontinuation of anticoagulation therapy for patients with intracranial hemorrhage and mechanical heart valves. Neurosurgery 1998; 42(4):769–73.

97. Tuhrim S, Horowitz DR, Sacher M, et al. Volume of ventricular blood is an important determinant of outcome in supratentorial intracerebral hemorrhage. Crit Care Med 1999;27(3):617–21.

98. Morgan T, Awad I, Keyl P, et al. Preliminary report of the clot lysis evaluating accelerated resolution of intraventricular hemorrhage (CLEAR-IVH) clinical trial. Acta Neurochir Suppl 2008; 105:217–20.

Management of Intracerebral Pressure in the Neurosciences Critical Care Unit

Scott A. Marshall, MD[a],*, Atul Kalanuria, MD[b],
Manjunath Markandaya, MBBS[c], Paul A. Nyquist, MD, MPH[b]

KEYWORDS

• Acquired brain injury • Intracranial pressure • Intracranial hypertension • ICP • Neuromonitoring

KEY POINTS

- The management of intracerebral hypertension is a mainstay of neurocritical care, although invasive monitoring remains controversial in certain populations of acquired brain injury.
- Conservative measures to promote improved intracranial compliance should be in place in all patients with acquired brain injury.
- The type of ongoing disease should determine the type of intracranial pressure monitor placed. Limited options exist for noninvasive monitors for intracranial pressure (ICP).
- Interventions for management of ICP involve hyperventilation, hyperosmolar therapy, $CMRO_2$ (cerebral metabolic rate of oxygen)-based strategies, surgical treatment options, and N-methyl-D-aspartate receptor antagonists.
- Individual intensive care units should have an established treatment algorithm in place to manage increased ICP.

BACKGROUND REGARDING INTRACRANIAL PRESSURE MONITORING

Introduction

Neurocritical care has evolved to include enhanced diagnostic and treatment options over the past several decades. Central to this care delivered in the neurosciences intensive care unit (ICU) is multimodality monitoring of patients with brain injury. Perhaps second to the bedside clinical examination, the most universal continuous neurologic monitor is likely the intracerebral pressure monitor. The management of increased intracranial pressure (ICP) is discussed.

Neuro-monitoring of patients with acquired brain injury is performed for patients most severely affected by their central nervous system injury. The Glasgow Coma Scale (GCS) allows rapid classification of the severity of the brain injury and fosters

Disclaimer: The opinions and views expressed herein belong solely to those of the authors. These opinions and views are not nor should they be implied as being endorsed by the Uniformed Services University of the Health Sciences, Department of the Army, Department of Defense, or any other branch of the Federal Government of the United States.
[a] Neurology and Critical Care, Department of Medicine, San Antonio Military Medical Center, 3551 Roger Brooke Drive, Fort Sam Houston, Texas, TX 78234, USA; [b] Departments of Anesthesia/Critical Care Medicine, Neurology, and Neurosurgery, The Johns Hopkins School of Medicine, 600 N Wolfe St, Baltimore, Maryland, MD 21290, USA; [c] Division(s) of Surgical/Trauma Critical Care, Neurosciences Critical Care, and Pulmonary/Critical Care Medicine, R Adams Cowley Shock Trauma Center, 22 S Greene St, University of Maryland, Baltimore, Maryland, MD 21201, USA
* Corresponding author.
E-mail address: Scott.A.Marshall1.mil@mail.mil

Neurosurg Clin N Am 24 (2013) 361–373
http://dx.doi.org/10.1016/j.nec.2013.03.004
1042-3680/13/$ – see front matter Published by Elsevier Inc.

improved communication regarding a patient's clinical status.[1] This scale classically describes patients with traumatic brain injury (TBI), but can be used to communicate the neurologic status of patients with brain injury from other causes (**Table 1**). Patients with GCS scores of 8 or less have significant neurologic injury. These patients often have abnormal neuroimaging to include computed tomography (CT) scan findings such as a skull fracture, traumatic intracranial hemorrhage, or contusional injury.[2] Rapid evacuation must occur from the point of injury to the ICU for management of the patient's critical care needs, including airway management, mechanical ventilation, neurosurgical evaluation, and neuromonitoring. These modalities may include jugular venous oximetry, brain tissue oxygenation (Pbto$_2$), cerebral microdialysis, electroencephalography (EEG), advanced neuroimaging, and ICP monitoring. Guidelines for the use of multimodality monitoring of patients with severe brain injury are published by the Brain Trauma Foundation and have been instrumental in improving care with evidence-based recommendations.[3] Guidelines are also available for the prehospital management of severe TBI, prehospital care of combat-related head trauma, and surgical management of TBI. These guidelines can be obtained online from the Brain Trauma Foundation at http://braintrauma.org. A tool to assess individual management compliance with published guidelines is available at http://tbiclickandlearn. com.[4] European guidelines for the management of severe head injury have been published by the European Brain Injury Consortium, which also discusses issues of neuromonitoring and ICP.[5] The recommendations in these guidelines have been suggested to serve as a general reference for the management of other mechanisms of brain injury in neurocritical care.[6]

Goals in the critical care management of patients who experience brain injury must address arrest of any ongoing injury, preservation of neurologic function, prevention of medical complications of critical illness, and improvement in overall outcome. These patients should be evaluated in a center with specialized neurologic care, such as neurosurgery and neurointensivist care, where decisions about neuromonitoring, including ICP monitoring, can be best made. Although still controversial, ICP monitoring is the only available technology shown to guide interventions and predict outcomes, especially in TBI.[7] Its use is widely considered a standard tool in the neurocritical care unit.[8] Information obtained by monitoring a patient's ICP can be used to prognosticate and to follow progression of intracranial disease. It also aids in the assessment of global perfusion metrics such as cerebral perfusion pressure (CPP). The merits of ICP monitoring-based treatment protocols and their influence on patient outcome have been recently investigated in a randomized trial,[8] which is further discussed.

Mechanism and Potential Conditions Associated with Increased ICP

Although TBI is the disease process commonly associated with alterations of ICP, different types of brain injury can result in increased ICP. Patients with ischemic and hemorrhagic stroke, aneurysmal subarachnoid hemorrhage, and noncommunicating hydrocephalus encounter issues with intracerebral hypertension.[3,6,9,10] Other critically ill populations with metabolic, infectious, or hemorrhagic space-occupying lesions, postcirculatory arrest, hyperthermia, or electrolyte abnormalities may also have increased ICP, with signs of poor intracranial compliance.[11] The relationship between intracranial volume and ICP was initially described by Monro[12] and later by Kellie[13] in 1783 and 1824, respectively. Given that the skull remains fixed and rigid with a static volume of brain, blood, and cerebrospinal fluid (CSF), any increase in 1 of these 3 components results in the

Table 1 GCS							
Eye		**Motor**		**Verbal**	
Eyes open spontaneously	4	Follows commands	6	Oriented, alert	5
		Localizes	5		
		Withdraws	4	Confused, appropriate	4
Eyes open to voice	3	Flexion	3	Disoriented, inappropriate	3
Eyes open to pain	2	Extension	2	Incomprehensible speech	2
No response	1	No response	1	No response	1

Data from Monro A. Observations on the structure and function of the nervous system. Edinburgh (United Kingdom): Creech & Johnson; 1783.

displacement of another of the 3 components outside the skull. As volume continues to increase, intracranial compliance, defined as the change in volume/change in pressure, moves from a near-linear relationship to an exponential relationship; small changes in volume result in large changes in pressure (**Fig. 1**). This situation results in alterations of the slope of the ICP waveform.[11] An example of an appropriate ICP waveform is shown in **Fig. 2**.

Basic Principles to Protect a Brain at Risk

A subset of patients in the neurosciences ICU may have clinical signs, a mechanism of injury, a pathophysiologic marker, or imaging findings that suggest that intracranial compliance is not ideal, and consideration should be given for invasive ICP monitoring. Clinical syndromes of increased ICP may be dramatic, such as new focal deficits referable to a localizable or falsely localizable lesion of descending motor tracts.[14] Worsening of ICP from spontaneous intracerebral hematomas can present with focal neurologic deficits such as unilateral motor or sensory findings.[15] Patients with brain injury who develop intracranial hypertension may progress to cerebral herniation. As mechanisms to compensate for increased ICP are exhausted, herniation may manifest in a variety of neurologic syndromes.[16] Although specific clinical presentations and focal findings may occur, patients essentially become more somnolent, with lower GCS scores. Paradoxic herniation, a unique herniation syndrome from a low-pressure phenomenon, has been reported with or without lumbar puncture after decompressive craniectomy (DC).[17,18] If the pressure change is a result of lumbar drainage and subsequent CSF leak, the use of a blood patch has been reported to be lifesaving.[19,20] In addition to the brain parenchymal damage that can occur from herniation, this phenomenon can result in cerebral infarcts secondary to compression of proximate vessels (eg, posterior cerebral artery infarction associated with uncal herniation).[21] These infarcts further increase edema and may affect long-term morbidity. Numerous investigators have published reports regarding outcome of patients with clinical and radiographic herniation from perturbations of ICP who have survived to discharge with variable disability. Prognostication for these patients should be performed after a trial of aggressive medical management has been completed to reduce their ICP.[19,20,22–24]

General measures for patients with acquired brain injury should be in place. For example, the head should be kept in midline position and increased 15° to 30°.[6] This strategy allows optimal venous drainage, which if compromised, can exacerbate intracranial hypertension. With traumatic acquired brain injury, patients often have cervical immobilization collars in place, because of the risk of concomitant cervical spine trauma.[25] If these collars are fitted properly, they assist in keeping the head midline and minimize jugular venous obstruction. Routine placement of internal jugular central lines has been discouraged, although at least 1 study suggests that brief access to the central circulation via the internal jugular vein is well tolerated by patients at risk for increased ICP.[26] The use of jugular venous bulb oximetry in neurotrauma patients ranges from 8% to 12% in the United States to 21% in Japan.[27,28] Because of the potential problems of internal jugular line-associated thrombosis, routine or nonemergent cannulation of the internal jugular vein is avoided (P Nyquist, personal communication, 2013). In addition, central lines that require the Trendelenburg position should not be used during herniation. Trendelenburg positioning may acutely increase ICP.[29]

Other conservative measures that may help protect the injured brain include avoidance of circumferential neck dressings, such as tracheostomy ties or other apparatus to secure the endotracheal tube, in patients on mechanical ventilation. This strategy allows maintenance of venous outflow from the intracranial circulation. Seizures, pain, agitation, and bladder or bowel distention should all be treated.[3] Patients with brain injury should not be overstimulated, because there is evidence to suggest that a quiet and therapeutic environment may improve sleep and restoration of normal circadian rhythms in some types of brain injury, and this may have secondary effects on outcome.[30] Fever should be controlled.[9,10,31] Mild hyperthermia has been shown to worsen proximal

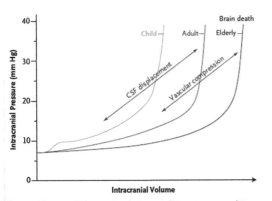

Fig. 1. Theoretic intracranial compliance curves. (*From* Ropper A. Hyperosmolar therapy for raised intracranial pressure. N Engl J Med 2012;367(8):748; with permission. Copyright © 2012 Massachusetts Medical Society.)

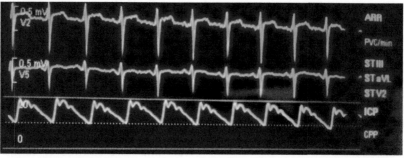

Fig. 2. Typical ICP waveform reading on the bedside monitor showing P1, P2, and P3 subpeaks of the ICP waveform. These waveforms are in descending order of amplitude. As intracranial compliance worsens, the P1 and P2 subpeaks may merge or the P2 subpeak may show a higher amplitude than the P1 subpeak. (*Data from* Asgari S, Bergsneider M, Hamilton R, et al. Consistent changes in intracranial pressure waveform morphology induced by acute hypercapnic cerebral vasodilatation. Neurocrit Care 2011;15(1):55–62.)

outcome in multiple mechanisms of brain injury, including TBI, ischemic stroke, hemorrhagic stroke, and subarachnoid hemorrhage.[31–35] It is reasonable to avoid hypotension and hypoxia in patients with acquired brain injury, because protective autoregulatory mechanisms are known to be abnormal in this setting.[36] Increases in ICP have been shown to worsen this phenomenon of impaired autoregulation.[36]

Indications for ICP Monitoring

Accurate monitoring of ICP is invasive and not without risk of complications. Specific to the setting of TBI, a level II recommendation to invasively monitor ICP given certain clinical and radiographic findings has been proposed. The merits of ICP monitoring as an evidence-based practice have been challenged. To answer the question of whether or not ICP should be treated, it is unlikely that a rigorous clinical trial will occur in which patients in whom ICP is known are randomized to receive or not receive treatment if they experience intracerebral hypertension. Regarding the question of monitoring, a recent trial was completed in South America[8] in which ICP monitoring is available but not routinely used. Patients with TBI were randomized to ICP-based treatment or to treatment decisions based on clinical examination and concurrent imaging findings. Intracranial hypertension was treated in both groups. The patients in the ICP monitoring group had a significantly shorter length of ICU stay and decreased times of ICU-administered brain-specific treatments, whereas the clinical and imaging-monitored group used significantly more mild hyperventilation (Pco$_2$ [partial pressure of carbon dioxide] 30–35 mm Hg) and more absolute hypertonic saline (HTS) for a longer period. The mortality, adverse events, and the primary outcome of functional and cognitive scores at 6 months

were not significantly different between monitoring groups. These conclusions regarding mortality are different from other prospective studies using ICP monitor-directed care.[37] Death and worsened outcomes in patients with brain trauma are often attributed to intractable ICP, and for critically ill patients at risk of increases in ICP, consideration for invasive monitoring and specific management based on monitored ICP are still recommended.[3,6,9,10,37]

Patients with severe acquired brain injury from any cause with a strong clinical suspicion of increased ICP and a nonreassuring clinical examination should be considered for ICP monitor placement.[3,6,9] Invasive monitoring devices include the extraventricular drain (EVD), intraparenchymal fiber-optic monitor, subdural bolt, and epidural fiber-optic catheters.

Types of Invasive Monitors

Monitoring of ICP is perhaps best achieved with the use of either ventriculostomy or an intraparenchymal monitor.[3,38] ICP monitoring is required for calculation of CPP (CPP = mean arterial blood pressure – ICP). The ventriculostomy or EVD is a fluid-coupled system that is accurate, inexpensive, and reliable. This modality allows measurement of ICP as well as the ability to reduce ICP by removal of CSF.[39] The EVD has a catheter attached to an external microstrain gauge and an external transducer, which allows intermittent ICP measurement. Pressure can be measured only when the drain is closed. Although imperfect, the recent development of in-line catheters that contain pressure transducers within their lumen allows simultaneous pressure monitoring and drainage.[40,41]

A variety of intraparenchymal monitors are in use. However, they are more expensive, have a shorter dwell time, and are believed to be less reliable than the EVD.[7] These devices are less technically challenging to place and can record pressure continuously, but cannot be rezeroed once inserted or used to drain CSF from the intracranial space. The technology used in these monitors varies, and they can incorporate either fiber-optic, strain gauge, or pneumatic technologies.[42] The placement of these monitors varies and depends on the site of the maximal injury in focal lesions. For example, in diffuse injury, the monitor is usually positioned in the frontal lobe of the nondominant hemisphere.[42] A small burr-hole is created to place these monitors, which may allow for the placement of other intraparenchymal monitors, such as brain tissue oxygen monitors or microdialysis probes. Some of the devices in use include the following[42]:

- Camino or Ventrix (Integra Neurosciences, Plainsboro, NJ)
- Codman microsensor (Codman, Raynham, MA)
- Spiegelberg ICP sensor and compliance device (Spiegelberg, Hamburg, Germany)
- Raumedic ICP sensor and multiparameter probe (Raumedic, Münchberg, Germany).

Subdural and extradural monitors were used in the past. These modalities are now less frequently used in modern neurocritical care units. Other invasive monitoring devices such as brain tissue oxygenation monitors, microdialysis catheters, and jugular venous saturation monitors can be used to tailor therapy and are described elsewhere in this issue Bullock et al. and LeRoux et al. Routine application of these devices awaits further study.[3] The use of brain tissue oxygen monitors has recently been reported to be associated with increased fluid and vasopressor use and pulmonary complications such as acute respiratory distress syndrome.[3] As with any monitor, the monitor itself does not alter outcome, but the information obtained influences the clinician's decisions and possibly outcome, a general principle most poignantly shown in the landmark ESCAPE (Evaluation Study of Congestive Heart Failure and Pulmonary Artery Catheterization Effectiveness) trial published in 2005.[43]

Noninvasive Measures of ICP

The search for an accurate and noninvasive monitor of ICP is ongoing. Two of the better options for nonabsolute measurement of ICP are the optic nerve sheath diameter (ONSD) and the pulsatility index (PI) calculated from transcranial Doppler studies (TCD). TCD is a portable and noninvasive tool widely used in the assessment of cerebral blood flow and screening for vasospasm in aneurysmal and traumatic subarachnoid hemorrhage.[10,44–46] Use of the PI can approximate a noncontinuous estimation of ICP, where an ispilateral/contralateral PI ratio greater than 1.25 is suspicious for compartmentalized ICP and mass effect.[47] Use of TCDs as a surrogate for ICP requires further study and is not routinely implemented.[48,49]

The use of ultrasonography in assessing the ONSD has also been studied.[50] In patients with increased ICP, the ONSD reliably increases as a result of its intimate relationship with CSF. Ultrasonography using a point-of-care linear array probe is placed on the superior and lateral aspect of the orbit against the upper eyelid. With the eye closed and angled slightly caudally and medially, the ONSD can be reliably measured.[51,52] For detection of ICP greater than 20 mm Hg, an ONSD greater than 0.48 cm has been found to have a sensitivity of 95% and specificity of 93%.[50,53] Trials are ongoing to further characterize this modality of monitoring ICP and clarify its role in ICP management.[54]

ICP Treatment Goals

The ICP goal in acquired brain injury is to maintain a normal pressure state, which is generally less than 20 cm H_2O or 15 mm Hg. Increased ICP is associated with poor outcome in TBI, ischemic stroke, subarachnoid hemorrhage, and intracerebral hemorrhage.[3,55–57] Current guidelines recommend instituting measures to control ICP when pressures of 20 mm Hg are reached, and to use aggressive means to prevent ICP increases to more than 25 mm Hg or CPP less than 60 mm Hg.[3,6,9] Awareness of CPP, as described earlier, is important, because many interventions to decrease ICP may also have systemic effects on peripheral hemodynamics. The maintenance of a CPP of at least 60 mm Hg with intravenous (IV) fluids or vasopressors is strongly recommended.[6,9] CPP goals may initially be satisfied with IV fluids, but if CPP cannot be maintained with a reasonable amount of IV fluids alone, norepinephrine and phenylephrine are commonly used. Overaggressive use of pressors and fluids to manipulate CPP greater than 70 mm Hg has been associated with increased incidence of pulmonary complications and acute lung injury.[58,59]

MANAGEMENT OF INCREASED ICP

Given the multiple different mechanisms by which ICP may be increased, its treatment can be nuanced with respect to different ongoing pathologic processes.[11] In general, treatment of intracranial hypertension is accomplished by manipulation of vasoreactivity, brain/blood osmotic gradient, metabolic rate of oxygen consumption, or physical/surgical means that affect intracranial compliance.

Hyperventilation

Hyperventilation may be a helpful short-lived and temporary intervention for increased ICP.[3,5,29] Prolonged hyperventilation has been associated with exacerbation of cerebral ischemia.[60] Short durations of mild hyperventilation (Pco_2 30–35 mm Hg) may be acceptable as a temporizing measure until other methods of managing ICP are available.[6] If hyperventilation is continued for longer than 12 hours, metabolic compensation negates any helpful effects of hyperventilation.[60] During a herniation event, hyperventilation acutely and reliably lowers Pco_2, as well as ICP, within seconds. The recommended Pco_2 goal is to maintain levels higher than 25 mm Hg.[3,61]

Conversely, hypoventilation must be monitored for its potential to increase ICP, a relationship that has been described in both preclinical and clinical models.[11] Procedures and different ventilator strategies have been shown to increase ICP via hypoventilation and hypercarbia.[62] Rescue ventilator modes (eg, airway pressure release ventilation) aimed at improving oxygenation at the expense of ventilation may require close monitoring of Pco_2, although success with 1 such mode in the setting of monitored ICP has been reported.[63,64] It may be helpful to use end-tidal CO_2 ($Etco_2$) monitoring in these patients, with the awareness that $Etco_2$ and Pco_2 may be discordant in the setting of chest trauma, hypotension, or metabolic acidosis.[65] Classically, a large pulmonary embolism or decreased cardiac output may also cause the $Etco_2$ to be lower than the Pco_2, in which case the latter may be higher than anticipated.[66,67] In these settings, it may be useful to correlate an arterial to alveolar CO_2 gap on a regular interval to assess for hypoventilation and hypercarbia (J Klein, personal communication, 2013).

Hyperosmolar Therapy

Creation of a relative increase in osmotic content in the bloodstream relative to the brain parenchyma causes efflux of fluid from intracellular and extracellular compartments of the brain into the vasculature. This situation effectually decreases the volume of the cranial compartment, thus reducing ICP and improving intracranial compliance.[29] Mannitol and HTS are the mainstays of hyperosmolar therapy.[3] Mannitol should be given IV via a peripheral or central IV line at a dose of 0.25 to 1.0 g/kg. Small doses of mannitol (0.25 g/kg) have been shown to effectively reduce ICP in patients with TBI.[68] Earlier data show that mannitol use in TBI correlates with decreased ICP and improved cerebral blood flow and CPP.[69] Mannitol can be given while following serum osmolality, and although a serum osmolality of 320 mOsm/L is generally accepted as a treatment end point, some investigators and experts advocate that higher levels can be obtained with caution.[70–72]

Concentrations of 1.5% to 23.4% HTS represent an option for osmotic therapy.[3] These varying concentrations of HTS have been studied versus mannitol, and the use of HTS seems to have better overall efficacy in terms of ICP control and avoidance of complications, such as hypotension. Two recent meta-analyses concerning the use of HTS in TBI, pediatrics, and nontraumatic acquired brain injury confirm the benefit of HTS over mannitol in reduction of ICP and improved CPP.[73,74] Bolus doses of 30 to 60 mL of 23.4% HTS have been used to emergently reverse a herniation event.[24] The ameliorative effect of 23.4% HTS on ICP has been shown to last longer than that of mannitol.[75] Such high concentrations of HTS must be administered via a central venous line during a 10-minute to 15-minute period to prevent phlebitis and hypotension. A reasonable initial treatment goal is to achieve supranormal serum sodium levels of 145 to 155 mEq/L, which is likely equivalent to a serum osmolality of 300 to 320 mOsm/L in most patients.[29] This level can then be titrated to effect to achieve optimal CPP and ICP goals. A 23.4% solution of HTS is effective in reducing ICP by a mean value of more than 8 mm Hg when given for ICP greater than 20 mm Hg and can increase CPP values by 6 mm Hg when pretreatment values are less than 70 mm Hg.[76] A continuous IV infusion of 1.5% to 3% HTS can be used to maintain high serum osmolality, as discussed earlier, but solutions of greater than 3% HTS should be given via a central line. If continuous infusions of HTS are used, serum sodium should be monitored every 4 hours, avoiding rapid changes in serum sodium so as not to precipitate cerebral edema or central pontine myelinolysis.[29] This complication is rare, likely because of clinician awareness regarding monitoring of serum sodium while patients are receiving HTS.[73] The phenomenon of rebound cerebral edema, which may occur with withdrawal of HTS, requires further study.[73] A recent review[72] discussed frequent questions that arise regarding the use of HTS in the setting of intracranial hypertension.

gents to Reduce the Cerebral Metabolic Rate of Oxygen (CMRo$_2$)

Despite optimal osmotic gradients and therapies, ICP may remain poorly controlled, and other options for treatment must be considered. Reductions in ICP may be achieved by alterations in the metabolic rate of the brain via induction of a pharmacologic coma.[77] The reduction in cerebral metabolism occurs through global reductions in cerebral blood flow and reduced tissue oxygen demand. Pentobarbital is in widespread use for induction of pharmacologic coma for this purpose.[28] This barbiturate is administered IV at a loading dose of 10 mg/kg during a 30-minute period, followed by a 5 mg/kg/h infusion for 3 hours, and maintenance therapy for 1 mg/kg/h titrated to therapeutic goals of either burst suppression on continuous EEG monitoring or a satisfactory reduction in ICP.[78] Smaller loading doses combined with an increase in the infusion dose can be given until burst suppression is seen or ICP is controlled. If ICP continues to increase and a patient has adequate burst suppression on EEG, further increases in pentobarbital may not be effective.[79] The use of pentobarbital coma can be associated with a large percentage of favorable outcomes in those patients who survive, although a recent Cochrane review was not supportive of this therapy to improve outcome.[80,81] Other barbiturates have been used in the past, such as the shorter-acting thiopental for acute exacerbations of ICP or during surgical procedures.[37] This medication is not currently available in the United States.

Another option for reducing CMRo$_2$ is the anesthetic propofol, which can be given at an IV loading dose of up to 2 mg/kg, followed by a titrated infusion of up to 2 to 75 μg/kg/min. The use of propofol for this indication is controversial and this drug has several side effects, the least of which includes dose-related hypotension. A study using propofol for ICP reduction showed a failure of an improvement in 6-month functional outcome, and long-term and high-dose propofol infusions have been associated with the development of propofol infusion syndrome (PRIS), which consists of renal failure, rhabdomyolysis, hyperkalemia, myocardial failure, metabolic acidosis, lipemia, hepatomegaly, and often death.[82] Patients receiving continuous infusions of propofol must be monitored for signs of PRIS, and long-term infusions more than 4 mg/kg should be avoided.[3,83] Laboratory monitoring for lactic acid, creatine kinase, and serum triglycerides to detect early signs of PRIS is recommended, although early detection and withdrawal of propofol does not guarantee survival if PRIS occurs.[83,84] Continuous EEG monitoring may be helpful to monitor for burst suppression or titrated control of ICP.

Induced hypothermia to improve outcomes in patients with intractable increases of ICP is promising but controversial. Preclinical data show induced hypothermia to be associated with improved neurophysiologic metrics in a hypoxic brain injury model, and there are randomized prospective data in TBI that induced mild hypothermia may improve outcome after TBI.[85,86] Hypothermia as a neuroprotectant strategy is appealing because of the multiple mechanisms by which hypothermia may protect the brain from secondary injury, including by the reduction of CMRo$_2$.[87,88] Current use of induced hypothermia for treatment of ICP in severe TBI is a second-tier therapy but may be helpful in refractory cases.[29] The potential of coagulopathy and antiplatelet effects of induced hypothermia should be considered, especially in the setting of hemorrhagic-acquired brain injury.[89–93] Shivering may negate the benefit from therapeutic hypothermia and must be controlled.[87] It is argued that induced hypothermia perhaps should be considered more of a first-tier therapy in some disease states that increase ICP, such as metabolic processes and fulminate liver failure.[94] If performed for ICP control, the optimal temperature may be closer to 35° rather than the typical 32° to 33°, although the optimal duration and depth of mild hypothermia remains unclear. It seems reasonable to use mild hypothermia for the period when ICP and cerebral edema are expected to peak, and rewarming from mild hypothermia should be performed sufficiently slowly (ie, 0.1° per hour). Infectious complications of prolonged mild hypothermia should not be dismissed, because the incidence of pulmonary infections (ie, ventilator-associated pneumonia) is high in some series.[95–97] Its use is advocated by some authorities because of strong evidence of its effectiveness on ICP, and although no clear consensus exists regarding whether there is an influence on long-term outcome for any treatment that reduces ICP, hypothermia is likely at least as effective at improving this metric in patients with acquired brain injury.[98] Two excellent review of the practical use of therapeutic hypothermia, including different modalities for the application of hypothermia, is referenced.[87,89]

Where great controversy seems to be lacking is the potential benefits of maintaining normothermia in patients with acquired brain injury. Avoiding hyperthermia in patients with severe acquired brain injury is recommended by numerous authorities.[9,10,31–35,99,100] Induced normothermia, just as therapeutic hypothermia, can be achieved in several ways, via antipyretics, ice-cold saline, airway cooling, invasive intravascular cooling, or various methods of surface cooling.[87,101–103]

Other Medial Options to Treat Increased ICP

Remote preclinical data suggest improved outcomes for females in some models of acquired brain injury.[104] Follow-up work has helped to define progesterone as a potentially protective compound from the standpoint of slowing the development of malignant cerebral edema and increased ICP.[105–108] The following 2 ongoing clinical trials are recruiting to examine the potential benefit of administered progesterone therapy in TBI: ProTECT III trial (Progesterone for Traumatic Brain Injury, Experimental Clinical Trial III) and SyNAPSe (Study of the Neuroprotective Activity of Progesterone in Severe Traumatic Brain Injury). Together, these 2 studies have a planned enrollment of more than 1100 patients, with expected completion dates of 2015 and 2013, respectively.[54] The use of progesterone outside the setting of Institutional Review Board-approved research protocols is not advocated.

The anesthetic ketamine offers yet another, if perhaps underused, option for the medical management of ICP. Ketamine, an inhibitor of the N-methyl-D-aspartate receptor, has long been reported to cause increases in ICP and was generally avoided in the anesthetic management of patients with acquired brain injury, although the validity of the science on which this practice was based has been subsequently questioned.[109–112] Perhaps because of its more generally prevalent use in children, research began to emerge in the pediatric critical care literature that ketamine appeared safe to use in patients with intracranial hypertension on controlled mechanical ventilation, and may even be beneficial for reducing ICP.[113] A large body of literature has helped to clarify the effects of ketamine on CMR_{O_2}, ICP, CPP, and cerebral blood flow in preclinical models, which seem favorable from a neuroprotectant standpoint in acquired brain injury.[114] However, the use of ketamine for control of ICP is not advocated in any of the published treatment guidelines for TBI, aneurysmal subarachnoid hemorrhage, ischemic stroke, or intracerebral hemorrhage.[3,6,9,10,100] If used, doses of 1 to 1.5 mg/kg may be appropriate in mechanically ventilated patients and followed for its effects on ICP.[113]

Surgical Treatment Options

In the setting of polytrauma, the phenomenon of ICP that does not respond to conventional treatment may represent a multiple compartment syndrome (MCS) of the intracranial, intraabdominal, and intrathoracic compartments.[115] Antecedent trauma or the required fluid or blood product resuscitation required to maintain CPP and mean arterial pressure (MAP) may play a role in the development of MCS. Published reports show that decompressive laparotomy performed in this setting resulted in improvements in intracranial compliance and ICP.[115–117] Whether decompressive laparotomy offers benefit to patients with intractable increases in ICP from other causes of acquired brain injury is unclear.

DC represents another clinical approach to the management of increased ICP. Reported results using this therapy are conflicting.[118–120] However, the role of DC in treating brief increases in ICP in TBI was evaluated in the recently published DECRA (Decompressive Craniectomy) trial.[121] ICP control was significantly improved in the surgical treatment arm, but 6-month outcome was worse compared with medical therapy. Patients with focal space-occupying lesions were excluded from the study, and the surgical arm cohort had a statistically significant difference in loss of pupil reactivity compared with the medically treated patients. This significant difference in the 2 treatment groups, combined with the choice of the surgical procedure performed, may limit the ability to generalize the conclusions of the study. Another study, RESCUEicp (Randomized Evaluation of Surgery with Craniectomy for Uncontrollable Increase of Intra-Cranial Pressure), may help further define the role of DC in the management of severe TBI.[122] RESCUEicp recently completed its enrollment of approximately 400 patients comparing DC with medical management (including barbiturates) in severe TBI.[122] The subject of the surgical management of increased ICP and the role for DC in other causes of refractory ICP is discussed in detail elsewhere in this issue.

Common clinical approaches for increased ICP management

Recognition of an ICP emergency should result in an algorithmic approach to treatment.[23] The management of acute increases in ICP initially involves ensuring that the waveform and ICP value are accurate. Respiratory derangements, ongoing seizure activity, hyperthermia, and metabolic causes need to be ruled out if suspected. Imaging with CT should be considered in any new episode of increased ICP without explanation. Physical interventions such as ensuring the head is midline and the head of the bed is up to at least 30°, establishing normothermia, and cessation of noxious stimuli such as suctioning may help to acutely lower temporary spikes in ICP. If this is unsuccessful and the ICP is believed to be accurate, brief hyperventilation of intubated patients may be performed to a P_{CO_2} of 30 to 35 mm Hg. If the ICP is measured with an EVD, then drainage of 5 to 10 mL of CSF may improve compliance and the overall treatment plan for ongoing drainage of CSF evaluated. If the patient with an intraparenchymal ICP monitor has moderately sized ventricles, then placement of an EVD should be considered. If central access exists, then 30–60 mL of 23.4% HTS may be given via a central line over a 15-minute period. This solution may need to be given faster, and if so, then a small dose of phenylephrine may help to augment the MAP so that the patient's CPP is maintained higher than 60 mm Hg. As an alternative to HTS, mannitol may be given via a peripheral line, with the dose tailored to the clinical situation. A dose of 1 g/kg is given for clinical signs of herniation and doses of 0.25 to 0.75 g/kg for less severe increases in ICP. In a herniation event, central access should be obtained, with consideration of a femoral central venous catheter or avoidance of extreme Trendelenburg positioning for subclavian lines.[29] If ICP continues to be increased after these maneuvers, then additional HTS can be given as well as further boluses of mannitol, treating up to a serum osmolality in the range of 320–340 mOsm/L. Standing infusions of 3% HTS can be used, with goal sodium values that may exceed 155 to 160 mEq/L if required. Further medical management includes use of bolus doses of propofol and consideration given to pharmacologic coma, induced hypothermia, ketamine, or surgical intervention.

SUMMARY

The management of patients with increased ICP in acquired brain injury from multiple potential causes may offer the potential to reduce secondary injury and improve outcomes. Controlling intracranial hypertension may maintain brain perfusion and alter the potential morbidity associated with acquired brain injury. Multimodality treatments in neurocritical care offer the potential to improve patient outcomes, both proximal and long-term.

REFERENCES

1. Teasdale G, Jennett B. Assessment of coma and impaired consciousness: a practical scale. Lancet 1974;2:81–4.
2. Geocadin R, Bhardwaj A, Mirski M, et al. Traumatic brain injury. Totowa (NJ): Humana Press; 2004.
3. Bratton SL, Chestnut RM, Ghajar J, et al. Guidelines for the management of severe traumatic brain injury. J Neurotrauma 2007;24(Suppl 1):S21–5.
4. BTF. Available at: http://braintrauma.org. Accessed November 22, 2012.
5. Maas A, Dearden M, Teasdale GM, et al. EBIC-guidelines for management of severe head injury in adults. European Brain Injury Consortium. Acta Neurochir (Wien) 1997;139(4):286–94.
6. Jauch E, Saver JL, Adams HP Jr, et al, American Heart Association Stroke Council, Council on Cardiovascular Nursing, Council on Peripheral Vascular Disease, and Council on Clinical Cardiology. Guidelines for the early management of patients with acute ischemic stroke: a guideline for healthcare professionals from the American Heart Association/American Stroke Association. Stroke 2013;44(3):870–947.
7. Farahvar A, Huang JH, Papadakos PJ. Intracranial monitoring in traumatic brain injury. Curr Opin Anaesthesiol 2011;24(2):209–13.
8. Chesnut R, Temkin N, Carney N, et al. A trial of intracranial-pressure monitoring in traumatic brain injury. N Engl J Med 2012;367(26):2471–81.
9. Morgenstern L, Hemphill JC 3rd, Anderson C, et al, American Heart Association Stroke Council and Council on Cardiovascular Nursing. Guidelines for the management of spontaneous intracerebral hemorrhage: a guideline for healthcare professionals from the American Heart Association/American Stroke Association. Stroke 2010;41(9):2108–29.
10. Connolly EJ, Rabinstein AA, Carhuapoma JR, et al. Guidelines for the management of aneurysmal subarachnoid hemorrhage: a guideline for healthcare professionals from the American Heart Association/American Stroke Association. Stroke 2012;43(6):1711–37.
11. Lee K, editor. The NeuroICU Book. 1st edition. New York: McGraw-Hill; 2012.
12. Monro A. Observations on the structure and function of the nervous system. Edinburgh (United Kingdom): Creech & Johnson; 1783.
13. Kellie G. An account of the appearances observed in the dissection of two of three individuals presumed to have perished in the storm of the 3rd, and whose bodies were discovered in the vicinity of Leith on the morning of the 4th, November 1821; with some reflections of the pathology of the brain. Transactions of the Medico-Chirurgical Society of Edinburgh 1824;1:84–169.
14. Schedler P, Geary S. Kernohan's notch phenomenon: a case study. J Neurosci Nurs 2002;34(3):158–9.
15. Ko S, Choi HA, Lee K. Clinical syndromes and management of intracerebral hemorrhage. Curr Atheroscler Rep 2012;14(4):307–13.
16. Brazis PW, Masdeu JC, Biller J. Localization in clinical neurology. Baltimore (MD): Lippincott Williams & Wilkins; 2007.

17. Vilela MD. Delayed paradoxical herniation after a decompressive craniectomy: case report. Surg Neurol 2008;69:293–6.

18. Reahme R, Bojanowski MW. Overt cerebrospinal fluid drainage is not a sine qua non for paradoxical herniation after decompressive craniectomy: case report. Neurosurgery 2010;67(1):214–5.

19. Seinfeld J, Sawyer M, Rabb CH. Successful treatment of paradoxical cerebral herniation by lumbar epidural blood patch placement: technical case report. Neurosurgery 2007;61(Suppl 3):E175.

20. Muehlschlegel S, Voetsch B, Sorond FA. Emergent epidural blood patch: lifesaving treatment of paradoxical herniation. Arch Neurol 2009;66:670–1.

21. Server A, Dullerud R, Haakonsen M, et al. Post-traumatic cerebral infarction. Neuroimaging findings, etiology and outcome. Acta Radiol 2001;42(3):254–60.

22. Stiver SI, Gean AD, Manley GT. Survival with good outcome after cerebral herniation and Duret hemorrhage caused by traumatic brain injury. J Neurosurg 2009;110:1242–6.

23. Qureshi AI, Suarez JI. More evidence supporting a brain code protocol for reversal of transtentorial herniation. Neurology 2008;70:990–1.

24. Koenig MA, Bryan M, Lewin JL III, et al. Reversal of transtentorial herniation with hypertonic saline. Neurology 2008;70:1023–9.

25. Bell RS, Vo AH, Neal CJ, et al. Military traumatic brain and spinal column injury: a 5 year study of the impact blast and other military grade weaponry on the central nervous system. J Trauma 2009;66(Suppl 4):S104–11.

26. Woda R, Miner ME, McCandless C, et al. The effect of right internal jugular vein cannulation on intracranial pressure. J Neurosurg Anesthesiol 1996;8(4):286–92.

27. Hesdorffer D, Ghajar J. Marked improvement in adherence to traumatic brain injury guidelines in the United States Trauma Centers. J Trauma 2007;63(4):841–7.

28. Suehiro E, Fujisawa H, Koizumi H, et al. Survey of current neurotrauma treatment practice in Japan. World Neurosurg 2011;75(3–4):563–8.

29. Raslan A, Bhardwaj A. Medical management of cerebral edema. Neurosurg Focus 2007;22:E12.

30. Dennis C, Lee R, Woodard EK, et al. Benefits of quiet time for neuro-intensive care patients. J Neurosci Nurs 2010;42(4):217–24.

31. Prasad K, Krishnan PR. Fever is associated with doubling of odds of short-term mortality in ischemic stroke: an updated meta-analysis. Acta Neurol Scand 2010;122(6):404–8.

32. Oh H, Jeong HS, Seo WS. Non-infectious hyperthermia in acute brain injury patients: relationships to mortality, blood pressure, intracranial pressure and cerebral perfusion pressure. Int J Nurs Pract 2012;18(3):295–302.

33. Douds G, Tadzong B, Agarwal AD, et al. Influence of fever and hospital-acquired infection on the incidence of delayed neurological deficit and poor outcome after aneurysmal subarachnoid hemorrhage. Neurol Res Int 2012;2012:479865.

34. Alberti A, Agnelli G, Caso V, et al. Non-neurological complications of acute stroke: frequency and influence on clinical outcome. Intern Emerg Med 2011;6(Suppl 1):119–23.

35. Rincon F, Lyden P, Mayer SA. Relationship between temperature, hematoma growth, and functional outcome after intracerebral hemorrhage. Neurocrit Care 2013;18(1):45–53.

36. Budohoski K, Czosnyka M, de Riva N, et al. The relationship between cerebral blood flow autoregulation and cerebrovascular pressure reactivity after traumatic brain injury. Neurosurgery 2012;71(3):652–60.

37. Farahvar A, Gerber LM, Chiu YL, et al. Increased mortality in patients with severe traumatic brain injury treated without intracranial pressure monitoring. J Neurosurg 2012;117(4):729–34.

38. Smith M. Monitoring intracranial pressure in traumatic brain injury. Anesth Analg 2008;106(1):240–8.

39. Timofeev I, Dahyot-Fizelier C, Keong N, et al. Ventriculostomy for control of raised ICP in acute traumatic brain injury. Acta Neurochir Suppl 2008;102:99–104.

40. Linsler S, Schmidtke M, Steudel WI, et al. Automated intracranial pressure-controlled cerebrospinal fluid external drainage with LiquoGuard. Acta Neurochir (Wien) 2012. [Epub ahead of print].

41. Birch A, Eynon CA, Schley D. Erroneous intracranial pressure measurements from simultaneous pressure monitoring and ventricular drainage catheters. Neurocrit Care 2006;5(1):51–4.

42. Le Roux P. Physiological monitoring of the severe traumatic brain injury patient in the intensive care unit. Curr Neurol Neurosci Rep 2013;13(3):331.

43. Binanay C, Califf RM, Hasselblad V, et al, ESCAPE Investigators and ESCAPE Study Coordinators. Evaluation study of congestive heart failure and pulmonary artery catheterization effectiveness: the ESCAPE trial. JAMA 2005;294(13):1625–33.

44. Armonda RA, Bell RS, Vo AH, et al. Wartime traumatic cerebral vasospasm: recent review of combat casualties. Neurosurgery 2006;59:1215–25.

45. Razumovsky A, Armonda RA. We still do not have a reliable and validated noninvasive technique that can provide an accurate quantitative measurement of intracranial pressure (ICP) that could replace invasive quantitative measurements of ICP. Neurosurgery 2011;68(1):E289–92.

46. Razumovsky A, Tigno T, Hochheimer SM, et al. Cerebral hemodynamic changes after wartime traumatic brain injury. Acta Neurochir Suppl 2013; 115:87–90.

47. Brandi G, Béchir M, Sailer S, et al. Transcranial color-coded duplex sonography allows to assess cerebral perfusion pressure noninvasively following severe traumatic brain injury. Acta Neurochir (Wien) 2010;152(6):965–72.

48. Zweifel C, Czosnyka M, Carrera E, et al. Reliability of the blood flow velocity pulsatility index for assessment of intracranial and cerebral perfusion pressures in head injured patients. Neurosurgery 2012;71(4):853–61.

49. de Riva N, Budohoski KP, Smielewski P, et al. Transcranial Doppler pulsatility index: what it is and what it isn't. Neurocrit Care 2012;17:58–66.

50. Rajajee V, Vanaman M, Fletcher JJ, et al. Optic nerve ultrasound for the detection of raised intracranial pressure. Neurocrit Care 2011;15(3): 506–15.

51. Amini A, Kariman H, Arhami Dolatabadi A, et al. Use of the sonographic diameter of optic nerve sheath to estimate intracranial pressure. Am J Emerg Med 2013;31(1):236–9.

52. Moretti R, Pizzi B, Cassini F, et al. Reliability of optic nerve ultrasound for the evaluation of patients with spontaneous intracranial hemorrhage. Neurocrit Care 2009;11(3):406–10.

53. Rajajee V, Fletcher J, Rochlen LR, et al. Comparison of accuracy of optic nerve ultrasound for the detection of intracranial hypertension in the setting of acutely fluctuating vs stable intracranial pressure: post-hoc analysis of data from a prospective, blinded single center study. Crit Care 2012; 16(3):R79.

54. Trials C. Available at: http://www.clinicaltrials.gov. Accessed February 7, 2013.

55. Fung C, Murek M, Z'Graggen WJ, et al. Decompressive hemicraniectomy in patients with supratentorial intracerebral hemorrhage. Stroke 2012; 43(12):3207–11.

56. Karnchanapandh K. Effect of increased ICP and decreased CPP on DND and outcome in ASAH. Acta Neurochir Suppl 2012;114:339–42.

57. Koennecke H, Belz W, Berfelde D, et al, Berlin Stroke Register Investigators. Factors influencing in-hospital mortality and morbidity in patients treated on a stroke unit. Neurology 2011;77(10): 965–72.

58. Fletcher JJ, Bergman K, Blostein PA, et al. Fluid balance, complications, and brain tissue oxygen tension monitoring following severe traumatic brain injury. Neurocrit Care 2010;13:47–56.

59. Contant CF, Valadka AB, Gopinath SP, et al. Adult respiratory distress syndrome: a complication of induced hypertension after severe head injury. J Neurosurg 2001;95:560–8.

60. Marion DW, Firlik A, McLaughlin MR. Hyperventilation therapy for severe traumatic brain injury. New Horiz 1995;3:439–47.

61. Stiver SI, Manley GT. Prehospital management of traumatic brain injury. Neurosurg Focus 2008; 33(Suppl 3):S228–40.

62. Kocaeli H, Korfali E, Taskapilioglu O, et al. Analysis of intracranial pressure changes during early versus late percutaneous tracheostomy in a neuro-intensive care unit. Acta Neurochir (Wien) 2008;150(12):1263–7.

63. Marik P, Young A, Sibole S, et al. The effect of APRV ventilation on ICP and cerebral hemodynamics. Neurocrit Care 2012;17(2):219–23.

64. Habashi NM. Other approaches to open-lung ventilation: airway pressure release ventilation. Crit Care Med 2005;33(Suppl 3):S228–40.

65. Lee S, Hong YS, Han C, et al. Concordance of end-tidal carbon dioxide and arterial carbon dioxide in severe traumatic brain injury. J Trauma 2009; 67(3):526–30.

66. Verschuren F, Liistro G, Coffeng R, et al. Volumetric capnography as a screening test for pulmonary embolism in the emergency department. Chest 2004;125(3):841–50.

67. Moon S, Lee SW, Choi SH, et al. Arterial minus end-tidal CO2 as a prognostic factor of hospital survival in patients resuscitated from cardiac arrest. Resuscitation 2007;72(2):219–25.

68. Mendelow AD, Teasdale GM, Russell T, et al. Effect of mannitol on cerebral blood flow and cerebral perfusion pressure in human head injury. J Neurosurg 1985;63:43–8.

69. Marshall LF, Smith RW, Rauscher LA, et al. Mannitol dose requirements in brain-injured patients. J Neurosurg 1978;48(2):169–72.

70. Ropper A. Hyperosmolar therapy for raised intracranial pressure. N Engl J Med 2012;367(8):746–52.

71. Diringer MN, Zazulia AR. Osmotic therapy: fact and fiction. Neurocrit Care 2004;1:219–33.

72. Marko N. Hyperosmolar therapy for intracranial hypertension: time to dispel antiquated myths. Am J Respir Crit Care Med 2012;185(5):467–8.

73. Mortazavi M, Romeo AK, Deep A, et al. Hypertonic saline for treating raised intracranial pressure: literature review with meta-analysis. J Neurosurg 2012; 116(1):210–21.

74. Kamel H, Navi BB, Nakagawa K, et al. Hypertonic saline versus mannitol for the treatment of elevated intracranial pressure: a meta-analysis of randomized clinical trials. Crit Care Med 2011;39(3):554–9.

75. Ware ML, Nemani VM, Meeker M, et al. Effects of 23.4% sodium chloride solution in reducing intracranial pressure in patients with traumatic brain

injury: a preliminary study. Neurosurgery 2005;57: 727–36.

76. Rockswold GL, Solid CA, Paredes-Andrade E, et al. Hypertonic saline and its effect on intracranial pressure, cerebral perfusion pressure, and brain tissue oxygen. Neurosurgery 2009;65:1035–41.

77. Nordström C, Messeter K, Sundbärg G, et al. Cerebral blood flow, vasoreactivity, and oxygen consumption during barbiturate therapy in severe traumatic brain lesions. J Neurosurg 1988;68(3): 424–31.

78. Ling GS, Marshall SA. Management of traumatic brain injury in the intensive care unit. Neurol Clin 2008;26:409–26.

79. Winer J, Rosenwasser RH, Jimenez F. Electroencephalographic activity and serum and cerebrospinal fluid pentobarbital levels in determining the therapeutic end point during barbiturate coma. Neurosurgery 1991;29(5):739–41.

80. Marshall G, James RF, Landman MP, et al. Pentobarbital coma for refractory intra-cranial hypertension after severe traumatic brain injury: mortality predictions and one-year outcomes in 55 patients. J Trauma 2010;69(2):275–83.

81. Roberts I, Sydenham E. Barbiturates for acute traumatic brain injury. Cochrane Database Syst Rev 2012;(12):CD000033.

82. Kelly DF, Goodale DB, Williams J, et al. Propofol in the treatment of moderate and severe head injury: a randomized, prospective double-blinded pilot trial. J Neurosurg 1999;90:1042–52.

83. Fudickar A, Bein B, Tonner PH. Propofol infusion syndrome in anesthesia and intensive care medicine. Curr Opin Anaesthesiol 2006;19(4):404–10.

84. Veldhoen E, Hartman BJ, van Gestel JP. Monitoring biochemical parameters as an early sign of propofol infusion syndrome: false feeling of security. Pediatr Crit Care Med 2009;10(2):19–21.

85. Marion DW, Penrod LE, Kelsey SF, et al. Treatment of traumatic brain injury with moderate hypothermia. N Engl J Med 1997;336:540–6.

86. Jia X. Improving neurological outcomes postcardiac arrest in a rat model: immediate hypothermia and quantitative EEG monitoring. Resuscitation 2008;90:1042–52.

87. Polderman KH. Induced hypothermia and fever control for prevention and treatment of neurological injuries. Lancet 2008;371:1955–69.

88. McIntyre L, Fergusson DA, Hébert PC, et al. Prolonged therapeutic hypothermia after traumatic brain injury in adults: a systematic review. JAMA 2003;289(22):2992–9.

89. Polderman KH. Application of therapeutic hypothermia in the intensive care unit. Opportunities and pitfalls of a promising treatment modality-part 2: practical aspects and side effects. Intensive Care Med 2004;30(5):757–69.

90. Watts DD, Trask A, Soeken K, et al. Hypothermic coagulopathy in trauma: effect of varying levels of hypothermia on enzyme speed, platelet function and fibrinolytic activity. J Trauma 1998;44:846–54.

91. Valeri CR, Feingold H, Cassidy G, et al. Hypothermia-induced reversible platelet dysfunction. Ann Surg 1987;205:175–81.

92. Mossad EB, Machado S, Apostolakis J. Bleeding following deep hypothermia and circulatory arrest in children. Semin Cardiothorac Vasc Anesth 2007;11:34–46.

93. Michelson AD, MacGregor H, Barnard MR, et al. Hypothermia-induced reversible platelet dysfunction. Thromb Haemost 1994;71:633–40.

94. Jalan R, Olde Damink SW, Deutz NE, et al. Moderate hypothermia in patients with acute liver failure and uncontrolled intracranial hypertension. Gastroenterology 2004;127(5):1338–46.

95. Moore E, Nichol AD, Bernard SA, et al. Therapeutic hypothermia: benefits, mechanisms and potential clinical applications in neurological, cardiac and kidney injury. Injury 2011;42(9):843–54.

96. Schwab S, Schwarz S, Bertram M, et al. Moderate hypothermia for the treatment of malignant middle cerebral artery infarct. Nervenarzt 1999;70(6): 539–46.

97. Delhaye C, Mahmoudi M, Waksman R. Hypothermia therapy: neurological and cardiac benefits. J Am Coll Cardiol 2012;59(3):197–210.

98. Schreckinger M, Marion D. Contemporary management of traumatic intracranial hypertension: is there a role for therapeutic hypothermia? Neurocrit Care 2009;11(3):427–36.

99. Maas AI, Stocchetti N, Bullock R. Moderate and severe traumatic brain injury in adults. Lance Neurol 2008;7:728–41.

100. Diringer M, Bleck TP, Claude Hemphill J 3rd, et al, Neurocritical Care Society. Critical care management of patients following aneurysmal subarachnoid hemorrhage: recommendations from the Neurocritical Care Society's Multidisciplinary Consensus Conference. Neurocrit Care 2011; 15(2):210–40.

101. Springborg J, Springborg KK, Romner B. First clinical experience with intranasal cooling for hyperthermia in brain-injured patients. Neurocrit Care 2013. [Epub ahead of print].

102. Diringer M, Neurocritical Care Fever Reduction Trial Group. Treatment of fever in the neurologic intensive care unit with a catheter-based heat exchange system. Crit Care Med 2004;32(2): 559–64.

103. Carhuapoma J, Gupta K, Coplin WM, et al. Treatment of refractory fever in the neurosciences critical care unit using a novel, water-circulating cooling device. A single-center pilot experience. J Neurosurg Anesthesiol 2003;15(4):313–8.

104. Attella MJ, Nattinville A, Stein DG. Hormonal state affects recovery from frontal cortex lesions in adult female rats. Behav Neural Biol 1987;48: 352–67.

105. Roof RL, Duvdevani R, Stein DG. Gender influences outcome of brain injury: progesterone plays a protective role. Brain Res 1993;607:333–6.

106. Stein DG, Wright DW, Kellermann AL. Does progesterone have neuroprotective properties? Ann Emerg Med 2008;51(2):164–72.

107. Maghool F, Khaksari M, Siahposht KA. Differences in brain edema and intracranial pressure following traumatic brain injury across the estrous cycle: involvement of female sex steroid hormones. Brain Res 2013;1497:61–72.

108. Shahrokhi N, Khaksari M, Soltani Z, et al. Effect of sex steroid hormones on brain edema, intracranial pressure, and neurologic outcomes after traumatic brain injury. Can J Physiol Pharmacol 2010;88(4): 414–21.

109. Schulte am Esch J, Pfeifer G, Thiemig I, et al. The influence of intravenous anaesthetic agents on primarily increased intracranial pressure. Acta Neurochir (Wien) 1978;45(1–2):15–25.

110. Schwedler M, Miletich DJ, Albrecht RF. Cerebral blood flow and metabolism following ketamine administration. Can Anaesth Soc J 1982;29(3): 222–6.

111. Schmittner M, Vajkoczy SL, Horn P, et al. Effects of fentanyl and S(+)-ketamine on cerebral hemodynamics, gastrointestinal motility, and need of vasopressors in patients with intracranial pathologies: a pilot study. J Neurosurg Anesthesiol 2007;19(4): 257–62.

112. Nimkoff L, Quinn C, Silver P, et al. The effects of intravenous anesthetics on intracranial pressure and cerebral perfusion pressure in two feline models of brain edema. J Crit Care 1997;12(3): 132–6.

113. Bar-Joseph G, Guilburd Y, Tamir A, et al. Effectiveness of ketamine in decreasing intracranial pressure in children with intracranial hypertension. J Neurosurg Pediatr 2009;4(1):40–6.

114. Hudetz J, Pagel PS. Neuroprotection by ketamine: a review of the experimental and clinical evidence. J Cardiothorac Vasc Anesth 2010;24(1):131–42.

115. Scalea T, Bochicchio GV, Habashi N, et al. Increased intra-abdominal, intrathoracic, and intracranial pressure after severe brain injury: multiple compartment syndrome. J Trauma 2007;62(3): 647–56.

116. Dorfman J, Burns JD, Green DM, et al. Decompressive laparotomy for refractory intracranial hypertension after traumatic brain injury. Neurocrit Care 2011;15(3):516–8.

117. Joseph D, Dutton RP, Aarabi B, et al. Decompressive laparotomy to treat intractable intracranial hypertension after traumatic brain injury. J Trauma 2004;57(4):687–93.

118. Albanese J, Leone M, Alliez JR, et al. Decompressive craniectomy for severe traumatic brain injury: evaluation of the effects at one year. Crit Care Med 2003;31:2535–8.

119. Guerra WK, Gaab MR, Dietz H, et al. Surgical decompression for traumatic brain swelling: indications and results. J Neurosurg 1999;90:187–96.

120. Pompucci A, Bonis PD, Pettorini B. Decompressive craniectomy for traumatic brain injury: patient age and outcome. J Neurotrauma 2007;24:1182.

121. Cooper DJ, Rosenfeld JV, Murray L, et al. Decompressive craniectomy in diffuse traumatic brain injury. N Engl J Med 2011;364:1493–502.

122. Current controlled trials. Available at: http:// controlled-trials.com/. Accessed February 8, 2013.

Surgical Treatment of Elevated Intracranial Pressure
Decompressive Craniectomy and Intracranial Pressure Monitoring

Tarek Y. El Ahmadieh, MD[a], Joseph G. Adel, MD[a],
Najib E. El Tecle, MD[a], Marc R. Daou, BA[a],
Salah G. Aoun, MD[b], Allan D. Nanney III, MD[a],
Bernard R. Bendok, MD, MSCI[a,*]

KEYWORDS

- Elevated intracranial pressure • Decompressive craniectomy • Intraventricular catheter
- Intracranial pressure monitoring • Intracranial mass • Intracranial hypertension hemicraniectomy

KEY POINTS

- Elevated intracranial pressure (ICP) is a relatively common complication of severe traumatic brain injury (TBI), intracranial hemorrhage, malignant middle cerebral artery (MCA) infarction, and high-grade subarachnoid hemorrhage (SAH). It is associated with high mortality and morbidity.
- Surgical interventions such as (1) insertion of intraventricular catheter, (2) removal of a space-occupying lesion, and (3) decompressive craniectomy can be life-saving in cases of refractory elevated ICP.
- Indications for ICP monitoring are summarized herein.
- Level I evidence obtained from 3 major randomized controlled trials (RCTs) (DECIMAL, DESTINY, and HAMLET) that supports decompressive craniectomy in young patients (≤60 years) with malignant MCA infarction is currently available.
- Recommendations for decompressive craniectomy in patients with severe TBI are currently being clarified. Data from the DECRA trial have shown increased unfavorable outcome in association with decompressive craniectomy. The RESCUEicp is an ongoing trial currently assessing the outcome of decompressive craniectomy in this setting.
- Recommendations for decompressive craniectomy in the setting of aneurysmal SAH are less clear. No RCTs are currently available.
- Although protocols are important, an individualized approach to all patients is crucial in the management of elevated ICP. It is important to balance the risks and potential outcomes of elevated ICP against those associated with any surgical intervention. Future RCTs should focus on functional outcome and quality of life of patients after surgery.

Disclosure: There are no conflicts of interest.
[a] Department of Neurological Surgery, McGaw Medical Center, Northwestern University Feinberg School of Medicine, 676 North Saint Clair Street, Suite 2210, Chicago, IL 60611, USA; [b] Department of Neurological Surgery, University of Texas Southwestern Medical Center, 5323 Harry Hines Blvd. Dallas, TX 75390-8855, USA
* Corresponding author.
E-mail address: bbendok@nmff.org

Neurosurg Clin N Am 24 (2013) 375–391
http://dx.doi.org/10.1016/j.nec.2013.03.003
1042-3680/13/$ – see front matter © 2013 Elsevier Inc. All rights reserved.

INTRODUCTION

Elevated intracranial pressure (ICP) is a relatively common and potentially devastating complication of a variety of cerebral pathologic conditions.[1] It occurs mainly as a result of large ischemic or hemorrhagic stroke, or following severe traumatic brain injury (TBI).[2,3] Current advances in technology, including modern neuroimaging and neuromonitoring techniques, allow early anticipation and detection of elevated ICP and hence more expeditious initiation of therapy.[4] First-line treatment for patients presenting with elevated ICP mainly involves noninvasive measures such as midline positioning and elevation of the head, hyperosmolar therapy, and, occasionally, hyperventilation and sedation in intubated patients.[5] In certain instances, however, the clinical impact of the primary or secondary brain injury can be severe, and patients may not respond well to conventional medical approaches. In such cases, more invasive techniques need to be implemented urgently to help immediately reduce elevated ICP. These techniques include (1) insertion of intraventricular catheter and cerebrospinal fluid (CSF) drainage, (2) removal of an intracranial space-occupying lesion (eg, hematoma), and (3) undergoing a decompressive craniectomy.[6] This review discusses the role of surgery in the management of elevated ICP, with special focus on the placement of intraventricular catheter and decompressive craniectomy. The authors describe the techniques and potential complications of each procedure, and review the existing evidence regarding the impact of these procedures on patient outcome. Surgical management of mass lesions and ischemic or hemorrhagic stroke occurring in the posterior fossa is not discussed herein.

NORMAL CEREBRAL DYNAMICS (MONRO-KELLIE DOCTRINE)

In a normal adult, the cranial vault can accommodate an average volume of approximately 1500 mL.[7] This volume is distributed among intracranial components as follows: brain tissue ($\approx$88%), blood ($\approx$7.5%), and CSF ($\approx$4.5%).[4,7] The cranium itself, however, is a closed container inside which the pressure depends on the sum of volumes of these components ($V_{Intracranial\ space} = V_{Brain} + V_{Blood} + V_{CSF}$). The normal ICP ranges between 10 and 15 mm Hg in an adult. For a normal ICP to be maintained, any increase in the volume of one of the intracranial components should be met with an equivalent decrease in one or both other components. This phenomenon is known as the Monro-Kellie doctrine.[8] Accordingly, in

cases of severe cerebral edema, brain swelling can lead to an uncompensated increase in the intracranial volume, resulting in elevated ICP and potential subsequent brain herniation. Elevated ICP can also lead to a decrease in cerebral blood flow (CBF) and a subsequent decrease in cerebral perfusion pressure (CPP).[9] In turn this can result in diffuse cerebral ischemia, which is one of the most important causes of secondary brain injury.[9]

CAUSES OF ELEVATED ICP

Based on the Monro-Kellie doctrine, any abnormality that leads to an uncompensated increase in intracranial volume can cause elevated ICP. One common cause of elevated ICP is severe TBI, which can result in primary or secondary brain edema.[10] Approximately 40% of patients with severe TBI develop brain edema and subsequent elevated ICP.[11] Other contributors to elevated ICP after severe TBI include: hyperemia (loss of vasomotor autoregulation); intracranial bleeding (eg, epidural hematoma, subdural hematoma, and intraparenchymal hemorrhage); hydrocephalus (eg, intraventricular hemorrhage and obstruction of CSF flow); and/or posttraumatic seizures (status epilepticus).[5] Large ischemic stroke, namely malignant middle cerebral artery (MCA) infarction, is another common cause of elevated ICP.[3,12] This type of stroke can lead to severe cytotoxic edema and reduction of regional CBF, and is associated with a mortality rate of approximately 80%.[13,14] Other clinical conditions that can lead to elevated ICP include brain tumors, abscesses, meningitis, hydrocephalus, aneurysmal subarachnoid hemorrhage (SAH), idiopathic intracranial hypertension, and venous sinus thrombosis.[4,5]

CLINICAL PRESENTATION

The clinical presentation of patients with elevated ICP can vary according to the nature of the underlying disorder as well as the severity and acuteness of symptoms. For example, patients who experience a severe TBI can present with an acute onset of elevated ICP caused by a rapidly expanding epidural hematoma. On the other hand, patients with slowly growing brain tumors may tolerate elevated ICP without showing any clinical manifestation. The classic signs and symptoms of elevated ICP include headache, vomiting, and papilledema.[1] Papilledema is a very reliable and specific sign of elevated ICP; however, it may not be evident in a large number of affected patients and is known to be observer dependent.[15] The Cushing triad, including hypertension, bradycardia, and respiratory irregularity (Cheyne-Stokes respiration), is a well-described phenomenon related to brainstem distortion or ischemia caused by elevated ICP.[16] The full triad, however, is only found in around 33% of cases. Cranial nerve palsies may also manifest in patients with elevated ICP.[17,18] Brain herniation syndromes, such as central and uncal herniation syndromes, can also occur as a result of elevated ICP, leading to progressive deterioration in the level of consciousness.

EVALUATION AND DIAGNOSIS

A high index of suspicion is crucial in the initial evaluation of patients at high risk of developing elevated ICP. Regardless of the underlying cause, assessment of the airway, breathing, and circulation (ABCs) should first take place in an acute setting. A full neurologic examination, particularly assessment of the Glasgow Coma Scale (GCS) score and bilateral pupils, should also be performed.[19] This neurologic assessment should be repeated frequently to detect early clinical deterioration. Any decrease in the patient's GCS score over the clinical course of the disease and/or development of pupillary asymmetry should be considered as a warning sign for an increasing ICP.[6] Endotracheal intubation should be considered in patients presenting with low levels of consciousness (GCS ≤8). In such scenarios, further clinical assessment of the patients is limited, and the use of radiologic studies, as well as direct ICP monitoring, becomes warranted. Unenhanced computed tomography (CT) of the brain can help support the diagnosis by detecting abnormalities that may be predictive of elevated ICP (eg, compression of basal cisterns and ventricles, effacement of sulci, and midline shift).[6,20,21] However, patients with no abnormal findings on initial CT scans may still have a 10% to 15% chance of developing elevated ICP.[22] Unenhanced CT of the brain can also help detect the underlying pathologic condition (eg, epidural hematoma). Magnetic resonance imaging (MRI), on the other hand, can help determine and calculate the stroke volume in patients presenting with large MCA infarcts.

MONITORING OF ICP
Methods

Two main methods of ICP monitoring are commonly used in clinical practice: (1) intraventricular catheters and (2) intraparenchymal microtransducer sensors.[23,24] Intraventricular catheters are considered the gold standard for ICP monitoring.[25] These catheters allow accurate measurement of the global ICP but also carry the advantage of therapeutic drainage of CSF.[24] The technique of intraventricular catheter insertion is described in the section on surgical management.

Indications for ICP Monitoring

Indications for ICP monitoring may include any clinical condition that carries an impending risk of elevated ICP (**Box 1**).[26] In 2007, the Brain Trauma Foundation guidelines recommended the use of ICP monitors in the management of patients with severe TBI.[10] These guidelines described level II evidence for ICP monitoring in all salvageable patients presenting with severe TBI (GCS 3–8) and an abnormal CT scan (defined as a scan that reveals an intracranial hematoma, contusion, swelling, herniation, or compressed basal cisterns).[10] In addition, level III evidence for ICP monitoring was described in patients presenting with severe TBI and a normal CT scan, but with 2 or more of the following: (1) age older than 40 years; (2) unilateral or bilateral motor posturing; or (3) systolic blood

---

Box 1
Potential indications for ICP monitoring

- According to Brain Trauma Foundation guidelines: All salvageable patients with Severe TBI (GCS 3–8) and
  - Abnormal CT scan (defined as scan that reveals intracranial hematoma, contusion, swelling, herniation, or compressed basal cistern) (level II evidence)
  - Normal CT scan, but with 2 or more of the following: (1) age older than 40 years, (2) unilateral or bilateral motor posturing, or (3) systolic blood pressure less than 90 mm Hg (level III evidence)
- Acute ischemic stroke (if surgical intervention is not feasible):
  - If patient is deteriorating clinically
  - If CT scan suggestive of mass effect
- Acute symptomatic hydrocephalus after SAH (level II evidence) and possibly in high-grade aneurysmal SAH
- Intubated patients in whom clinical assessment is not feasible
- After surgical removal of intracranial mass
- Central nervous system infections such as meningitis and encephalitis

Abbreviations: CT, computed tomography; GCS, Glasgow Coma Scale; ICP, intracranial pressure; SAH, subarachnoid hemorrhage; TBI, traumatic brain injury.

pressure less than 90 mm Hg.[10] Despite these recommendations, there has been significant variability in practice of ICP monitoring among practitioners worldwide.[27] In the authors' practice, the need for ICP monitoring is dictated by the clinical presentation of the patient and imaging findings, even in patients younger than 40 years. A case-by-case approach to all patients is therefore critical in the ICP management issues related to TBI. In a recently published multicenter controlled trial, Chesnut and colleagues[28] noted no significant improvement in outcomes in patients who presented with severe TBI and were managed according to the ICP monitoring guidelines, in comparison with those who were managed based on follow-up imaging and clinical examination (P = .49). This observation raises intriguing and counterintuitive questions about the true role of ICP monitoring in TBI.

Indications for ICP monitoring in other clinical settings are not well defined, and vary depending on individual and institutional protocols. According to the 2012 guidelines for management of aneurysmal SAH, insertion of an intraventricular catheter and diversion of CSF are recommended in patients presenting with acute symptomatic hydrocephalus after SAH (level II evidence).[29] In addition, significant support exists in the literature for ICP monitoring in patients presenting with high-grade aneurysmal SAH (Hunt and Hess grades III–V),[30] especially because elevated ICP in such patients is associated with poor outcome.[24,26,31,32] ICP monitoring has also been suggested in SAH cases where serial clinical assessment of patients is not feasible.[26] In the setting of acute ischemic stroke, it may be appropriate to monitor ICP in patients who are deteriorating clinically and in those with CT scans suggestive of mass effect.[4] However, it remains unclear whether ICP monitoring can improve clinical outcome in this particular setting.[24,33] Other indications of ICP monitoring may include central nervous system infections such as meningitis and encephalitis.[24]

Multimodal Neuromonitoring

A patient-specific multimodal intracranial monitoring approach has been suggested in the management of patients at increased risk of elevated ICP.[4,23,24,34–37] This approach includes: (1) monitoring of ICP and CPP; (2) monitoring of cerebral oxygenation (jugular bulb venous oximetry, or cerebral oxygen partial pressure); (3) monitoring of the metabolic status (cerebral microdialysis); and (4) monitoring of electrophysiologic brain activity (electroencephalography and somatosensory evoked potentials). It is thought that ICP monitoring alone may not reflect the full neurologic picture of patients at increased risk of elevated ICP. Consequently, ICP-driven therapy alone may not be able to address all the underlying pathophysiologic processes that can cause brain injury.[23,38] Furthermore, in their review of 70 patients who presented with severe TBI (GCS <8), Spiotta and colleagues[36] reported a significant decrease in the mortality rate among patients who received cerebral oxygen–driven therapy (25.7%) compared with those who received ICP-CPP–driven therapy alone (45.3%, P<.05). A similar decrease in the mortality rate was noted in several other studies comparing cerebral oxygen–driven therapy with ICP-CPP–driven therapy alone.[35,37] The studies suggested implementation of oxygen-driven therapy into the management of elevated ICP. Nevertheless, given the current lack of randomized controlled trials (RCTs) addressing this issue, definitive conclusions based on single-center experiences cannot be drawn.

Monitoring of the brain metabolic status using cerebral microdialysis techniques has also been suggested in the multimodal monitoring of patients at increased risk of elevated ICP.[39,40] Microdialysis catheters can detect intraparenchymal glucose and lactate concentrations in the brain, and are thought to reflect brain metabolic status. However, the role of microdialysis in the management of patients with elevated ICP remains to be defined.[41] Monitoring of the electrophysiologic activity of the brain can also be used in the management of patients at increased risk of elevated ICP.[4,34,42]

MANAGEMENT OF ELEVATED ICP

The main goal in the management of elevated ICP is to recognize and address the underlying pathology while at the same time applying measures to rapidly reduce ICP. In cases where the underlying pathology requires urgent surgery, for example in a patient presenting with a large epidural hematoma, it is important to move the patient to the operating room in a timely fashion. Meanwhile, noninvasive measures such as elevation of the head, mannitol administration, and even hyperventilation may be implemented to reduce ICP. In such cases, however, surgical evacuation of the hematoma may be the only definitive treatment for elevated ICP. In other cases where the underlying pathology is essentially nonsurgical, for example in a patient presenting with a mild to moderate cerebral edema from TBI or stroke, conservative (medical) therapy should be the primary treatment of choice, until further intervention becomes indicated.

Threshold Values for Treatment

According to the Brain Trauma Foundation guidelines, treatment of patients with elevated ICP caused by TBI should be initiated when ICP measurement exceeds 20 mm Hg (level II evidence).[10] Data from the literature have shown that patients with a mean ICP greater than 20 mm Hg have a significantly higher mortality rate than those with lower ICP values.[10,43,44] The mortality rate has also been shown to further increase in patients with prolonged, refractory elevated ICP.[45] Nonetheless, in the setting of less acute conditions, such as brain tumors, it has been suggested that patients may be able to tolerate higher ICP values, for longer periods of time, without significant complications.[6,11] Unfortunately, there are currently no well-defined thresholds for the treatment of elevated ICP caused by clinical conditions other than severe TBI. Most medical centers, however, initiate therapy when the ICP measurement exceeds 20 to 25 mm Hg.[5,6] The Brain Trauma Foundation guidelines also recommend treatment of patients with CPP values lower than 50 mm Hg (level III evidence).[10] Fluid resuscitation and vasopressors are typically used in such cases to induce hypertension, and therefore prevent cerebral ischemia that can result from low CBF and CPP.[24,46] It has been suggested, however, according to the same guidelines, to maintain a CPP value lower than 70 mm Hg to prevent the advent of life-threatening conditions such as secondary brain edema and/or adult respiratory distress syndrome, which can be induced by the excessive administration of vasopressors and fluids to raise CPP.[10,47,48]

Medical Management

When a patient is suspected clinically to have an elevated ICP confirmed by imaging, the treatment dictated by the clinical scenario should be initiated. Ordinarily, the head is elevated greater than 45° and sometimes up to 90° off the bed. The head is also maintained in midline and, if the patient has a neck collar, it is important to ensure that it is not compressing the jugular venous system in the neck area. The goal of these measures is to optimize the venous drainage of the brain and thus help decrease intracranial blood volume and ICP. Hyperosmolar therapy can then be implemented using diuretics, mannitol, and/or hypertonic saline. Mannitol is given at a bolus dose of 1 g/kg body weight followed by a maintenance dose of 0.5 g/kg every 6 hours, weaned over 2 to 3 days.[10] Serum osmolality is usually checked before every dose to maintain an osmolality of 310 to 320 mOsm/kg. Occasionally, a diuretic (eg, furosemide) may be used as needed to maintain a negative total daily balance. Meanwhile, mean arterial pressure is monitored to maintain CPP at 50 mm Hg or greater. A hypertonic saline (1.5% or 3% NaCl) drip may also be used, targeting a sodium level of 145 to 155 mEq/L. Serum sodium level should be monitored closely every 4 to 6 hours to ensure that the change in serum sodium level does not exceed 12 mEq/L/d. In the case of acute herniation, a sodium bullet (23.4%) may be used.

In the setting of an intracranial tumor with concern of associated elevated ICP, steroids may help decrease vasogenic edema by decreasing brain volume. On the other hand, if a patient has presented with a low GCS score that required intubation, the insertion of an ICP monitor may be warranted. In such cases, additional maneuvers such as short-term hyperventilation can be used to treat spikes of elevated ICP (target $Paco_2$: 30–35 mm Hg or even lower).[49] In patients with an intraventricular catheter, CSF drainage may be used as well. In cases where medical management fails and surgical intervention is not feasible, barbiturates can be used to induce a pharmacologic coma, which usually controls ICP by decreasing the metabolic demand and sympathetic response.[10]

Surgical Management

Although medical treatment may in certain instances reduce elevated ICP, medical management alone may not be sufficient to affect a normal ICP. Clinical conditions including severe TBI, large ischemic stroke, and high-grade SAH, as well as large subdural, epidural, and intraparenchymal hematomas, can result in a propagating a vicious cycle of brain edema, elevated ICP, reduced CBF, hypoxemia/ischemia, and further edema, eventually leading to severe brain injury.[50] Breaking this vicious cycle may require an urgent surgical intervention that allows complete removal of the underlying pathology or provides more room for brain swelling. Surgical management of elevated ICP includes: (1) insertion of intraventricular catheter and CSF drainage; (2) removal of an intracranial space-occupying lesion; and (3) undergoing a decompressive craniectomy.

Insertion of intraventricular catheter and CSF drainage

The earliest report on surgical cannulation of the lateral ventricle dates back to the late 1800s, when Keen first described the anatomic landmarks used in the procedure to treat hydrocephalus.[51,52] In 1908, Anton and Von Bramann described the first corpus callosum puncture technique, which aimed at connecting the lateral ventricle to the subarachnoid space.[53,54] Ten years later, Dandy described his technique of intraventricular catheterization of the lateral ventricle, which involved anterior and occipital ventricular horn punctures to obtain an air ventriculography.[55,56] Guillaume and Janny[57,58] eventually introduced the concept of ICP monitoring using intraventricular catheters in the early 1950s. Currently, with proper training and experience, placement of external ventricular drains in most patients can be achieved safely and quickly at the bedside.[59] In addition, intraventricular catheters are now considered the gold standard for measurement and monitoring of elevated ICP, and are also an important component of its management.

Indications In addition to their previously described role in ICP monitoring, intraventricular catheters are used in the treatment of various clinical conditions associated with elevated ICP. These catheters allow temporary drainage of CSF from the ventricular system, resulting in an immediate reduction of the intracranial volume and ICP. Indications for insertion of an intraventricular catheter and CSF drainage include elevated ICP attributable to a variety of causes including acute or subacute hydrocephalus, severe TBI, subarachnoid hemorrhage (Hunt and Hess grades 3–5), intraventricular hemorrhage, and meningitis.[6] Intraventricular catheters can further serve as a means for direct injection of tissue plasminogen activator (tPA) into the ventricular system in cases of severe hemorrhage (casted ventricles). Studies on intraventricular injection of tPA have shown promising results in terms of clot resolution and reduction in mortality rate.[60–63] In the recently published CLEAR-IVH trial (Clot Lysing: Evaluating Accelerated Resolution of Intraventricular Hemorrhage), tPA was found to significantly accelerate the resolution of intraventricular hemorrhage in a dose-dependent manner ($P<.0001$).[64] Drainage of CSF using an intraventricular catheter can provide brain relaxation, and may therefore be beneficial during aneurysm surgery. Indications for the insertion of an intraventricular catheter and ICP monitoring in TBI are summarized in **Box 1**.

Surgical technique Before the insertion of an intraventricular catheter, it is important to assess the size of the lateral ventricles to determine whether an adequate volume of CSF is available. Placement of a catheter into severely compressed ventricles can be technically challenging, and may lead to devastating complications such as hemorrhage.[6] Neurosurgical navigation can be helpful in cases of slit ventricles or shifted ventricles caused by mass effect.[6,52] It is also important to study intracranial abnormality before inserting an intraventricular catheter, to avoid passing through lesions lying in the trajectory of the catheter (eg, arteriovenous malformation).[52] Intraventricular catheters are usually inserted into the frontal horn of the lateral ventricle through a burr hole made at the Kocher point (usually the nondominant side), which is located 11 cm posterior to the nasion and 2 to 3 cm from the midline (approximately at the midpupillary line). After defining the anatomic landmarks, proper prepping and draping of the surgical site should be performed. A 1-cm linear skin incision is made, and a self-retaining retractor is used to hold the skin edges. A twist drill is then used to access the dura. After the drilling is completed, bone-wax may be placed on bone edges to stop the bleeding. A small incision in the dura is made. The catheter is then inserted perpendicular to the brain surface for a depth of 5 to 6 cm (from the brain surface) aiming at the ipsilateral medial epicanthus in the coronal plane and external auditory meatus in the sagittal plane, until CSF is obtained.[56] Deeper insertion of the catheter ($\geq$8 cm from the brain surface) often results in undesirable positioning and should therefore be avoided. This procedure can be performed free-handedly or using stereotactic guidance. The catheter is tunneled subcutaneously around 3 to 5 cm away from the burr hole, and is attached to an external pressure transducer with a 3-way stopcock and a draining bag. In the case of a ruptured aneurysm, care should be taken to avoid any rapid drainage. The authors open the drain at 20 cm H_2O in such cases. For most other indications the drainage threshold is typically set at 10 cm H_2O. The patient's head is elevated at an angle of approximately 30° and the zero-line, located at the ICP monitor scale, is placed at the level of the tragus (equivalent to foramen of Monroe). The setting for CSF drainage can be adjusted based on clinical and imaging response. In cases of trauma-induced elevated ICP, once a normal ICP is maintained for 48 to 72 hours the draining tube is clamped and the ICP monitored, with serial neurologic examinations being performed. If the patient does not show any signs or symptoms of elevated ICP for 12 to 24 hours, the catheter may be removed.

Outcomes In terms of clinical outcomes, external ventricular drainage has been shown to result in immediate reduction in ICP and has been deemed to be a highly effective measure for controlling ICP in multiple clinical settings.[65–68] Evidence of improved neurologic outcomes at 6 months has been reported following ICP control with intraventricular catheters in patients presenting with TBI.[6,65] Improvement in the neurologic status of patients presenting with aneurysmal SAH has also been noted after insertion of an intraventricular catheter.[68]

Complications Three main complications are associated with the insertion of intraventricular catheters: (1) intracranial bleeding, (2) infection, and (3) obstruction.[6] In their meta-analysis of hemorrhagic complications associated with insertion of intraventricular catheters, Binz and colleagues[69] reported an overall hemorrhagic risk of 5.7% and a clinically significant hemorrhagic risk of less than 1%. The risk of intracranial bleeding is found to increase in patients with coagulation disorders, and may be influenced by technique. Subdural hematoma is another potential complication.[70,71] Rebleeding from a ruptured intracranial aneurysm can occur following the insertion of an intraventricular catheter, possibly due to changes in the pressure gradients across the aneurysm wall.[72] Infection related to insertion of intraventricular catheters is another potential complication that may result in ventriculitis, meningitis, formation of brain abscess, and empyema. The rate of infection associated with intraventricular catheters ranges between 0% and 22%.[52,73,74] Catheter infection can be minimized by ensuring a sterile insertion technique with appropriate catheter tunneling and antibiotic administration.[75] In addition, proper wound care and minimum interruption of the closed system (eg, frequent flushing) may help reduce infection rates.[52,75] The use of antibiotic-impregnated catheters has been suggested as a way to reduce the risk of infection.[76,77] In their review of the literature, Gutierrez-Gonzalez and Boto[76] reported a decrease in device-related infection rate and hospital costs in patients with antibiotic-impregnated catheters, compared with those with standard catheters. The review included 3 retrospective cohorts, 1 retrospective review of a prospective database, and 1 prospective RCT.[76] However, in a recently published prospective RCT, these catheters did not a show significant reduction in infection risk when compared with standard catheters.[78] Silver-impregnated catheters have been shown to significantly reduce the infection rate in comparison with standard catheters in a double-blind RCT.[79] Obstruction of CSF drainage is a commonly encountered complication of intraventricular catheters, which can be caused by a blood clot obstructing the catheter.[6] Flushing the catheter with normal saline or tPA, in cases of hemorrhage, may clear the pathway and retain function. If patency cannot be established with flushing, the catheter may be replaced by a new catheter, typically with a "soft-pass technique."

Removal of intracranial space-occupying lesions

The most effective and definitive treatment for elevated ICP caused by a space-occupying lesion is surgical removal. Of note, the insertion of an intraventricular catheter can also be helpful in detecting secondary increases in ICP and can be an important component of the surgical management.[6,10,80] Intracranial hematomas are by far the most common cause of elevated ICP in patients presenting with severe TBI, complicating around 25% to 45% of cases.[81] According to the Brain Trauma Foundation guidelines, surgical evacuation of acute epidural hematomas is indicated if the hematoma is greater than 30 cm³, regardless of the patient's GCS.[82] However, nonsurgical measures and serial CT scans may be implemented in the management of epidural hematomas that are smaller than 30 cm³ and have the following features: (1) a thickness less than 15 mm, (2) a midline shift less than 5 mm, and (3) a GCS greater than 8.[82] Evacuation of subdural hematomas is also indicated in cases where a hematoma thickness greater than 10 mm or a midline shift greater than 5 mm is noted on CT scan.[80] Comatose patients with smaller hematomas may also need surgical evacuation if they deteriorate clinically between the time of injury and hospital admission: (1) GCS decrease by 2 or more points, (2) and/or asymmetric or fixed, dilated pupils, (3) and/or ICP increase more than 20 mm Hg.[80]

In contrast to epidural and subdural hematomas, for which clear evidence supporting surgical evacuation is available, surgical management of traumatic intraparenchymal mass lesions remains a subject of controversy.[6,83–85] The Surgical Trial in Traumatic Intracerebral Hemorrhage (STITCH) is a multicenter RCT that is currently comparing outcomes of early surgical treatment of patients with traumatic intracerebral hemorrhage with those of conservative (medical) therapy.[83] Until prospective data are obtained from this trial, evidence regarding the management of patients with traumatic intracerebral hemorrhage remains dependent on single-center retrospective studies.[6,86,87] Based on the available studies, the Brain Trauma Foundation guidelines recommended surgical evacuation of intraparenchymal hematomas in clinically deteriorating patients, and in patients who are not responding to medical therapy or who have a clear evidence of mass effect on imaging.[88] Patients with frontal or temporal contusions greater than 50 cm³ should also be treated surgically.[88] Similarly, patients with contusions greater than 20 cm³, who have a GCS score of 6 to 8 and an additional midline shift of at least 5 mm and/or cisternal compression, may be considered for surgical treatment.[88]

Indications for surgical evacuation of spontaneous intracerebral hematomas remain controversial. In the Surgical Trial in Intracerebral Hemorrhage (STICH), 1033 patients presenting with spontaneous intracerebral hemorrhage were randomized to one of two treatment arms: (1) early surgery or (2) initial conservative therapy.[84] The results of the trial showed no overall benefit from early surgery (468 patients) in comparison with conservative treatment (496 patients) ($P =$ .414).[84] The mortality rate at 6 months for surgically treated patients was 36%, compared with 37% for conservatively treated patients. A trend toward favorable outcome from early surgery was noted in patients with superficial (cortical) intracerebral hematomas 1 cm or less from the cortical surface in comparison with deeper hematomas.[84] In current practice, whether an intracerebral hematoma should be surgically evacuated depends largely on the clinical condition of each patient and the treatment protocol at each institution. Surgical management of patients with spontaneous intracerebral hematomas may include the insertion of an intraventricular catheter in the contralateral lateral ventricle to help monitor and control ICP. This action can be of particular importance in patients who present with an intraventricular extension of the bleed.

Indications for surgical removal of other space-occupying lesions, such as brain tumors or abscesses, in the setting of elevated ICP are not well defined and may therefore vary according to the inherent features of the lesion itself, the clinical condition of the patient, and the experience at each center. In general, any abnormal intracranial mass resulting in elevated ICP should be considered for surgery, especially after failure of medical therapy.

Decompressive craniectomy

The practice of craniectomy dates back to the prehistoric age.[89] In an interesting observation, human skulls from the Paleolithic Period were found to have bony defects suggestive of human interventions.[89] These defects were recognized by Broca, in the late 1800s, to have been created in subjects who subsequently survived.[90,91] It remains unclear, however, whether these procedures were performed as part of old rituals or in attempts to treat patients with disorders. The modern description of craniectomy goes back to the time of 2 famous neurosurgeons, Theodor Kocher (1901) and Harvey Cushing (1905), who were the first to report surgical decompression techniques as a measure to effectively reduce elevated ICP.[92] It was suggested that surgical removal of part of the skull provides room for the brain to swell and therefore reduces ICP. Over the past century, however, management of elevated ICP with decompressive craniectomy has been a subject of extensive scrutiny and controversy. It was not until 1999, after Guerra and colleagues[93] published their experience of 20 years, that decompressive craniectomy regained wide acceptance. At present, decompressive craniectomy is being implemented in various treatment protocols for the management of elevated ICP and has been part of several RCTs.[12,93,94]

Indications Three main indications, of variable levels of evidence, exist for the use of decompressive craniectomy in the management of elevated ICP: (1) severe TBI, (2) malignant MCA infarction, and (3) aneurysmal SAH.[50,92] According to the Brain Trauma Foundation guidelines, bifrontal decompressive craniectomy is indicated within 48 hours of injury for patients with diffuse, posttraumatic cerebral edema and medically refractory elevated ICP.[88] In addition, according to the same guidelines, subtemporal decompression, temporal lobectomy, and hemispheric decompressive craniectomy can be considered as treatment options for patients who present with diffuse parenchymal injury and refractory elevated ICP who also have clinical and radiographic evidence for impending transtentorial brain herniation.[88] Despite these guidelines, there has been a continuous debate regarding the optimal timing of the procedure, and its effect on patient outcome and quality of life.[6] Many argue that the obtained results may not justify the treatment, especially if the reduction in the mortality rate is to be associated with an increase in the rate of severe disability.[50,92] Furthermore, long-term functional outcomes of patients undergoing decompressive craniectomy after TBI remain to be determined.

A higher level of evidence is currently available for the use of decompressive craniectomy in patients with malignant MCA infarction.[95] This evidence is based on data obtained from 3 major RCTs: DECIMAL,[96] DESTINY,[97] and HAMLET (**Table 1**).[98] Indications for decompressive craniectomy in patients with malignant MCA infarction are well described in the 2008 guidelines of the United Kingdom National Institute for Health and Clinical Excellence.[99] Decompressive craniectomy is recommended in patients who present within 24 hours of the onset of symptoms and meet all of the following criteria: (1) age younger than 60 years, (2) National Institute of Health Stroke Scale (NIHSS) score higher than 15, and (3) infarct of at least 50% of the MCA territory or infarct volume greater than

Table 1
Randomized controlled trials conducted on decompressive craniectomy in the management of malignant MCA infarction

Study	Study Type	No. of Patients	Time Interval from Symptom Onset to Surgery (h)	Follow-Up	Treatment Arms	Primary Outcome (mRS <4) (%)	Severe Disability (mRS 4–5) (%)	Mortality (mRS 6) (%)
HeADDFIRST (Frank et al)[133]	Multicenter RCT	26	96	180 d	DC / Conservative	Awaiting publication	—	35.3 / 40.0
HeMMI (Jamora et al)[134]	Single-center RCT	—	72	6 mo	DC / Conservative	Recruitment started in 2004, awaiting publication	—	—
DECIMAL (Vahedi et al,[96] 2007)	Multicenter RCT	38	24	12 mo (stopped)	DC (n = 20) / Conservative (n = 18)	50.0 / 22.2	25.0 / 0	25.0 / 77.8
DESTINY (Jüttler et al)[97]	Multicenter RCT	32	12–36	12 mo (stopped)	DC (n = 17) / Conservative (n = 15)	47.1 / 26.7	35.3 / 20.0	17.6 / 53.0
HAMLET (Hofmeijer et al,[98] 2006)	Multicenter RCT	64	96	12 mo (stopped)	DC (n = 32) / Conservative (n = 32)	25.0	53.1 / 15.6	21.9 / 59.4
POOLED ANALYSIS (Vahedi et al,[95] 2007)	Multicenter RCT: enrollment in DECIMAL, DESTINY, or HAMLET	93	48	12 mo	DC (n = 51) / Conservative (n = 42)	43.1 / 21.4	35.3 / 7.2	21.6 / 71.4

Abbreviations: DC, decompressive craniectomy; MCA, middle cerebral artery; mRS, modified Rankin Scale; RCT, randomized controlled trial.

145 cm^3 as shown on diffusion-weighted MRI.[99] The procedure is likely best performed within a maximum of 48 hours after the onset of symptoms.[99] In a pooled analysis combining data from the 3 RCTs, decompressive craniectomy done within 48 hours of stroke onset was associated with lower mortality and more favorable outcomes (see **Table 1**).[95] Whether the outcome scales used in clinical trials truly reflect the quality of life of patients after surgery remains a subject of controversy. Decompressive craniectomy may still be considered in patients older than 60 years; however, the likelihood of a good outcome is less than in younger individuals. In their literature review on decompressive craniectomy performed in patients with malignant MCA infarction, Arac and colleagues[13] reported significantly higher rates of poor outcomes in the patient group older than 60 years (81.8%) compared with patients 60 years or younger (33.1%) ($P<.0001$).

Evidence for the use of decompressive craniectomy in the setting of aneurysmal SAH is limited to single-center experiences.[32,94,100–102] In one study by Buschmann and colleagues,[102] 38 patients who presented with aneurysmal SAH were treated with surgical clipping of the aneurysm and concomitant decompressive hemicraniectomy. Of the 38 patients, 31 presented with a high-grade SAH (Hunt and Hess grade 4–5). Indications for the hemicraniectomy included: (1) intraoperative signs of brain edema (group 1); (2) elevated ICP with epidural, subdural, or intracerebral hematoma after surgery (group 2); (3) elevated ICP and cerebral edema without radiologic signs of infarction (group 3); and (4) elevated ICP and cerebral edema with radiologic signs of infarction (group 4).[102] At 12-month follow-up, a good functional outcome was noted in 52.4% of patients in group 1, 60% in group 2, 83.3% in group 3, and 16.7% in group 4.[102] The study concluded that more than half of the patients with aneurysmal SAH can benefit from decompressive craniectomy, and recommended early surgical intervention in patients who present with aneurysmal SAH and refractory elevated ICP.[102] Another study by Smith and colleagues[32] reported good outcomes in patients who presented with a high-grade SAH (Hunt and Hess grade 4–5) and large Sylvian fissure hematoma, and who were treated with decompressive hemicraniectomy and surgical evacuation of the hematoma. The study suggested that a decompressive hemicraniectomy may be of benefit in a carefully selected group of patients with aneurysmal SAH.[32]

Other indications for decompressive craniectomy may include intracerebral hemorrhage,[103,104] subdural empyema,[105] meningitis,[106] encephalitis,[107] toxoplasmosis,[108] encephalopathy caused by Reye syndrome,[109] and severe cerebral venous and dural sinus thrombosis.[110]

Surgical technique Two main types of decompressive craniectomy are currently used in clinical practice: (1) unilateral craniectomy and (2) bilateral craniectomy.[50,92,111–114] Unilateral craniectomy, or decompressive hemicraniectomy, is usually performed in patients presenting with unilateral brain edema and midline shift caused by TBI, malignant MCA infarction, or SAH.[6,12,102] The presence of midline shift is an important factor that dictates the side on which the craniectomy should be performed. A thorough evaluation of the patient should be conducted prior to the procedure. Once in the operating room, the patient is placed in the supine position after induction of general anesthesia. The head is elevated and turned laterally, such that the craniectomy side faces upward, and is then fixed with a head frame. If needed, a shoulder roll may be used to elevate the ipsilateral shoulder and assist positioning. It is important to avoid excessive rotation of the head and neck so as not to compress the jugular venous system. After proper shaving, a marker is used to align the surface anatomy of important structure, such as the sagittal and transverse sinuses, and to draw the incision line. The incision line is "question mark" in shape, starting approximately 1 cm anterior to the tragus and moving up toward the area just above the ear pinna, then turning posteriorly toward the external occipital protuberance (**Fig. 1**). The line is then curved superiorly and anteriorly to end just behind the hairline. It is important to ensure that the curvature extends posterior enough to allow for a minimum craniectomy size of 12 cm.[12,115] Local anesthesia is injected along the incision line, and appropriate prepping and draping is performed. The incision is made, and the skin flap and underlying temporalis muscle are reflected anteriorly. Five burr holes are made in the following locations: (1) temporal squamous bone superior to the zygomatic process inferiorly, (2) keyhole area behind the zygomatic arch anteriorly, (3) along the superior temporal line posteroinferiorly, and in the (4) parietal and (5) frontal parasagittal areas (see **Fig. 1**). The burr holes are then connected with a footplated bit. Careful attention should be given to avoid laceration of the superior sagittal sinus. The bone flap can then be removed and stored either in the subcutaneous tissue of the abdominal wall or in a freezer ($-20°$ to $-70°C$).[92,116] Further removal of bone from the sphenoid wing of the temporal bone can help provide access to the temporal lobe. A stellate-shaped durotomy is then made slowly and carefully to avoid injury to

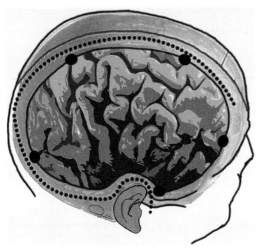

Fig. 1. Unilateral craniectomy or decompressive hemicraniectomy. Question mark–shaped skin incision (*dotted line*). Five burr holes made in the temporal squamous bone superior to the zygomatic process inferiorly, keyhole area behind the zygomatic arch anteriorly, along the superior temporal line posteroinferiorly, and in the parietal and frontal parasagittal areas.

the underlying brain tissue. It is important to extend the durotomy inferiorly to the skull base, to decompress the middle cranial fossa.[111] After the durotomy is completed, a drain may be placed if indicated. A duraplasty is performed, and a layer of Surgicel (Johnson and Johnson Medical, Inc., Arlington, TX, USA) left on the brain surface. The temporalis muscle and fascia are left unsutured to allow expansion of the brain, whereas the galea and skin are sutured in layers. Reconstruction with autologous or synthetic bone is often performed 5 to 8 weeks after the procedure.[92]

Bilateral craniectomy is usually indicated in patients who present with diffuse brain edema without a focal lesion (eg, contusions due to severe TBI).[6,117] This procedure can be performed by either decompressive hemicraniectomies on both sides, or a bifrontal craniectomy.[92,117] The same surgical principles, previously described for the unilateral craniectomy, apply for the bifrontal craniectomy. However, in the latter the head should be fixed in the neutral position, and the incision should extend from the area anterior to the tragus on both sides. The curve should be made parallel and 2 to 3 cm posterior to the coronal suture. Burr holes are made in keyhole areas on both sides, in both squamous temporal bones, and in the parietal area just behind the coronal suture and 1 cm from the midline.[111] The burr holes are connected, and the bone flap carefully removed. The area overlying the superior sagittal sinus should be

manipulated carefully, as the dura may be adherent to the scalp. A rim of bone may be preserved over the sinus to avoid bleeding complications.[93] The durotomy may be performed in a bilateral stellate, U-shaped, or "fish-mouth" fashion.[50,111,116]

Outcomes Over the past few years, several single-center studies have been conducted to assess the outcome of decompressive craniectomy in the setting of TBI.[118–120] However, variations in patient selection, outcome scoring, and the timing and techniques of surgery have made it difficult to reach conclusions. In one of the largest studies, Williams and colleagues[118] retrospectively reviewed 171 patients who presented with severe TBI and elevated ICP and underwent decompressive craniectomy. The study used the Glasgow Outcome Scale Extended (GOSE), and reported good outcomes (GOSE 5–8) in 56% of the patients. This outcome was noted in younger individuals and in patients who achieved higher ICP reduction.[118] More recently, the outcome of decompressive craniectomy after TBI has been assessed in RCTs (**Table 2**). In the DEcompressive CRAniectomy (DECRA) trial, published in 2011, 155 adult patients presenting with severe TBI and refractory elevated ICP were randomized to one of two treatment arms: (1) early bifrontotemporoparietal decompressive craniectomy (within 72 hours) and standard care; or (2) standard care alone.[117] The study showed that early decompressive craniectomy is associated with more unfavorable outcomes at 6 months than is standard care ($P = .02$).[117] However, decompressive craniectomy was found to significantly decrease ICP and the length of stay in the intensive care unit. Mortality rates were similar in both treatment arms (19% in craniectomy group vs 18% in standard-care group).[117] At present, another ongoing RCT (RESCUEicp: Randomized Evaluation of Surgery with Craniectomy for Uncontrollable Elevation of intracranial pressure) is evaluating the role of decompressive craniectomy in the management of patients with severe TBI and refractory elevated ICP.[121] This study is expected to provide additional insight regarding the long-term outcome of decompressive craniectomy in the setting of severe TBI. Other issues, such as the timing of surgery and the optimal technique to be used, also need to be clarified.

The effect of decompressive craniectomy on outcome of patients with malignant MCA infarction has been assessed in multiple retrospective and nonrandomized prospective studies.[122–125] Most studies showed a significant decrease in mortality when compared with medical management. However, some uncertainty remains regarding the impact on functional outcome and quality of life.

Table 2
Randomized controlled trials conducted on decompressive craniectomy in the management of traumatic brain injury

Study	Study Type	Inclusion Criteria	Treatment Arms	Follow-Up	Outcome
DECRA trial (Cooper et al,[117] 2011)	Multicenter RCT	Severe diffuse TBI and intracranial hypertension refractory to first-tier therapies	Two arms: 1. DC + standard care (n = 73) vs 2. Standard care alone (n = 82)	6 mo	DC group had less time in ICU and less time with high ICP. On Extended Glasgow Outcome Scale DC patients performed worse than patients who received standard care (OR 1.84) and had a greater risk of unfavorable outcome (OR 2.21). Death rate in DC group (19%) and in standard-care group (18%) was comparable
RESCUEicp (Hutchinson et al,[121] 2006)	Multicenter RCT	Severe TBI; ICP refractory to optimal, protocol-driven conservative therapy	Two arms: 1. DC vs 2. Medical management	—	Ongoing

Abbreviations: DC, decompressive craniectomy; ICP, intracranial pressure; ICU, intensive care unit; OR, odds ratio; RCT, randomized controlled trial; TBI, traumatic brain injury.

In an attempt to better define the role of decompressive craniectomy in the management of malignant MCA infarction, 3 RCTs were conducted: DECIMAL,[96] DESTINY,[97] and HAMLET (see **Table 1**).[98] In their pooled analysis of the 3 trials, Vahedi and colleagues[95] reported on 93 patients, of whom 51 were randomized to decompressive craniectomy and 42 to medical treatment. The study noted a higher number of patients in the surgical arm who had a modified Rankin Scale (mRS) score of 4 or less (75% vs 24% in the medical arm), mRS score of 3 or less (43% vs 21% in the medical arm), and who survived (78% vs 29% in the medical arm).[95] Data obtained from the 3 randomized trials and the pooled analysis suggests that decompressive craniectomy can significantly decrease mortality and increase the number of patients with a favorable outcome. However, it must be noted that the number of patients with moderately severe disability (mRS ≤4) is also increased.[95] In addition, the long-term functional and psychosocial outcome, as well as the effect of decompressive craniectomy on elderly patients, remained undefined. Recently, in their systematic review of the literature, Rahme and colleagues[126] assessed functional outcome, depression, quality of life, and mortality rates in patients who underwent decompressive craniectomy in the treatment of malignant MCA infarction. Their study included 3 major RCTs, 3 prospective cohorts, and 10 retrospective studies. The mortality rate was 24.3% among the 382 patients reviewed. Favorable functional outcome was reported in 41% of the 156 survivors (mRS score ≤3); however, 47% of the patients experienced moderately severe disability (mRS score ≤4).[126] The quality of life was also assessed despite significant variations in assessment tools and reporting among studies. The mean overall reduction in quality of life after decompressive craniectomy was 45.2% of the 157 survivors with available quality-of-life data. The mean physical and psychosocial reductions in quality of life were 66.9% and 36.8%, respectively.[126] In terms of depression outcomes, 25% of the 80 survivors with available data were diagnosed with moderate or severe depression. It is interesting that despite the high number of patients with moderate disability, 76.6% of the 209 survivors with available patient feedback after surgery were satisfied with their lives and announced they would again give their consent for decompressive craniectomy.[126]

The outcome of decompressive craniectomy in patients presenting with SAH and refractory elevated ICP has been assessed in several studies.[94,101,102] In their review of 16 patients with aneurysmal SAH who underwent decompressive craniectomy, Schirmer and colleagues[94] reported good functional outcomes in 7 patients (64%; mRS ≤3). Eleven patients in this study had a Hunt and Hess score of 4 to 5. The median follow-up duration was approximately 15 months.[94] Decompressive craniectomy performed within 48 hours after SAH was the only factor significantly associated with better outcomes ($P<.01$). The study suggested early surgery in patients with high-grade aneurysmal SAH.[94] Ziai and colleagues,[101] on the other hand, reported poor outcome in 3 of 4 patients with aneurysmal SAH who underwent decompressive craniectomy, and death in 1 patient. Because of the lack of clear guidelines recommending decompressive craniectomy in this particular setting, a careful case-by-case approach to all patients with aneurysmal SAH is advised. The pros and cons of surgical intervention and the possibility of a poor prognosis should be discussed with the family.

Complications The most common complication following decompressive craniectomy is the formation of a subdural fluid collection or hygroma.[93,127–129] In their review of 57 patients who underwent decompressive craniectomy after TBI, Guerra and colleagues[93] reported the occurrence of postoperative hygromas in 15 patients (26%). Kilincer and colleagues[128] also reported contralateral subdural effusion in a patient who presented with aneurysmal SAH and underwent surgical clipping and decompressive craniectomy. Brain herniation through the cranial defect is another potential complication that can occur as a result of inadequate decompression.[115,130] In their review of 60 patients who presented with right MCA infarctions and underwent decompressive hemicraniectomy, Wagner and colleagues[115] reported a higher rate of bleeding complications and mortality in association with small-sized craniectomies, and recommended a craniectomy size of at least 12 cm to achieve an adequate decompressive volume and reduction in ICP.[115] Other complications may include infections such as meningitis or osteomyelitis of the bone flap,[129,131] postoperative seizures,[132] and hydrocephalus.

REFERENCES

1. Dunn LT. Raised intracranial pressure. J Neurol Neurosurg Psychiatry 2002;73(Suppl 1):i23–7.
2. Jennett B. Epidemiology of head injury. Arch Dis Child 1998;78(5):403–6.
3. Hacke W, Schwab S, Horn M, et al. 'Malignant' middle cerebral artery territory infarction: clinical course and prognostic signs. Arch Neurol 1996;53(4):309–15.
4. Wolfe TJ, Torbey MT. Management of intracranial pressure. Curr Neurol Neurosci Rep 2009;9(6): 477–85.
5. Rangel-Castilla L, Gopinath S, Robertson CS. Management of intracranial hypertension. Neurol Clin 2008;26(2):521–41, x.
6. Li LM, Timofeev I, Czosnyka M, et al. Review article: the surgical approach to the management of increased intracranial pressure after traumatic brain injury. Anesth Analg 2010;111(3):736–48.
7. Doczi T. Volume regulation of the brain tissue–a survey. Acta Neurochir 1993;121(1–2):1–8.
8. Sankhyan N, Vykunta Raju KN, Sharma S, et al. Management of raised intracranial pressure. Indian J Pediatr 2010;77(12):1409–16.
9. Mangat HS. Severe traumatic brain injury. Continuum (Minneap Minn) 2012;18(3):532–46.
10. Brain Trauma Foundation, American Association of Neurological Surgeons, Congress of Neurological Surgeons. Guidelines for the management of severe traumatic brain injury. J Neurotrauma 2007; 24(Suppl 1):S1–106.
11. Miller JD, Becker DP, Ward JD, et al. Significance of intracranial hypertension in severe head injury. J Neurosurg 1977;47(4):503–16.
12. Arnaout OM, Aoun SG, Batjer HH, et al. Decompressive hemicraniectomy after malignant middle cerebral artery infarction: rationale and controversies. Neurosurg Focus 2011;30(6):E18.
13. Arac A, Blanchard V, Lee M, et al. Assessment of outcome following decompressive craniectomy for malignant middle cerebral artery infarction in patients older than 60 years of age. Neurosurg Focus 2009;26(6):E3.
14. Hofmeijer J, Schepers J, Veldhuis WB, et al. Delayed decompressive surgery increases apparent diffusion coefficient and improves peri-infarct perfusion in rats with space-occupying cerebral infarction. Stroke 2004;35(6):1476–81.
15. Selhorst JB, Gudeman SK, Butterworth JF, et al. Papilledema after acute head injury. Neurosurgery 1985;16(3):357–63.
16. Wan WH, Ang BT, Wang E. The Cushing response: a case for a review of its role as a physiological reflex. J Clin Neurosci 2008;15(3):223–8.
17. Sperry B. Benign intracranial hypertension associated with palsy of the third cranial nerve. J Am Osteopath Assoc 1979;78(11):816–21.
18. Patton N, Beatty S, Lloyd IC. Bilateral sixth and fourth cranial nerve palsies in idiopathic intracranial hypertension. J R Soc Med 2000;93(2):80–1.
19. Jennett B, Teasdale G, Braakman R, et al. Predicting outcome in individual patients after severe head injury. Lancet 1976;1(7968):1031–4.

20. Miller MT, Pasquale M, Kurek S, et al. Initial head computed tomographic scan characteristics have a linear relationship with initial intracranial pressure after trauma. J Trauma 2004;56(5):967–72 [discussion: 972–3].

21. Kishore PR, Lipper MH, Becker DP, et al. Significance of CT in head injury: correlation with intracranial pressure. AJR Am J Roentgenol 1981;137(4):829–33.

22. Eisenberg HM, Gary HE Jr, Aldrich EF, et al. Initial CT findings in 753 patients with severe head injury. A report from the NIH Traumatic Coma Data Bank. J Neurosurg 1990;73(5):688–98.

23. Kirkman MA, Smith M. Multimodal intracranial monitoring: implications for clinical practice. Anesthesiol Clin 2012;30(2):269–87.

24. Smith M. Monitoring intracranial pressure in traumatic brain injury. Anesth Analg 2008;106(1):240–8.

25. Maniker AH, Vaynman AY, Karimi RJ, et al. Hemorrhagic complications of external ventricular drainage. Neurosurgery 2006;59(4 Suppl 2):ONS419–24 [discussion: ONS424–5].

26. Jantzen JP. Prevention and treatment of intracranial hypertension. Best Pract Res Clin Anaesthesiol 2007;21(4):517–38.

27. Sahjpaul R, Girotti M. Intracranial pressure monitoring in severe traumatic brain injury—results of a Canadian survey. Can J Neurol Sci 2000;27(2):143–7.

28. Chesnut RM, Temkin N, Carney N, et al. A trial of intracranial-pressure monitoring in traumatic brain injury. N Engl J Med 2012;367(26):2471–81.

29. Connolly ES Jr, Rabinstein AA, Carhuapoma JR, et al. Guidelines for the management of aneurysmal subarachnoid hemorrhage: a guideline for healthcare professionals from the American Heart Association/American Stroke Association. Stroke 2012;43(6):1711–37.

30. Spiotta AM, Provencio JJ, Rasmussen PA, et al. Brain monitoring after subarachnoid hemorrhage: lessons learned. Neurosurgery 2011;69(4):755–66 [discussion: 766].

31. Heuer GG, Smith MJ, Elliott JP, et al. Relationship between intracranial pressure and other clinical variables in patients with aneurysmal subarachnoid hemorrhage. J Neurosurg 2004;101(3):408–16.

32. Smith ER, Carter BS, Ogilvy CS. Proposed use of prophylactic decompressive craniectomy in poor-grade aneurysmal subarachnoid hemorrhage patients presenting with associated large sylvian hematomas. Neurosurgery 2002;51(1):117–24 [discussion: 124].

33. Schwab S, Aschoff A, Spranger M, et al. The value of intracranial pressure monitoring in acute hemispheric stroke. Neurology 1996;47(2):393–8.

34. Amantini A, Fossi S, Grippo A, et al. Continuous EEG-SEP monitoring in severe brain injury. Neurophysiol Clin 2009;39(2):85–93.

35. Stiefel MF, Spiotta A, Gracias VH, et al. Reduced mortality rate in patients with severe traumatic brain injury treated with brain tissue oxygen monitoring. J Neurosurg 2005;103(5):805–11.

36. Spiotta AM, Stiefel MF, Gracias VH, et al. Brain tissue oxygen-directed management and outcome in patients with severe traumatic brain injury. J Neurosurg 2010;113(3):571–80.

37. Narotam PK, Morrison JF, Nathoo N. Brain tissue oxygen monitoring in traumatic brain injury and major trauma: outcome analysis of a brain tissue oxygen-directed therapy. J Neurosurg 2009;111(4):672–82.

38. Oddo M, Villa F, Citerio G. Brain multimodality monitoring: an update. Curr Opin Crit Care 2012;18(2):111–8.

39. Tisdall MM, Smith M. Cerebral microdialysis: research technique or clinical tool. Br J Anaesth 2006;97(1):18–25.

40. Chen JW, Rogers SL, Gombart ZJ, et al. Implementation of cerebral microdialysis at a community-based hospital: a 5-year retrospective analysis. Surg Neurol Int 2012;3:57.

41. Hillered L, Persson L, Nilsson P, et al. Continuous monitoring of cerebral metabolism in traumatic brain injury: a focus on cerebral microdialysis. Curr Opin Crit Care 2006;12(2):112–8.

42. Amantini A, Amadori A, Fossi S. Evoked potentials in the ICU. Eur J Anaesthesiol Suppl 2008;42:196–202.

43. Juul N, Morris GF, Marshall SB, et al. Intracranial hypertension and cerebral perfusion pressure: influence on neurological deterioration and outcome in severe head injury. The Executive Committee of the International Selfotel Trial. J Neurosurg 2000;92(1):1–6.

44. Balestreri M, Czosnyka M, Hutchinson P, et al. Impact of intracranial pressure and cerebral perfusion pressure on severe disability and mortality after head injury. Neurocrit Care 2006;4(1):8–13.

45. Treggiari MM, Schutz N, Yanez ND, et al. Role of intracranial pressure values and patterns in predicting outcome in traumatic brain injury: a systematic review. Neurocrit Care 2007;6(2):104–12.

46. Rosner MJ, Rosner SD, Johnson AH. Cerebral perfusion pressure: management protocol and clinical results. J Neurosurg 1995;83(6):949–62.

47. Robertson CS, Valadka AB, Hannay HJ, et al. Prevention of secondary ischemic insults after severe head injury. Crit Care Med 1999;27(10):2086–95.

48. Vespa P. What is the optimal threshold for cerebral perfusion pressure following traumatic brain injury? Neurosurg Focus 2003;15(6):E4.

49. Muizelaar JP, Marmarou A, Ward JD, et al. Adverse effects of prolonged hyperventilation in patients with severe head injury: a randomized clinical trial. J Neurosurg 1991;75(5):731–9.

50. Hutchinson P, Timofeev I, Kirkpatrick P. Surgery for brain edema. Neurosurg Focus 2007;22(5):E14.

51. Keen WW. Surgery of the lateral ventricles of the brain. Lancet 1890;136(3498):553–5.

52. Dey M, Jaffe J, Stadnik A, et al. External ventricular drainage for intraventricular hemorrhage. Curr Neurol Neurosci Rep 2012;12(1):24–33.

53. Anton G, Von Bramann FG. Balkenstich bei Hydrozephalien, tumoren und bei Epilepsie. Medizinische Wochenschrift 1908;55:1673.

54. Chesler DA, Pendleton C, Jallo GI, et al. "Colossal" breakthrough: the callosal puncture as a precursor to third ventriculostomy. Minim Invasive Neurosurg 2011;54(5–6):243–6.

55. Dandy WE. Ventriculography following the injection of air into the cerebral ventricles. Ann Surg 1918; 68(1):5–11.

56. Ghajar J. Intracranial pressure monitoring techniques. New Horiz 1995;3(3):395–9.

57. Guillaume J, Janny P. Continuous intracranial manometry; importance of the method and first results. Rev Neurol 1951;84(2):131–42.

58. Guillaume J, Janny P. Continuous intracranial manometry; physiopathologic and clinical significance of the method. Presse Med 1951;59(45): 953–5.

59. Kakarla UK, Kim LJ, Chang SW, et al. Safety and accuracy of bedside external ventricular drain placement. Neurosurgery 2008;63(1 Suppl 1): ONS162–6 [discussion: ONS166–7].

60. Naff NJ, Carhuapoma JR, Williams MA, et al. Treatment of intraventricular hemorrhage with urokinase: effects on 30-Day survival. Stroke 2000; 31(4):841–7.

61. Coplin WM, Vinas FC, Agris JM, et al. A cohort study of the safety and feasibility of intraventricular urokinase for nonaneurysmal spontaneous intraventricular hemorrhage. Stroke 1998;29(8):1573–9.

62. Ronning P, Sorteberg W, Nakstad P, et al. Aspects of intracerebral hematomas—an update. Acta Neurol Scand 2008;118(6):347–61.

63. Jaffe J, Melnychuk E, Muschelli J, et al. Ventricular catheter location and the clearance of intraventricular hemorrhage. Neurosurgery 2012;70(5): 1258–63 [discussion: 1263–4].

64. Webb AJ, Ullman NL, Mann S, et al. Resolution of intraventricular hemorrhage varies by ventricular region and dose of intraventricular thrombolytic: the Clot Lysis: Evaluating Accelerated Resolution of IVH (CLEAR IVH) program. Stroke 2012;43(6): 1666–8.

65. Timofeev I, Dahyot-Fizelier C, Keong N, et al. Ventriculostomy for control of raised ICP in acute traumatic brain injury. Acta Neurochir Suppl 2008; 102:99–104.

66. Fortune JB, Feustel PJ, Graca L, et al. Effect of hyperventilation, mannitol, and ventriculostomy drainage on cerebral blood flow after head injury. J Trauma 1995;39(6):1091–7 [discussion: 1097–9].

67. Kerr ME, Weber BB, Sereika SM, et al. Dose response to cerebrospinal fluid drainage on cerebral perfusion in traumatic brain-injured adults. Neurosurg Focus 2001;11(4):E1.

68. Suzuki M, Otawara Y, Doi M, et al. Neurological grades of patients with poor-grade subarachnoid hemorrhage improve after short-term pretreatment. Neurosurgery 2000;47(5):1098–104 [discussion: 1104–5].

69. Binz DD, Toussaint LG 3rd, Friedman JA. Hemorrhagic complications of ventriculostomy placement: a meta-analysis. Neurocrit Care 2009;10(2): 253–6.

70. Carmel PW, Albright AL, Adelson PD, et al. Incidence and management of subdural hematoma/hygroma with variable- and fixed-pressure differential valves: a randomized, controlled study of programmable compared with conventional valves. Neurosurg Focus 1999;7(4):e7.

71. Lang SS, Kofke WA, Stiefel MF. Monitoring and intraoperative management of elevated intracranial pressure and decompressive craniectomy. Anesthesiol Clin 2012;30(2):289–310.

72. Gigante P, Hwang BY, Appelboom G, et al. External ventricular drainage following aneurysmal subarachnoid haemorrhage. Br J Neurosurg 2010; 24(6):625–32.

73. Park P, Garton HJ, Kocan MJ, et al. Risk of infection with prolonged ventricular catheterization. Neurosurgery 2004;55(3):594–9 [discussion: 599–601].

74. Dasic D, Hanna SJ, Bojanic S, et al. External ventricular drain infection: the effect of a strict protocol on infection rates and a review of the literature. Br J Neurosurg 2006;20(5):296–300.

75. Schade RP, Schinkel J, Visser LG, et al. Bacterial meningitis caused by the use of ventricular or lumbar cerebrospinal fluid catheters. J Neurosurg 2005;102(2):229–34.

76. Gutierrez-Gonzalez R, Boto GR. Do antibiotic-impregnated catheters prevent infection in CSF diversion procedures? Review of the literature. J Infect 2010;61(1):9–20.

77. Zabramski JM, Whiting D, Darouiche RO, et al. Efficacy of antimicrobial-impregnated external ventricular drain catheters: a prospective, randomized, controlled trial. J Neurosurg 2003;98(4):725–30.

78. Pople I, Poon W, Assaker R, et al. Comparison of infection rate with the use of antibiotic-impregnated vs standard extraventricular drainage devices: a prospective, randomized controlled trial. Neurosurgery 2012;71(1):6–13.

79. Keong N, Bulters D, Richards H, et al. The SILVER (Silver-Impregnated Line Vs EVD Randomized) Trial: a double-blind, prospective, randomized controlled trial of an intervention to reduce the rate of external ventricular drain infection. Neurosurgery 2012;71(2):349–403.

80. Bullock MR, Chesnut R, Ghajar J, et al. Surgical management of acute subdural hematomas. Neurosurgery 2006;58(Suppl 3):S16–24 [discussion: Si–iv].

81. Thurman D, Guerrero J. Trends in hospitalization associated with traumatic brain injury. JAMA 1999;282(10):954–7.

82. Bullock MR, Chesnut R, Ghajar J, et al. Surgical management of acute epidural hematomas. Neurosurgery 2006;58(Suppl 3):S7–15 [discussion: Si-iv].

83. Gregson BA, Rowan EN, Mitchell PM, et al. Surgical Trial in Traumatic Intracerebral Hemorrhage (STITCH(Trauma)): study protocol for a randomized controlled trial. Trials 2012;13:193.

84. Mendelow AD, Gregson BA, Fernandes HM, et al. Early surgery versus initial conservative treatment in patients with spontaneous supratentorial intracerebral haematomas in the International Surgical Trial in Intracerebral Haemorrhage (STICH): a randomised trial. Lancet 2005;365(9457):387–97.

85. Seelig JM, Becker DP, Miller JD, et al. Traumatic acute subdural hematoma: major mortality reduction in comatose patients treated within four hours. N Engl J Med 1981;304(25):1511–8.

86. Choksey M, Crockard HA, Sandilands M. Acute traumatic intracerebral haematomas: determinants of outcome in a retrospective series of 202 cases. Br J Neurosurg 1993;7(6):611–22.

87. Zumkeller M, Hollerhage HG, Proschl M, et al. The results of surgery for intracerebral hematomas. Neurosurg Rev 1992;15(1):33–6.

88. Bullock MR, Chesnut R, Ghajar J, et al. Surgical management of traumatic parenchymal lesions. Neurosurgery 2006;58(Suppl 3):S25–46 [discussion: Si-iv].

89. Apuzzo ML, Liu CY, Sullivan D, et al. Surgery of the human cerebrum—a collective modernity. Neurosurgery 2007;61(Suppl 1):28 [discussion: 28–31].

90. Broca P. La trépanation chez les Incas. Bull Acad Natl Med 1867;(32):866–71.

91. Clower WT, Finger S. Discovering trepanation: the contribution of Paul Broca. Neurosurgery 2001; 49(6):1417–25 [discussion: 1425–6].

92. Schirmer CM, Ackil AA Jr, Malek AM. Decompressive craniectomy. Neurocrit Care 2008;8(3): 456–70.

93. Guerra WK, Gaab MR, Dietz H, et al. Surgical decompression for traumatic brain swelling: indications and results. J Neurosurg 1999;90(2):187–96.

94. Schirmer CM, Hoit DA, Malek AM. Decompressive hemicraniectomy for the treatment of intractable intracranial hypertension after aneurysmal subarachnoid hemorrhage. Stroke 2007;38(3):987–92.

95. Vahedi K, Hofmeijer J, Juettler E, et al. Early decompressive surgery in malignant infarction of the middle cerebral artery: a pooled analysis of three randomised controlled trials. Lancet Neurol 2007;6(3):215–22.

96. Vahedi K, Vicaut E, Mateo J, et al. Sequential-design, multicenter, randomized, controlled trial of early decompressive craniectomy in malignant middle cerebral artery infarction (DECIMAL Trial). Stroke 2007;38(9):2506–17.

97. Juttler E, Schwab S, Schmiedek P, et al. Decompressive Surgery for the Treatment of Malignant Infarction of the Middle Cerebral Artery (DESTINY): a randomized, controlled trial. Stroke 2007;38(9):2518–25.

98. Hofmeijer J, Amelink GJ, Algra A, et al. Hemicraniectomy after middle cerebral artery infarction with life-threatening Edema trial (HAMLET). Protocol for a randomised controlled trial of decompressive surgery in space-occupying hemispheric infarction. Trials 2006;7:29.

99. Tyrrell P, Rudd A, Cullen K, et al. In: Stroke: National clinical guideline for diagnosis and initial management of acute stroke and transient ischaemic attack (TIA). London: Royal college of physicians of London; 2008.

100. D'Ambrosio AL, Sughrue ME, Yorgason JG, et al. Decompressive hemicraniectomy for poor-grade aneurysmal subarachnoid hemorrhage patients with associated intracerebral hemorrhage: clinical outcome and quality of life assessment. Neurosurgery 2005;56(1):12–9 [discussion: 19–20].

101. Ziai WC, Port JD, Cowan JA, et al. Decompressive craniectomy for intractable cerebral edema: experience of a single center. J Neurosurg Anesthesiol 2003;15(1):25–32.

102. Buschmann U, Yonekawa Y, Fortunati M, et al. Decompressive hemicraniectomy in patients with subarachnoid hemorrhage and intractable intracranial hypertension. Acta Neurochir 2007;149(1):59–65.

103. Murthy JM, Chowdary GV, Murthy TV, et al. Decompressive craniectomy with clot evacuation in large hemispheric hypertensive intracerebral hemorrhage. Neurocrit Care 2005;2(3):258–62.

104. Maira G, Anile C, Colosimo C, et al. Surgical treatment of primary supratentorial intracerebral hemorrhage in stuporous and comatose patients. Neurol Res 2002;24(1):54–60.

105. Wada Y, Kubo T, Asano T, et al. Fulminant subdural empyema treated with a wide decompressive craniectomy and continuous irrigation–case report. Neurol Med Chir 2002;42(9):414–6.

106. Baussart B, Cheisson G, Compain M, et al. Multimodal cerebral monitoring and decompressive surgery for the treatment of severe bacterial meningitis with increased intracranial pressure. Acta Anaesthesiol Scand 2006;50(6):762–5.

107. Schwab S, Junger E, Spranger M, et al. Craniectomy: an aggressive treatment approach in severe encephalitis. Neurology 1997;48(2):412–7.

108. Agrawal D, Hussain N. Decompressive craniectomy in cerebral toxoplasmosis. Eur J Clin Microbiol Infect Dis 2005;24(11):772–3.

109. Ausman JI, Rogers C, Sharp HL. Decompressive craniectomy for the encephalopathy of Reye's syndrome. Surg Neurol 1976;6(2):97–9.

110. Keller E, Pangalu A, Fandino J, et al. Decompressive craniectomy in severe cerebral venous and dural sinus thrombosis. Acta Neurochir Suppl 2005;94:177–83.

111. Quinn TM, Taylor JJ, Magarik JA, et al. Decompressive craniectomy: technical note. Acta Neurol Scand 2011;123(4):239–44.

112. Johnson RD, Maartens NF, Teddy PJ. Technical aspects of decompressive craniectomy for malignant middle cerebral artery infarction. J Clin Neurosci 2011;18(8):1023–7.

113. Whitfield PC, Patel H, Hutchinson PJ, et al. Bifrontal decompressive craniectomy in the management of posttraumatic intracranial hypertension. Br J Neurosurg 2001;15(6):500–7.

114. Timofeev I, Santarius T, Kolias AG, et al. Decompressive craniectomy—operative technique and perioperative care. Adv Tech Stand Neurosurg 2012;38:115–36.

115. Wagner S, Schnippering H, Aschoff A, et al. Suboptimum hemicraniectomy as a cause of additional cerebral lesions in patients with malignant infarction of the middle cerebral artery. J Neurosurg 2001;94(5):693–6.

116. Winter CD, Adamides A, Rosenfeld JV. The role of decompressive craniectomy in the management of traumatic brain injury: a critical review. J Clin Neurosci 2005;12(6):619–23.

117. Cooper DJ, Rosenfeld JV, Murray L, et al. Decompressive craniectomy in diffuse traumatic brain injury. N Engl J Med 2011;364(16):1493–502.

118. Williams RF, Magnotti LJ, Croce MA, et al. Impact of decompressive craniectomy on functional outcome after severe traumatic brain injury. J Trauma 2009;66(6):1570–4 [discussion: 1574–6].

119. Howard JL, Cipolle MD, Anderson M, et al. Outcome after decompressive craniectomy for the treatment of severe traumatic brain injury. J Trauma 2008;65(2):380–5 [discussion: 385–6].

120. Bell RS, Mossop CM, Dirks MS, et al. Early decompressive craniectomy for severe penetrating and closed head injury during wartime. Neurosurg Focus 2010;28(5):E1.

121. Hutchinson PJ, Corteen E, Czosnyka M, et al. Decompressive craniectomy in traumatic brain injury: the randomized multicenter RESCUEicp study (www.RESCUEicp.com). Acta Neurochir Suppl 2006;96:17–20.

122. Lee SC, Wang YC, Huang YC, et al. Decompressive surgery for malignant middle cerebral artery syndrome. J Clin Neurosci 2013;20(1):49–52.

123. Carter BS, Ogilvy CS, Candia GJ, et al. One-year outcome after decompressive surgery for massive nondominant hemispheric infarction. Neurosurgery 1997;40(6):1168–75 [discussion: 1175–6].

124. Kilincer C, Asil T, Utku U, et al. Factors affecting the outcome of decompressive craniectomy for large hemispheric infarctions: a prospective cohort study. Acta Neurochir 2005;147(6):587–94 [discussion: 594].

125. Uhl E, Kreth FW, Elias B, et al. Outcome and prognostic factors of hemicraniectomy for space occupying cerebral infarction. J Neurol Neurosurg Psychiatry 2004;75(2):270–4.

126. Rahme R, Zuccarello M, Kleindorfer D, et al. Decompressive hemicraniectomy for malignant middle cerebral artery territory infarction: is life worth living? J Neurosurg 2012;117(4):749–54.

127. Aarabi B, Hesdorffer DC, Ahn ES, et al. Outcome following decompressive craniectomy for malignant swelling due to severe head injury. J Neurosurg 2006;104(4):469–79.

128. Kilincer C, Simsek O, Hamamcioglu MK, et al. Contralateral subdural effusion after aneurysm surgery and decompressive craniectomy: case report and review of the literature. Clin Neurol Neurosurg 2005;107(5):412–6.

129. Kakar V, Nagaria J, John Kirkpatrick P. The current status of decompressive craniectomy. Br J Neurosurg 2009;23(2):147–57.

130. Wirtz CR, Steiner T, Aschoff A, et al. Hemicraniectomy with dural augmentation in medically uncontrollable hemispheric infarction. Neurosurg Focus 1997;2(5):E3 [discussion: 1 p following E3].

131. Albanese J, Leone M, Alliez JR, et al. Decompressive craniectomy for severe traumatic brain injury: evaluation of the effects at one year. Crit Care Med 2003;31(10):2535–8.

132. Pillai A, Menon SK, Kumar S, et al. Decompressive hemicraniectomy in malignant middle cerebral artery infarction: an analysis of long-term outcome and factors in patient selection. J Neurosurg 2007;106(1):59–65.

133. Frank JI CD, Thisted R, Kordeck C, et al. HeADDFIRST Trialists. Hemicraniectomy and durotomy upon deterioration from infarction related swelling trial (HeADDFIRST): First public presentation of the primary study findings. Abstract and Scientific Session, 55th Annual Meeting of the American Academy of Neurology, March 19–April 5, 2003.

134. Jamora R, Nigos J, Collantes M, et al. Hemicraniectomy for malignant middle cerebral artery infarcts (HeMMI). Paper presented at: 29th International Stroke Conference (February 2004). Available at: www.strokecenter.org/trials/TrialDetail.aspx.

Seizures and the Neurosurgical Intensive Care Unit

Panayiotis N. Varelas, MD, PhD[a,b],*,
Marianna V. Spanaki, MD, PhD, MBA[a],
Marek A. Mirski, MD, PhD[c,d]

KEYWORDS

• Seizures • Neurosurgical intensive care unit • Antiepileptic drugs

KEY POINTS

- Although prophylaxis is often not recommended, prompt treatment of seizures, especially recurrent or prolonged, improves the clinical outcome.
- Seizures occurring in the neurosurgical intensive care unit (NICU) are of diverse structural causes and metabolic disturbances, each with a distinct risk of seizures.
- Several, but not all, new anticonvulsants hold promise as successful agents to treat NICU-related seizures.

INTRODUCTION

The neurosurgical intensive care unit (NICU) is a complex environment. Seizures occur more often in this unit than in general or other specialty ICUs, partly because of the patient population but also because of the enhanced neurologic monitoring undertaken in such units with specialty trained personnel. Both primary neurologic as well as non-neurologic causes of seizures may occur, often in combination, leading to complex clinical evaluations to ascertain the probable cause. Therefore, to avoid confusion and frustration, the neurosurgeon, neuro-intensivist, or consulting neurologist should have an algorithmic approach to the problem.

This topic is vast. In this review, the authors present the most common causes of seizures encountered in the NICU, suggest treatment algorithms, and end with the most recent information regarding the newest antiepileptic drugs (AEDs). The interested reader can find additional information in other review articles[1] or specialized textbooks on this subject.[2]

INCIDENCE

The incidence of seizures in the general ICUs ranges from 3.3% to 34.0%, depending on the ICU population and the detection method. When a routine electroencephalogram (EEG) is used, the incidence is lower than when continuous EEG monitoring is used. Varelas and colleagues[3] reported that out of 129 emergent EEGs ordered in ICUs, 49 (38%) showed some ictal (12%) or interictal (26%) epileptiform activity. Independent variables predicting seizures in the ICU were age, cardiopulmonary arrest, and use of prolonged EEG for detection.

The specific patient population admitted to the ICU may also play a role. For example, in an NICU, 34% of patients had nonconvulsive seizures on continuous EEG, and 76% of them were in nonconvulsive status epilepticus (NCSE).[4]

[a] Department of Neurology, Henry Ford Hospital, 2799 West Grand Boulevard, Detroit, MI 48202-2689, USA; [b] Department of Neurosurgery, Henry Ford Hospital, 2799 West Grand Boulevard, Detroit, MI 48202-2689, USA; [c] Department of Neurology, Johns Hopkins Hospital, 600 North Wolfe Street, Meyer 8-140, Baltimore, MD 21287, USA; [d] Department of Anesthesiology and Critical Care, Johns Hopkins Hospital, 600 North Wolfe Street, Meyer 8-140, Baltimore, MD 21287, USA
* Corresponding author. Department of Neurology, Henry Ford Hospital, 2799 West Grand Boulevard, K-11, Detroit, MI 48202-2689.
E-mail address: varelas@neuro.hfh.edu

Neurosurg Clin N Am 24 (2013) 393–406
http://dx.doi.org/10.1016/j.nec.2013.03.005
1042-3680/13/$ – see front matter © 2013 Elsevier Inc. All rights reserved.

Box 1
Common causes of critical care seizures

Neurologic pathology

Neurovascular

Ischemic stroke

Hemorrhagic stroke

Subarachnoid hemorrhage

Intracerebral hemorrhage

Arteriovenous malformation

Cerebral sinus thrombosis

Hyperperfusion syndrome

Tumor

Primary

Metastatic

Central nervous system (CNS) infection

Abscess

Meningitis

Encephalitis

Encephalitis (noninfectious)

Paraneoplastic limbic

N-methyl-d-aspartate–receptor antibodies

Nonparaneoplastic limbic

Voltage–gated K+ channel antibodies (VGKC/LGII)

Inflammatory disease

Vasculitis

Acute disseminated encephalomyelitis

Traumatic head injury

Depressed skull fragments

Cerebral contusion

Extra-axial hemorrhage

Subdural hematoma

Epidural hematoma

Hygroma (?)

Primary epilepsy

Primary CNS metabolic disturbance (inherited)

Complications of critical illness

Hypoxia/ischemia

Drug/substance toxicity

Antibiotics

Antiviral agents

Antidepressants

Antipsychotics

Bronchodilators

Local anesthetics

Immunosuppressives

Cocaine

Amphetamines

Phencyclidine

Drug/substance withdrawal

Barbiturates

Benzodiazepines

Opioids

Alcohol

Infection (febrile seizures)

Metabolic abnormalities

Hypophosphatemia

Hyponatremia

Hypoglycemia

Renal/hepatic dysfunction

Data from Mirski MA, Varelas PN. Seizures and status epilepticus in the critically ill. Crit Care Clin 2008;24:115–47, ix.

CAUSE AND PATHOPHYSIOLOGY

Seizures in the NICU can be caused either by primary neurologic pathology or as a complication of critical illness (**Box 1**). Although in general ICUs the latter may be more common, in neurologic and neurosurgical patients, structural pathology may be the leading cause. In several patients, however, both can be present. In this case, it is difficult to decide which one of the two is the major contributor, but correcting the nonstructural disorder usually brings seizures under control.

The mechanisms by which nonstructural abnormalities induce seizures are, in many cases, unknown. Drugs precipitate seizures by either preventing γ-aminobutyric acid (GABA) binding to the $GABA_A$ receptor,[5] such as with antibiotics, or via antagonism at the Na^+ channels, such as with the local anesthetics. Depending on the level of potassium, hyperkalemia may depolarize the neuronal membranes or inactivate the Na^+ and Ca^{++} channels, leading to an increased threshold for membrane depolarization. Hyponatremia and low osmolarity, as a consequence of increased cellular edema and increased neuronal excitability, may also lead to seizures. During alkalosis, increased inward Na^+ and Ca^{++} channel currents and during hypomagnesemia decreased N-methyl-d-aspartate receptor antagonism promote cell depolarization.[6]

SEIZURES AFTER STROKE
Seizures after Ischemic Stroke

The most common cause of seizures in patients older than 60 years is ischemic stroke,[7] although the overall risk is fairly low, ranging from 4.4% to 13.8% depending on the subgroups of patients included in the analysis and the follow-up period.[8,9] These seizures can be divided into early (24 hours to 4 weeks, depending on the definition used by the study) and late (usually after the first 4 weeks). Early seizures occur in 1.8% to 15.0% of patients[10,11] and are thought to be caused by excitatory or inhibitory alterations in the penumbral tissue.[12] They are not associated with higher mortality at 1 month and 1 year or with an unfavorable functional outcome, as in a large recent registry from France.[13] Thrombolysis with tissue plasminogen activator (t-PA), however, may lead to worse outcomes in 3 months in the group with seizures compared with the group without seizures.[14] Additionally, patients receiving endovascular treatment and developing early poststroke seizures have worse outcomes and higher mortality compared with seizure-free patients.[15] Late seizures (after 4 weeks) have been reported in 2.5% to 15.0% of poststroke cases[16–18] and are thought to emanate from gliosis and the development of a meningo-cerebral cicatrix. These patients with late-onset seizures are at an almost 3 times higher risk for subsequent stroke.[19]

Status epilepticus (SE) comprises one-fourth to one-sixth of poststroke seizures and is significantly correlated with infarcts in the posterior temporal region.[20] Interestingly, if SE is the first epileptic manifestation after stroke, it is usually not followed by other seizures. If, however, SE follows early or late seizures, the chances are high that it will recur as SE or seizures.[21] Using data from the Nationwide Inpatient Sample, Bateman and colleagues[22] estimated that generalized convulsive SE developed in 0.2% of the acute ischemic strokes, in 0.3% of the intracerebral hemorrhages, and was associated with higher rates of adverse outcomes.

Management of patients with ischemic stroke and seizures in the NICU should not be different than that for seizures from other causes. The most recent guidelines from the American Heart Association and the American Stroke Association do not recommend prophylactic use of AEDs and recognize that there are few data pertaining to the efficacy of these drugs in the treatment of poststroke seizures.[23] Some studies report protection from seizures with AEDs only during the period that these drugs are administered but have no carryover effect in preventing late-onset seizures following AED discontinuation.[24] However, some patients may be at a higher risk for seizures, such as those with stroke after cardioembolism (seizures occurring within the first 24 hours),[9] those with high admission glucose[13] or after thrombolysis with t-PA,[14] with large infarcts, cortical involvement or hemorrhagic component,[8,11,17,25] with watershed distributions[26] and affecting temporal and parietal branches of the middle cerebral artery (late seizures) or temporal and occipital branches of the middle cerebral artery (early seizures).[20] Additional factors for poststroke seizures and a possible need for longer AED administration are preexisting dementia,[27] late poststroke seizures (an independent predictor of epilepsy),[8,17] and SE following poststroke seizures.[21] In a study of 204 patients with stroke-related seizures, seizure recurrence was observed in 13.8% of the early seizure (<15 days), in 54.7% of the late-seizure (1–24 months), and in 34.0% of the very-late-seizure (>24 months) group. Interestingly, 25% of the very late seizures were related to lacunar strokes and very mild disability.[28]

Regarding the choice of AEDs, the available data are also not very helpful; randomized studies comparing AEDs to placebo for primary or secondary prevention of seizures are missing.[29] New-generation AEDs, such as lamotrigine, gabapentin, and levetiracetam, in low doses would be reasonable choices, especially for elderly patients, because of their improved safety profile and fewer interactions with other drugs, including anticoagulants, compared with first-generation AEDs.[24] Topiramate may have additional neuroprotective properties against cerebral ischemia,[30] in contrast with phenytoin, barbiturates, and benzodiazepines, that may have a negative effect on recovery from stroke.[31] Overall, poststroke seizures are usually easily controlled and monotherapy usually suffices.[24]

Seizures after Intracerebral Hemorrhage

The risk for seizures is 2 to 7 times higher with intracerebral hemorrhage (ICH) than with ischemic stroke.[8,25,32] This difference was evident in the study by Vespa and colleagues,[33] whereby 28% of patients with ICH developed seizures despite being given prophylactic AEDs. Only 6% of those with ischemic stroke had seizures in the absence of AEDs.

The incidence of post-ICH seizures varies between 0% and 28%, with studies using continuous EEG monitoring (CEEG) reporting higher range percentages.[33–36] In patients with electrographic seizures, CEEG will detect them within 1 hour in

56% and within 2 days in 94% of the time.[36] Supporting cortical localization as a principal risk, lobar or subcortical ICHs have the highest incidence of seizures; those in the posterior fossa have almost zero.[8,34] In a large Italian study, hyperlipidemia conferred a lower risk for seizures after ICH.[25] After surgical evacuation of the hematoma, seizures occur even more frequently. In a study of 110 patients with evacuated thrombus, 41.8% of patients had seizures, 29.6% of which were clinical and 16.3% were electrographic. ICH volume, presence of subarachnoid hemorrhage (SAH) and subdural hemorrhage predicted early seizures; subdural hematoma and increased admission international normalized ratio predicted late seizures.[37]

As with ischemic stroke, it is unclear if seizures should be treated prophylactically. The current guidelines suggest administration of AEDs only if clinical or electrographic seizures occur. They also recommend CEEG in patients with depressed mental status out of proportion to the degree of brain injury to detect them.[38] Patients with alcoholism with ICH who have a 3-fold increased risk for SE[39] should also be treated with AEDs that increase GABAergic inhibition (for example, benzodiazepines). If late seizures occur (after 2 weeks from onset), long-term AEDs should be prescribed because of the greater risk of epilepsy.[40–42] However, it is unknown which AEDs should be used. In a prospective study of 98 patients with ICH, phenytoin (and not levetiracetam) was associated with more fever, worse National Institute of Health's stroke scale at 14 days, and worse modified Rankin scale up to 3 months. Interestingly, even excluding the 7 patients who did have seizures from the analysis did not change the results.[43]

Seizures after SAH

At the onset of SAH, many patients have motor manifestations and loss of consciousness, which may not be seizures but represent opisthotonos or posturing from acute hydrocephalus or loss of cerebral blood flow momentarily.[2,44] However, early seizures in 1.1% to 16.0% and late seizures in 5.1% to 14.0% of patients with SAH have also been reported.[45–47] In a recent review of 25 studies with 7000 patients, early postoperative seizures occurred in 2.3% and late postoperative seizures in 5.5% of patients (on average 7.45 months after the bleed). Late seizures were more likely with middle cerebral artery aneurysms, Hunt/Hess grade III, and clipping.[48] Because rebleeding from an unprotected aneurysm during seizures is a serious concern, most neurosurgeons prefer to administer AEDs until the aneurysm is secured. However, rebleeding may also manifest as a new seizure.[45,49] Therefore, if there is a prolonged change in the neurologic status or new blood in the ventriculostomy after a seizure, imaging of the brain should be considered. Because CEEG detects NCSE in 8% of patients with SAH, it should be used in those NICU patients with otherwise unexplained coma or neurologic deterioration after SAH[50] or if sedated. In a recent study from Sweden, 7% of sedated patients had seizures, and one was in NCSE for 5 hours.[51]

The therapeutic management of the ruptured aneurysm may also correlate with the incidence of seizures. Coiling, theoretically, may be associated with a lower risk for seizures because of less cortical injury. In a large prospective study, no seizures were witnessed in the periprocedural period (within 30 days) and only 1.7% patients developed late de novo seizures.[52] Further data from the International Subarachnoid Aneurysm Trial have shown a relative risk for seizures of 0.52 with coiling compared with clipping.[53] However, others have found that treatment of only unruptured aneurysms with clipping was associated with a higher risk of seizures or epilepsy compared with coiling, but this difference was not evident in ruptured aneurysms.[54]

The evidence for prophylactic use of AEDs is not compelling.[55] Some experts advocate withholding AEDs on several grounds in the early period because many seizures are unpreventable (occur at onset or during the prehospital period).[56] AED use may precipitate fever, and their use has been correlated to a worse Glasgow Outcome Scale–measured outcome, higher incidence of cerebral vasospasm, neurologic deterioration or cerebral infarction,[57] as well as cognitive and functional disability with phenytoin.[58] Additionally, early perioperative seizures are not predictive of subsequent epilepsy,[59] and such seizures do not lead to a worse outcome after a minimum 1-year follow-up.[60] Others, however, advocate AED use for patients with onset seizures (given only during the hospitalization period),[45,47] rebleeding,[47] subdural hematoma or cerebral infarction at any time point,[61] thick subarachnoid clot, or just periprocedurally[62] but not after coiling of the aneurysm.[52] In a recent review, a 3-day treatment seems to provide similar seizure prevention with better outcome than longer treatment.[63] The American Heart Association's most recent guidelines support prophylactic AEDs in the immediate posthemorrhagic period and routine use of AEDs only in patients with high risk for delayed seizures, such as prior seizure, intracerebral hematoma, intractable hypertension, infarction, or middle cerebral artery aneurysm.[64]

It is also unclear which AED should be preferred when seizures occur. Most of the data are derived from phenytoin use, an AED that can reduce the bioavailability of nimodipine, a drug frequently used in these patients.[65] Despite fewer available data, newer AEDs may have a similar[66] or improved profile.[67,68]

The recently reported association of cortical spreading depolarizations (recorded via electrocorticography) with delayed ischemic neurologic deficits despite the absence of vasospasm, opens new horizons in our understanding of electric epiphenomena after SAH.[69–71] The clinical improvement with hypertension in patients with SAH and vasospasm may also be related to spreading depolarizations, because, in animals, a reverse correlation between spreading depression and blood pressure has been reported.[72]

Seizures and Cerebral Venous and Sinus Thrombosis

Seizures are very common after cerebral venous and sinus thrombosis, occurring in 29% to 50% of patients, frequently as an inaugural manifestation.[73,74] Early seizures (within 2 weeks from onset) occur in 34% to 44% of patients and are predicted by presenting seizures, motor or sensory deficits, parenchymal lesion on admission (hemorrhage, infarct, focal edema), and the presence of cortical vein thrombosis.[73–75] Late seizures occur in 9.5% of patients and may be more common in those patients with early seizures.[74] Although randomized controlled studies for prophylactic use of AEDs are not available, these drugs may be prescribed in those patients at high risk for early seizures because they may be associated with higher morbidity and early mortality.[73–75] In a recent retrospective study, however, whereby all patients with seizures received AEDs, seizures were not associated with death or 6-month worse outcomes.[76]

Reperfusion-Hyperperfusion Syndrome and Seizures

Reperfusion-hyperperfusion syndrome (RHS) is an uncommon complication of carotid endarterectomy, carotid angioplasty, and stenting.[77,78] Seizures occur either immediately after revascularization procedures (usually because of distal embolization) or later (7 hours to 14 days)[77–81] and are considered a delayed manifestation of RHS. Transient periodic lateralizing epileptiform discharges have also been reported after internal carotid stenting in a patient with previous ICH[82] and NCSE after superficial temporal to middle cerebral artery anastomosis, successfully treated with AEDs.[83] The use of prophylactic AEDs remains controversial; early onset seizures are treated almost without exception in addition to tight blood pressure control as an adjunct to a likely procedural complication (ICH, severe edema, ischemic stroke). The management of late seizures also includes AEDs in addition to tight blood pressure control, to a level of equalizing transcranial Doppler-measured velocities ipsilateral and contralateral to the treated carotid artery.[79]

TRAUMATIC BRAIN INJURY AND SEIZURES

The incidence of posttraumatic seizures varies widely, with estimates of 2% to 12% in civilian populations and up to 53% in military populations.[84,85] Traumatic brain injury (TBI) accounts for 10% to 20% of symptomatic epilepsy in the general population and 5% of epilepsy in general.[86,87] In a study, however, using CEEG in the NICU, 22% of post-TBI patients had seizures (52% of which were nonconvulsive). One-third of these patients were in SE with minimal clinical signs, such as facial twitching or eye fluttering, and all died.[88] Hippocampal atrophy on volumetric magnetic resonance imaging (MRI), suggesting an anatomic damaging effect, has also been associated with nonconvulsive posttraumatic seizures.[89]

Clinical studies divide seizures into immediate (<24 hours), early (within 1 week, with a seizure incidence of 2.1%–16.9%), or late (with an incidence of 1.9% to >30.0%).[86,87,90] Independent risk factors for late seizures or posttraumatic epilepsy include early seizures, coma or loss of consciousness for more than 24 hours, dural penetration, biparietal or multiple contusions, intracranial hemorrhage, depressed skull fracture not surgically treated, and at least one nonreactive pupil.[87,91] In a recent study, diffuse axonal injury on MRI was not correlated with posttraumatic epilepsy, but cerebral contusions were.[92] Early seizures occur in 25% of patients not treated with AEDs and are associated with seizures immediately following trauma, depressed skull fracture, intracerebral hematoma, or subdural hematoma. The risk is lower (15%–20% range) if the patients had a penetrating head injury, epidural hematoma, cortical contusion, and had a Glasgow Coma scale score of 10 or less.[91] Although early seizures are independently associated with an unfavorable outcome, their effect is much lower than other variables, such as severity of brain injury or older age.[93] Injury surrogate markers have been associated with seizures. In a study of 20 patients with moderate to severe TBI monitored with microdialysis and CEEG, 10 patients had post-TBI seizures, which resulted in episodic increases in intracranial pressure (ICP) and lactate/pyruvate ratio. Both remained elevated beyond postinjury hour 100 in the subgroup with seizures (compared with the subgroup without), suggesting long-lasting effects.[94]

If early and, especially, late posttraumatic seizures occur, AEDs should be used. The treatment of post-TBI seizures in the ICU is not different from the treatment of any other seizures. Prophylactic AED administration is more controversial. In a systematic review of randomized trials, prophylactic AEDs were effective in reducing early seizures; but there was no evidence that they reduced the occurrence of late seizures or had any effect on death and neurologic disability.[95] The current practice parameters by the American Academy of Neurology (AAN)[96] and the Brain Trauma Foundation[97] advocate prophylactic treatment only during the first 7 days from a head injury. Regarding the choice of AEDs, phenytoin has been shown to decrease the incidence of early posttraumatic seizures[97] and be more cost-effective than levetiracetam.[98] Levetiracetam was equally effective as phenytoin in preventing early seizures in a prospective study of 32 patients with severe TBI but was associated with an increased seizure tendency on 1-hour EEG.[99] Valproic acid, compared with phenytoin, did not seem to benefit and actually showed a trend toward higher mortality.[100] Lastly, vagus nerve stimulation may reduce seizures in patients with refractory posttraumatic epilepsy.[101]

BRAIN TUMORS AND SEIZURES

Many patients admitted to the NICU with brain tumors have seizures (in up to 35% of all tumor cases[102]) and the incidence is both pathology and location dependent. In high-grade, rapidly progressive tumors, such as glioblastoma, or metastatic tumors, seizures occur in 25% to 35% of cases, which is lower than the reported 70% incidence in slower-growing tumors, such as astrocytomas or meningiomas, and 90% in oligodendrogliomas. The locations with the highest incidence are the temporoparietal regions with cortical gray involvement.[103]

Although patients with brain tumors and seizures should be treated with AEDs, prophylactic treatment is controversial. AEDs may interfere with corticosteroids, chemotherapy, and radiation treatment and induce more frequent and serious allergic reactions in such patients.[104] Therefore, the AAN's practice parameter does not support prophylactic AEDs in patients with newly diagnosed brain tumors. Postoperatively, patients who have not experienced a seizure should have tapering and discontinuation of AEDs within a week (particularly those patients who are medically stable and have AED-related side effects).[10] Patients who have brain metastases may have less propensity to develop seizures; based on recently published guidelines, they should also not be on prophylactic AEDs.[106,107]

If seizures occur, the newer-generation AEDs such as gabapentin, lacosamide, levetiracetam, oxcarbazepine, pregabalin, topiramate, and zonisamide, are preferred because they have fewer drug interactions, especially with chemotherapy and cause fewer side effects.[108] In a small case series of 25 patients with brain tumor–related epilepsy, oxcarbazepine monotherapy at a mean dosage of 1230 mg/d led to significant improvement in mood and seizure-freedom rate.[109] Perioperative oral or intravenous (IV) levetiracetam administration in patients with primary brain tumors also led to seizure freedom 100% in the presurgery and 84% to 88% in the early late postsurgery phases.[110]

If a primary or metastatic brain tumor is causing SE, a combination of IV phenytoin, IV levetiracetam (median dosage 3 g/d), and by-mouth pregabalin (median dosage 375 mg/d) led to 70% control, on average, 24 hours after the addition of the third AED.[111] In another small case series pregabalin controlled non-convulsive (NC) seizures or NCSE in 67% of 9 patients with brain tumors.[112]

Older AEDs may also have a role in treating brain tumor–related seizures. In a recent study of patients with glioblastoma, valproic acid improved the survival of patients on temozolomide/radiotherapy compared with those receiving an enzyme-inducing AED or no AED.[113] It is unclear if this valproic effect is through increased temozolomide bioavailability or its action as a histone deacetylase inhibitor.[114]

DRUG-INDUCED SEIZURES

Drugs rank low as precipitants of seizures in the NICU.[5,115] Antibiotics, such as the penicillins, cephalosporins, carbapenems (especially imipenem), aztreonam, fluoroquinolones, isoniazid, and metronidazole, can precipitate seizures when administered intrathecally[116] or at high doses in patients with renal insufficiency[5] or undergoing continuous renal replacement therapy.[117] Peak concentration periods of the drug may also provoke electrographic changes. During infusion of cefepime and CEEG, 23.7% of patients had continuous epileptiform discharges compared with only 3.75% during meropenem infusion.[118] Because of their specific action through GABA receptors, it is important to remember that first-line

AEDs should be GABAergic agonists, such as benzodiazepines or barbiturates. In case of isoniazid intoxication, the addition of IV pyridoxine is important because the drug antagonizes B6 transformation to pyridoxal phosphate, an essential cofactor for GABA synthesis.[5]

Intrathecal administration of baclofen may provoke seizures or convulsive or nonconvulsive SE in patients with multiple sclerosis.[119] Similarly, intrathecal absorption of the locally used hemostatic agent tranexamic acid can lead to seizures.[120] These seizures are self-limiting and easily controlled with AEDs.

Rapid opioid withdrawal may provoke seizures, which appear on average, 2 to 4 days following discontinuation.[121] Normeperidine, a metabolite of meperidine, is a strong proconvulsant. This drug should probably be avoided in the NICU.[122]

ELECTROLYTE AND METABOLIC ABNORMALITIES

Hyponatremia is the most frequent ICU electrolyte abnormality associated with new-onset seizures (in 18.2% of ICU patients[121]). Acute hyponatremia is associated with a higher risk for seizures than chronic hyponatremia.[123] Correction of Na^+ levels is adequate treatment if structural intracranial pathology is not present. The rate of Na^+ correction with hypertonic solutions can be faster in acute cases (up to 1–2 mEq/L/h of Na^+ increase until seizures are under control) than in chronic cases, when it should be less than 0.5 mEq/L/h.[124]

Disturbances in glucose levels have become common in NICU patients with implementation of tighter glucose control than in the past. Both focal and generalized seizures can be caused by hyperglycemia and hypoglycemia. Seizures related to nonketotic hyperosmolar hyperglycemia may present as speech arrest, visual disturbances, or be related to limb movement (reflex seizures).[125,126] Seizures associated with hypoglycemia are frequently preceded by signs of sympathetic excitation. There is no role for AEDs, and only correction of the glucose abnormality will bring the seizures under control.[2]

TREATMENT OF NICU SEIZURES

Seizures complicating critically ill neurosurgical patients should not be considered benign phenomena. During seizures or SE, ICP increases in parallel with cerebral blood flow, brain temperature, and lactate/pyruvate ratio and is correlated with dramatic reductions of brain tissue oxygen tension.[94,127] Although there is no broad acceptance that seizures lead to worse outcomes, most intensivists will treat NICU seizures emergently targeting the ensuing immediate brain metabolic stress and potentially the long-standing secondary effects.

The management of NICU seizures basically follows the same general rules, which guide treatment of noncritically ill patients (Box 2). A new staged approach to the treatment of SE has been proposed and included in Box 2.[128–131] Because the NICU admits the most resistant-to-treatment seizures, familiarity of the medical and nursing staff with the process of diagnosis and treatment is essential. Urgency without panic is important when seizures are recurrent or SE is present because the duration of seizures is related to resistance to treatment and overall outcome.[132]

Newer Antiepileptic Agents and Their Potential Use in the NICU

Several newer AEDs have currently found their place in the epileptologist's armamentarium. Their use in the NICU is limited because of a lack of parenteral preparations and no approved status beyond adjunct therapy. Therefore, their use should be limited to those patients who are able to swallow or with a nasogastric tube and with proven gastric emptying and absorption of the drug. Indications for their administration include (1) continuation of home regimen; (2) adjunct treatment to older parenteral AEDs, when there is a failure to control seizures; (3) specific organ dysfunction or disease prohibiting the use of other parenteral AEDs; (4) proven allergy to older AEDs; and (5) reason for limited interactions with other crucial drugs, such as chemotherapeutic or immunosuppressive agents, as in patients with brain tumors[108] or after transplantation.[133]

Gabapentin is renally metabolized and has moderate anticonvulsant effects. In the ICU, gabapentin may be considered in patients with hepatic failure or porphyria.[134] Used as a monotherapy, in a dose range from 900 mg/d for patients weighing less than 75 kg to 1200 mg/d for patients weighing more than 75 kg, gabapentin controlled late poststroke seizures in 82% of cases, with higher success among patients who had partial seizures as compared with those with generalized seizures.[135]

Lamotrigine has been approved as an adjunctive therapy or monotherapy in partial or generalized epilepsy and in the Lennox-Gastaut syndrome. Few human data regarding its use in SE exist, and caution should be exerted because cases of new-onset NCSE[136] and myoclonic SE[137] have been reported with its use.

Box 2
Management of seizures in the ICU

1. Brief single seizure (<60 seconds)

   Observe; eliminate cause if identified. Consider a course of chronic therapy: phenytoin 15 to 20 mg/kg or fosphenytoin 15 to 20 mg/kg phenytoin equivalents (PE) loading dose and 300 to 400 mg/d. The goal serum level is 10 to 20 mcg/mL or free level 1 to 2 mcg/mL. Consider IV/oral valproic acid 600 to 3000 mg/d or oral carbamezapine 600 to 1200 mg/d for patients who are phenytoin intolerant. Seizure precautions include padding bed rails and increased observation.

2. Prolonged or more than 1 seizure

   Check oxygen saturation and vital signs. Immediately administer IV benzodiazepine-lorazepam 1 to 2 mg, diazepam 10 to 20 mg, or midazolam 2 to 5 mg with concurrent loading dose phenytoin or fosphenytoin (PE) 15 to 20 mg/kg and maintenance as discussed earlier. Administer valproic acid IV 400 to 600 mg every 6 hours if patients are phenytoin intolerant. Perform similar seizure precautions.

3. Recurrent or refractory seizures of more than 5 minutes or more than 2 discrete seizures between which there is no recovery of consciousness (meeting criteria for SE)

   Stage 1: Emergent initial measures

   Preserve airway and oxygenation by oxygen face mask or intubation, as needed.

   Establish IV access.

   Order EEG to be available during therapy.

   Measure finger-stick blood glucose. Administer 1 A of DW 50% IV if less than 60 mg/100 dL and 100 mg thiamine IV.

   Send to the laboratory the following: antiepileptic blood levels, electrolytes, complete blood count, liver function tests, arterial blood gases, toxicology screen (urine and blood).

   At the same time with the abovementioned stage, complete the following: immediate benzodiazepines (IV lorazepam 0.07–0.1 mg/kg or diazepam 0.15–0.25 mg/kg IV). If there is no IV access, administer diazepam 20 mg per rectum or midazolam 10 mg intramuscularly, buccally, or intranasally.

   Stage 2: Urgent control

   The phenytoin loading dose is 20 mg/kg IV at 50 mg/min or fosphenytoin 20 mg/kg PE IV at 150 mg/min.

   If patients are allergic to phenytoin, administer valproate 25 to 40 mg/kg IV load at 1.5 to 3.0 mg/kg/min or levetiracetam 30 to 70 mg/kg IV (500 mg/min) or phenobarbital 20 mg/kg IV (rate 100 mg/min).

   If the seizures continue, administer phenytoin or fosphenytoin (additional 5 mg/kg–10 mg/kg or 5 mg/kg–10 mg/kg PE). The goal serum level is 20 mg dL to 25 mg/dL. If there is a phenytoin allergy, administer an additional valproate load of 20 mg/kg IV.

   The EEG is connected and running.

   Stage 3: Refractory SE

   If patients are NCSE and not yet intubated, one or more of phenytoin, valproic acid, levetiracetam, phenobarbital (that has not been administered in stage 2), or lacosamide can be tried.

   Perform intubation and mechanical ventilation.

   Provide hemodynamic support by pressors and IV fluid boluses.

   Administer propofol 2 mg/kg IV bolus and 150 μg/kg/min to 200 μg/kg/min infusion, or thiopental 2 to 3 mg/kg IV bolus and 0.3 mg/kg/min to 0.4 mg/kg/min infusion, or midazolam 0.2 mg/kg IV bolus, which can be repeated every 5 minutes up to a total of 2 mg/kg, followed by an infusion of 0.1 to 0.2 mg/kg/h.

   If seizures continue, administer pentobarbital 10 mg/kg IV load at up to 50 mg/min, which can be repeated several times until an EEG burst-suppression pattern with 20 to 30 seconds suppression goal is achieved. Start at the same time continuous infusion 1 mg/kg/h and titrate up to 10 mg/kg/h for the same goal.

Stage 4: Alternative therapies for super-refractory SE (in order from the first to the last resort)

Ketamine 0.5 to 4.5 mg/kg bolus IV and up to 5 mg/kg/h infusion

Isoflurane, desflurane, gabapentin, or levetiracetam (in acute intermittent porphyria)

Topiramate 2 to 25 mg/kg/d (children) or up to 300 to 1600 mg/d (adults) per orogastric tube

Magnesium infusion 4 g bolus IV, 2 to 6 g/h infusion

Pyridoxine 180 to 600 mg/d IV or per orogastric tube

Steroids 1 g/d IV for 3 days, followed by 1 mg/kg/d for 1 week or

Intravenous immunoglobulin 0.4 g/kg/d IV for 5 days or plasmapheresis

Hypothermia 32°C to 35°C for less than 48 hours

Ketogenic diet 4:1

Neurosurgical resection of epileptic focus

Electroconvulsive therapy

Vagal nerve or deep brain stimulation or transcranial magnetic stimulation

Data from Refs.[2,128–131]

Topiramate is used in both children and adults with SE.[138,139] The dose administered in adults via nasogastric tube is high, ranging from 300 mg/d to 1600 mg/d. In a recent study of 35 patients with refractory SE treated with topiramate as an adjunct AED, the response rate was 86% (as the third AED) and remained stable at 67% after administration as the fourth, fifth, sixth, or seventh AED. Overall, SE was terminated in 71% of patients within 72 hours after the first administration of topiramate.[140]

Zonisamide controlled intractable SE in siblings with Lafora body disease[141]; but because no parenteral form is available in the United States, its use is limited in the adult NICU as an adjunctive treatment of resistant partial seizures.[142]

Oxcarbazepine is a 10-keto carbamazepine analogue, with a safer clinical profile than carbamazepine. There are no data to support its use in the NICU, and the higher risk for hyponatremia may also be a limiting factor. However, it has been successfully used to treat seizures associated with porphyria cutanea tarda.[143]

Oxcarbazepine monotherapy may improve seizure freedom rate in patients with brain tumor–related epilepsy.[109]

Levetiracetam has a distinct advantage for the ICU use because it is not metabolized through the cytochrome P450 system and its metabolites are inactive and renally excreted. There is no need for drug level monitoring, and there are no significant interactions with other common ICU medications, including other AEDs. It may be used either as an approved adjunct therapy or as an alternative AED in the setting of hepatic insufficiency or porphyria.[144] In renal failure, a 50% dosage is suggested. Levetiracetam may be used to control seizures or SE, and there are some data showing comparable effects with benzodiazepines without the risk for artificial ventilation or hypotension common with the latter. For example, in a recent open-label randomized study of 79 patients with convulsive SE or subtle SE that compared levetiracetam 20 mg/kg IV over 15 minutes with lorazepam 0.1 mg/kg over 2 to 4 minutes, SE was controlled by levetiracetam in 76.3% and by lorazepam in 75.6% of patients.[145] In a review of studies using levetiracetam after benzodiazepines in 334 patients with SE, its efficacy ranged from 44% to 94%.[146] Overall, more than 700 patients with SE have been treated with an initial dosage of 2 to 3 g/d and an estimated success rate around 70%.[147] In a retrospective study of 181 episodes of SE not responding to the benzodiazepine first-line treatment, however, levetiracetam failed more often than valproic acid as a second-line AED in controlling SE.[148]

Lacosamide is also available in an IV formulation and may be a safe and effective alternative for the treatment of seizures in the ICU, based on a series of 24 critically ill patients treated for seizures or refractory SE.[149] In a recent review of 136 episodes of refractory SE, it had a success rate of 56% after a bolus dose of 200 to 400 mg over 3 to 5 minutes.[150] In an accidental intrathecal administration of 60 mg baclofen, lacosamide, in addition to levetiracetam, controlled seizures that occurred in the ICU.[151]

Pregabalin (a renally excreted, orally administered antiepileptic), when added as the second to fourth AED, controlled NC seizures or NCSE in 52% of 21 critically ill patients with NC seizures or NCSE. In this study, 67% of patients with brain tumors responded compared with none after a hypoxic injury.[112]

Retigabine is a unique AED because it opens voltage-gated K+ channels of the Kv7 subfamily. Because it is not metabolized through cytochrome P450, it has limited interaction with other hepatically metabolized drugs.[152]

REFERENCES

1. Mirski MA, Varelas PN. Seizures and status epilepticus in the critically ill. Crit Care Clin 2008; 24:115–47, ix.

2. Varelas PN. Seizures in critical care. A guide to diagnosis and therapeutics. 2nd edition. Humana Press; 2010.

3. Varelas PN, Hacein-Bey L, Hether T, et al. Emergent electroencephalogram in the intensive care unit: indications and diagnostic yield. Clin EEG Neurosci 2004;35:173–80.

4. Jordan KG. Continuous EEG monitoring in the neuroscience intensive care unit and emergency department. J Clin Neurophysiol 1999;16:14–39.

5. Wallace KL. Antibiotic-induced convulsions. Crit Care Clin 1997;13:741–62.

6. Somjen GG. Ion regulation in the brain: implications for pathophysiology. Neuroscientist 2002;8: 254–67.

7. Hauser WA, Kurland LT. The epidemiology of epilepsy in Rochester, Minnesota, 1935 through 1967. Epilepsia 1975;16:1–66.

8. Bladin CF, Alexandrov AV, Bellavance A, et al. Seizures after stroke: a prospective multicenter study. Arch Neurol 2000;57:1617–22.

9. Szaflarski JP, Rackley AY, Kleindorfer DO, et al. Incidence of seizures in the acute phase of stroke: a population-based study. Epilepsia 2008;49:974–81.

10. Arboix A, Comes E, Massons J, et al. Relevance of early seizures for in-hospital mortality in acute cerebrovascular disease. Neurology 1996;47:1429–35.

11. Reith J, Jorgensen HS, Nakayama H, et al. Seizures in acute stroke: predictors and prognostic significance. The Copenhagen Stroke Study. Stroke 1997;28:1585–9.

12. Sun DA, Sombati S, DeLorenzo RJ. Glutamate injury-induced epileptogenesis in hippocampal neurons: an in vitro model of stroke-induced "epilepsy". Stroke 2001;32:2344–50.

13. Hamidou B, Aboa-Eboule C, Durier J, et al. Prognostic value of early epileptic seizures on mortality and functional disability in acute stroke: the Dijon Stroke Registry (1985-2010). J Neurol 2012. [Epub ahead of print].

14. Alvarez V, Rossetti AO, Papavasileiou V, et al. Acute seizures in acute ischemic stroke: does thrombolysis have a role to play? J Neurol 2013; 260:55–61.

15. Jung S, Schindler K, Findling O, et al. Adverse effect of early epileptic seizures in patients receiving endovascular therapy for acute stroke. Stroke 2012;43:1584–90.

16. Lancman ME, Golimstok A, Norscini J, et al. Risk factors for developing seizures after a stroke. Epilepsia 1993;34:141–3.

17. Lamy C, Domigo V, Semah F, et al. Early and late seizures after cryptogenic ischemic stroke in young adults. Neurology 2003;60:400–4.

18. Berges S, Moulin T, Berger E, et al. Seizures and epilepsy following strokes: recurrence factors. Eur Neurol 2000;43:3–8.

19. Cleary P, Shorvon S, Tallis R. Late-onset seizures as a predictor of subsequent stroke. Lancet 2004; 363:1184–6.

20. De Reuck J, De Groote L, Van Maele G, et al. The cortical involvement of territorial infarcts as a risk factor for stroke-related seizures. Cerebrovasc Dis 2008;25:100–6.

21. Rumbach L, Sablot D, Berger E, et al. Status epilepticus in stroke: report on a hospital-based stroke cohort. Neurology 2000;54:350–4.

22. Bateman BT, Claassen J, Willey JZ, et al. Convulsive status epilepticus after ischemic stroke and intracerebral hemorrhage: frequency, predictors, and impact on outcome in a large administrative dataset. Neurocrit Care 2007;7:187–93.

23. Jauch EC, Saver JL, Adams HP Jr, et al. Guidelines for the early management of patients with acute ischemic stroke: a guideline for healthcare professionals from the American Heart Association/American Stroke Association. Stroke 2013;44:870–947.

24. Gilad R. Management of seizures following a stroke: what are the options? Drugs Aging 2012; 29:533–8.

25. Beghi E, D'Alessandro R, Beretta S, et al. Incidence and predictors of acute symptomatic seizures after stroke. Neurology 2011;77:1785–93.

26. Denier C, Masnou P, Mapoure Y, et al. Watershed infarctions are more prone than other cortical infarcts to cause early-onset seizures. Arch Neurol 2010;67:1219–23.

27. Cordonnier C, Henon H, Derambure P, et al. Influence of pre-existing dementia on the risk of post-stroke epileptic seizures. J Neurol Neurosurg Psychiatry 2005;76:1649–53.

28. De Reuck J, Sieben A, Van Maele G. Characteristics and outcomes of patients with seizures according to the time of onset in relation to stroke. Eur Neurol 2008;59:225–8.

29. Kwan J, Wood E. Antiepileptic drugs for the primary and secondary prevention of seizures after stroke. Cochrane Database Syst Rev 2010;(1):CD005398.

30. Leker RR, Neufeld MY. Anti-epileptic drugs as possible neuroprotectants in cerebral ischemia. Brain Res Brain Res Rev 2003;42:187–203.

31. Goldstein LB. Potential effects of common drugs on stroke recovery. Arch Neurol 1998;55:454–6.
32. Giroud M, Gras P, Fayolle H, et al. Early seizures after acute stroke: a study of 1,640 cases. Epilepsia 1994;35:959–64.
33. Vespa PM, O'Phelan K, Shah M, et al. Acute seizures after intracerebral hemorrhage: a factor in progressive midline shift and outcome. Neurology 2003;60:1441–6.
34. Faught E, Peters D, Bartolucci A, et al. Seizures after primary intracerebral hemorrhage. Neurology 1989;39:1089–93.
35. Tatu L, Moulin T, El Mohamad R, et al. Primary intracerebral hemorrhages in the Besancon stroke registry. Initial clinical and CT findings, early course and 30-day outcome in 350 patients. Eur Neurol 2000;43:209–14.
36. Claassen J, Jette N, Chum F, et al. Electrographic seizures and periodic discharges after intracerebral hemorrhage. Neurology 2007;69:1356–65.
37. Garrett MC, Komotar RJ, Starke RM, et al. Predictors of seizure onset after intracerebral hemorrhage and the role of long-term antiepileptic therapy. J Crit Care 2009;24:335–9.
38. Morgenstern LB, Hemphill JC 3rd, Anderson C, et al. Guidelines for the management of spontaneous intracerebral hemorrhage: a guideline for healthcare professionals from the American Heart Association/American Stroke Association. Stroke 2010;41:2108–29.
39. Passero S, Rocchi R, Rossi S, et al. Seizures after spontaneous supratentorial intracerebral hemorrhage. Epilepsia 2002;43:1175–80.
40. Cervoni L, Artico M, Salvati M, et al. Epileptic seizures in intracerebral hemorrhage: a clinical and prognostic study of 55 cases. Neurosurg Rev 1994;17:185–8.
41. Qureshi AI, Tuhrim S, Broderick JP, et al. Spontaneous intracerebral hemorrhage. N Engl J Med 2001;344:1450–60.
42. Yang TM, Lin WC, Chang WN, et al. Predictors and outcome of seizures after spontaneous intracerebral hemorrhage. Clinical article. J Neurosurg 2009;111:87–93.
43. Naidech AM, Garg RK, Liebling S, et al. Anticonvulsant use and outcomes after intracerebral hemorrhage. Stroke 2009;40:3810–5.
44. Haines SJ. Decerebrate posturing misinterpreted as seizure activity. Am J Emerg Med 1988;6:173–7.
45. Pinto AN, Canhao P, Ferro JM. Seizures at the onset of subarachnoid haemorrhage. J Neurol 1996;243:161–4.
46. Hasan D, Schonck RS, Avezaat CJ, et al. Epileptic seizures after subarachnoid hemorrhage. Ann Neurol 1993;33:286–91.
47. Butzkueven H, Evans AH, Pitman A, et al. Onset seizures independently predict poor outcome after subarachnoid hemorrhage. Neurology 2000;55:1315–20.
48. Raper DM, Starke RM, Komotar RJ, et al. Seizures after aneurysmal subarachnoid hemorrhage: a systematic review of outcomes. World Neurosurg 2012. [Epub ahead of print].
49. Hart RG, Byer JA, Slaughter JR, et al. Occurrence and implications of seizures in subarachnoid hemorrhage due to ruptured intracranial aneurysms. Neurosurgery 1981;8:417–21.
50. Dennis LJ, Claassen J, Hirsch LJ, et al. Nonconvulsive status epilepticus after subarachnoid hemorrhage. Neurosurgery 2002;51:1136–43 [discussion: 44].
51. Lindgren C, Nordh E, Naredi S, et al. Frequency of non-convulsive seizures and non-convulsive status epilepticus in subarachnoid hemorrhage patients in need of controlled ventilation and sedation. Neurocrit Care 2012;17:367–73.
52. Byrne JV, Boardman P, Ioannidis I, et al. Seizures after aneurysmal subarachnoid hemorrhage treated with coil embolization. Neurosurgery 2003;52:545–52 [discussion: 50–2].
53. Molyneux AJ, Kerr RS, Yu LM, et al. International subarachnoid aneurysm trial (ISAT) of neurosurgical clipping versus endovascular coiling in 2143 patients with ruptured intracranial aneurysms: a randomised comparison of effects on survival, dependency, seizures, rebleeding, subgroups, and aneurysm occlusion. Lancet 2005;366:809–17.
54. Hoh BL, Nathoo S, Chi YY, et al. Incidence of seizures or epilepsy after clipping or coiling of ruptured and unruptured cerebral aneurysms in the nationwide inpatient sample database: 2002-2007. Neurosurgery 2011;69:644–50 [discussion: 50].
55. Naval NS, Stevens RD, Mirski MA, et al. Controversies in the management of aneurysmal subarachnoid hemorrhage. Crit Care Med 2006;34:511–24.
56. Rhoney DH, Tipps LB, Murry KR, et al. Anticonvulsant prophylaxis and timing of seizures after aneurysmal subarachnoid hemorrhage. Neurology 2000;55:258–65.
57. Rosengart AJ, Huo JD, Tolentino J, et al. Outcome in patients with subarachnoid hemorrhage treated with antiepileptic drugs. J Neurosurg 2007;107:253–60.
58. Naidech AM, Kreiter KT, Janjua N, et al. Phenytoin exposure is associated with functional and cognitive disability after subarachnoid hemorrhage. Stroke 2005;36:583–7.
59. Lin CL, Dumont AS, Lieu AS, et al. Characterization of perioperative seizures and epilepsy following aneurysmal subarachnoid hemorrhage. J Neurosurg 2003;99:978–85.
60. Lin YJ, Chang WN, Chang HW, et al. Risk factors and outcome of seizures after spontaneous

aneurysmal subarachnoid hemorrhage. Eur J Neurol 2008;15:451–7.

61. Claassen J, Peery S, Kreiter KT, et al. Predictors and clinical impact of epilepsy after subarachnoid hemorrhage. Neurology 2003;60:208–14.

62. Baker CJ, Prestigiacomo CJ, Solomon RA. Short-term perioperative anticonvulsant prophylaxis for the surgical treatment of low-risk patients with intracranial aneurysms. Neurosurgery 1995;37:863–70 [discussion: 70–1].

63. Lanzino G, D'Urso PI, Suarez J. Seizures and anticonvulsants after aneurysmal subarachnoid hemorrhage. Neurocrit Care 2011;15:247–56.

64. Connolly ES Jr, Rabinstein AA, Carhuapoma JR, et al. Guidelines for the management of aneurysmal subarachnoid hemorrhage: a guideline for healthcare professionals from the American Heart Association/American Stroke Association. Stroke 2012;43:1711–37.

65. Wong GK, Poon WS. Use of phenytoin and other anticonvulsant prophylaxis in patients with aneurysmal subarachnoid hemorrhage. Stroke 2005; 36:2532 [author reply].

66. Mink S, Muroi C, Seule M, et al. Levetiracetam compared to valproic acid: plasma concentration levels, adverse effects and interactions in aneurysmal subarachnoid hemorrhage. Clin Neurol Neurosurg 2011;113:644–8.

67. Szaflarski JP, Sangha KS, Lindsell CJ, et al. Prospective, randomized, single-blinded comparative trial of intravenous levetiracetam versus phenytoin for seizure prophylaxis. Neurocrit Care 2010;12: 165–72.

68. Shah D, Husain AM. Utility of levetiracetam in patients with subarachnoid hemorrhage. Seizure 2009;18:676–9.

69. Bosche B, Graf R, Ernestus RI, et al. Recurrent spreading depolarizations after subarachnoid hemorrhage decreases oxygen availability in human cerebral cortex. Ann Neurol 2010;67:607–17.

70. Sakowitz OW, Santos E, Nagel A, et al. Clusters of spreading depolarizations are associated with disturbed cerebral metabolism in patients with aneurysmal subarachnoid hemorrhage. Stroke 2013;44:220–3.

71. Woitzik J, Dreier JP, Hecht N, et al. Delayed cerebral ischemia and spreading depolarization in absence of angiographic vasospasm after subarachnoid hemorrhage. J Cereb Blood Flow Metab 2012;32:203–12.

72. Sukhotinsky I, Yaseen MA, Sakadzic S, et al. Perfusion pressure-dependent recovery of cortical spreading depression is independent of tissue oxygenation over a wide physiologic range. J Cereb Blood Flow Metab 2010;30:1168–77.

73. Masuhr F, Busch M, Amberger N, et al. Risk and predictors of early epileptic seizures in acute cerebral venous and sinus thrombosis. Eur J Neurol 2006;13:852–6.

74. Ferro JM, Correia M, Rosas MJ, et al. Seizures in cerebral vein and dural sinus thrombosis. Cerebrovasc Dis 2003;15:78–83.

75. Ferro JM, Canhao P, Bousser MG, et al. Early seizures in cerebral vein and dural sinus thrombosis risk factors and role of antiepileptics. Stroke 2008;39:1152–8.

76. Kalita J, Chandra S, Misra UK. Significance of seizure in cerebral venous sinus thrombosis. Seizure 2012;21:639–42.

77. Coutts SB, Hill MD, Hu WY. Hyperperfusion syndrome: toward a stricter definition. Neurosurgery 2003;53:1053–8 [discussion: 1058–60].

78. Breen JC, Caplan LR, DeWitt LD, et al. Brain edema after carotid surgery. Neurology 1996;46: 175–81.

79. Jorgensen LG, Schroeder TV. Defective cerebrovascular autoregulation after carotid endarterectomy. Eur J Vasc Surg 1993;7:370–9.

80. Ho DS, Wang Y, Chui M, et al. Epileptic seizures attributed to cerebral hyperperfusion after percutaneous transluminal angioplasty and stenting of the internal carotid artery. Cerebrovasc Dis 2000;10: 374–9.

81. Kieburtz K, Ricotta JJ, Moxley RT 3rd. Seizures following carotid endarterectomy. Arch Neurol 1990;47:568–70.

82. Marino D, Vatti G, Rufa A, et al. Transient periodic lateralised epileptiform discharges (PLEDs) following internal carotid artery stenting. Epileptic Disord 2012;14:85–9.

83. Hamamura T, Morioka T, Sayama T, et al. Cerebral hyperperfusion syndrome associated with nonconvulsive status epilepticus following superficial temporal artery-middle cerebral artery anastomosis. Case report. Neurol Med Chir (Tokyo) 2010;50:1099–104.

84. Salazar AM, Jabbari B, Vance SC, et al. Epilepsy after penetrating head injury. I. Clinical correlates: a report of the Vietnam Head Injury Study. Neurology 1985;35:1406–14.

85. Lee ST, Lui TN, Wong CW, et al. Early seizures after moderate closed head injury. Acta Neurochir (Wien) 1995;137:151–4.

86. Herman ST. Epilepsy after brain insult: targeting epileptogenesis. Neurology 2002;59:S21–6.

87. Pitkanen A, Bolkvadze T. Head trauma and epilepsy. In: Noebels JL, Avoli M, Rogawski MA, Olsen RW, Delgado-Escueta AV, editors. Source Jasper's Basic Mechanisms of the Epilepsies [Internet]. 4th edition. Bethesda (MD): National Center for Biotechnology Information (US); 2012.

88. Vespa PM, Nuwer MR, Nenov V, et al. Increased incidence and impact of nonconvulsive and convulsive seizures after traumatic brain injury as

detected by continuous electroencephalographic monitoring. J Neurosurg 1999;91:750–60.

89. Vespa PM, McArthur DL, Xu Y, et al. Nonconvulsive seizures after traumatic brain injury are associated with hippocampal atrophy. Neurology 2010;75: 792–8.

90. Frey LC. Epidemiology of posttraumatic epilepsy: a critical review. Epilepsia 2003;44(Suppl 10):11–7.

91. Temkin NR. Risk factors for posttraumatic seizures in adults. Epilepsia 2003;44(Suppl 10):18–20.

92. Scheid R, von Cramon DY. Clinical findings in the chronic phase of traumatic brain injury: data from 12 years' experience in the Cognitive Neurology Outpatient Clinic at the University of Leipzig. Dtsch Arztebl Int 2010;107:199–205.

93. Wiedemayer H, Triesch K, Schafer H, et al. Early seizures following non-penetrating traumatic brain injury in adults: risk factors and clinical significance. Brain Inj 2002;16:323–30.

94. Vespa PM, Miller C, McArthur D, et al. Nonconvulsive electrographic seizures after traumatic brain injury result in a delayed, prolonged increase in intracranial pressure and metabolic crisis. Crit Care Med 2007;35:2830–6.

95. Schierhout G, Roberts I. Prophylactic antiepileptic agents after head injury: a systematic review. J Neurol Neurosurg Psychiatry 1998;64:108–12.

96. Chang BS, Lowenstein DH. Practice parameter: antiepileptic drug prophylaxis in severe traumatic brain injury: report of the Quality Standards Subcommittee of the American Academy of Neurology. Neurology 2003;60:10–6.

97. Bratton SL, Chestnut RM, Ghajar J, et al. Guidelines for the management of severe traumatic brain injury. XIII. Antiseizure prophylaxis. J Neurotrauma 2007;24(Suppl 1):S83–6.

98. Cotton BA, Kao LS, Kozar R, et al. Cost-utility analysis of levetiracetam and phenytoin for posttraumatic seizure prophylaxis. J Trauma 2011;71: 375–9.

99. Jones KE, Puccio AM, Harshman KJ, et al. Levetiracetam versus phenytoin for seizure prophylaxis in severe traumatic brain injury. Neurosurg Focus 2008;25:E3.

100. Temkin NR, Dikmen SS, Anderson GD, et al. Valproate therapy for prevention of posttraumatic seizures: a randomized trial. J Neurosurg 1999;91: 593–600.

101. Englot DJ, Rolston JD, Wang DD, et al. Efficacy of vagus nerve stimulation in posttraumatic versus nontraumatic epilepsy. J Neurosurg 2012;117:970–7.

102. Le Blanc FE, Rasmussen T. Cerebral seizures and brain tumors. In: Magnus O, de Haas AM, Vinken PJ, et al, editors. Handbook of clinical neurology. Amsterdam: North-Holland Publishing; 1974. p. 295–301.

103. Sirven JI, Wingerchuk DM, Drazkowski JF, et al. Seizure prophylaxis in patients with brain tumors: a meta-analysis. Mayo Clin Proc 2004; 79:1489–94.

104. Aguiar D, Pazo R, Duran I, et al. Toxic epidermal necrolysis in patients receiving anticonvulsants and cranial irradiation: a risk to consider. J Neurooncol 2004;66:345–50.

105. Glantz MJ, Cole BF, Forsyth PA, et al. Practice parameter: anticonvulsant prophylaxis in patients with newly diagnosed brain tumors. Report of the Quality Standards Subcommittee of the American Academy of Neurology. Neurology 2000;54: 1886–93.

106. Bhangoo SS, Linskey ME, Kalkanis SN. Evidence-based guidelines for the management of brain metastases. Neurosurg Clin N Am 2011;22:97–104, viii.

107. Mikkelsen T, Paleologos NA, Robinson PD, et al. The role of prophylactic anticonvulsants in the management of brain metastases: a systematic review and evidence-based clinical practice guideline. J Neurooncol 2010;96:97–102.

108. Maschio M. Brain tumor-related epilepsy. Curr Neuropharmacol 2012;10:124–33.

109. Maschio M, Dinapoli L, Sperati F, et al. Oxcarbazepine monotherapy in patients with brain tumor-related epilepsy: open-label pilot study for assessing the efficacy, tolerability and impact on quality of life. J Neurooncol 2012;106:651–6.

110. Bahr O, Hermisson M, Rona S, et al. Intravenous and oral levetiracetam in patients with a suspected primary brain tumor and symptomatic seizures undergoing neurosurgery: the HELLO trial. Acta Neurochir (Wien) 2012;154:229–35 [discussion: 35].

111. Swisher CB, Doreswamy M, Gingrich KJ, et al. Phenytoin, levetiracetam, and pregabalin in the acute management of refractory status epilepticus in patients with brain tumors. Neurocrit Care 2012; 16:109–13.

112. Swisher CB, Doreswamy M, Husain AM. Use of pregabalin for nonconvulsive seizures and nonconvulsive status epilepticus. Seizure 2013;22:116–8.

113. Weller M, Gorlia T, Cairncross JG, et al. Prolonged survival with valproic acid use in the EORTC/NCIC temozolomide trial for glioblastoma. Neurology 2011;77:1156–64.

114. Tsai HC, Wei KC, Tsai CN, et al. Effect of valproic acid on the outcome of glioblastoma multiforme. Br J Neurosurg 2012;26:347–54.

115. Rhoney DH, Varelas PN. Drug-induced seizures in critically ill patients. In: Varelas PN, editor. Seizures in critical care. A guide to diagnosis and therapeutics. 2nd edition. New York: Humana Press; 2010. p. 307–40.

116. Boswell MV, Wolfe JR. Intrathecal cefazolin-induced seizures following attempted discography. Pain Physician 2004;7:103–6.

117. Smith NL, Freebairn RC, Park MA, et al. Therapeutic drug monitoring when using cefepime in

continuous renal replacement therapy: seizures associated with cefepime. Crit Care Resusc 2012; 14:312–5.

118. Naeije G, Lorent S, Vincent JL, et al. Continuous epileptiform discharges in patients treated with cefepime or meropenem. Arch Neurol 2011;68:1303–7.

119. Schuele SU, Kellinghaus C, Shook SJ, et al. Incidence of seizures in patients with multiple sclerosis treated with intrathecal baclofen. Neurology 2005; 64:1086–7.

120. Yeh HM, Lau HP, Lin PL, et al. Convulsions and refractory ventricular fibrillation after intrathecal injection of a massive dose of tranexamic acid. Anesthesiology 2003;98:270–2.

121. Wijdicks EF, Sharbrough FW. New-onset seizures in critically ill patients. Neurology 1993;43:1042–4.

122. Armstrong PJ, Bersten A. Normeperidine toxicity. Anesth Analg 1986;65:536–8.

123. Cluitmans FH, Meinders AE. Management of severe hyponatremia: rapid or slow correction? Am J Med 1990;88:161–6.

124. Soupart A, Decaux G. Therapeutic recommendations for management of severe hyponatremia: current concepts on pathogenesis and prevention of neurologic complications. Clin Nephrol 1996;46:149–69.

125. Hennis A, Corbin D, Fraser H. Focal seizures and non-ketotic hyperglycaemia. J Neurol Neurosurg Psychiatry 1992;55:195–7.

126. Tiras R, Mutlu A, Ozben S, et al. Forced eye closure-induced reflex seizure and non-ketotic hyperglycemia. Ann Saudi Med 2009;29:313–5.

127. Ko SB, Ortega-Gutierrez S, Choi HA, et al. Status epilepticus-induced hyperemia and brain tissue hypoxia after cardiac arrest. Arch Neurol 2011;68: 1323–6.

128. Shorvon S. Super-refractory status epilepticus: an approach to therapy in this difficult clinical situation. Epilepsia 2011;52(Suppl 8):53–6.

129. Shorvon S, Ferlisi M. The treatment of super-refractory status epilepticus: a critical review of available therapies and a clinical treatment protocol. Brain 2011;134:2802–18.

130. Shorvon S, Ferlisi M. The outcome of therapies in refractory and super-refractory convulsive status epilepticus and recommendations for therapy. Brain 2012;135:2314–28.

131. Trinka E, Hofler J, Zerbs A. Causes of status epilepticus. Epilepsia 2012;53(Suppl 4):127–38.

132. Towne AR, Pellock JM, Ko D, et al. Determinants of mortality in status epilepticus. Epilepsia 1994;35:27–34.

133. Shepard PW, St Louis EK. Seizure treatment in transplant patients. Curr Treat Options Neurol 2012;14:332–47.

134. Pandey CK, Singh N, Bose N, et al. Gabapentin and propofol for treatment of status epilepticus in acute intermittent porphyria. J Postgrad Med 2003;49:285.

135. Alvarez-Sabin J, Montaner J, Padro L, et al. Gabapentin in late-onset poststroke seizures. Neurology 2002;59:1991–3.

136. Trinka E, Dilitz E, Unterberger I, et al. Non convulsive status epilepticus after replacement of valproate with lamotrigine. J Neurol 2002;249:1417–22.

137. Guerrini R, Belmonte A, Parmeggiani L, et al. Myoclonic status epilepticus following high-dosage lamotrigine therapy. Brain Dev 1999;21:420–4.

138. Towne AR, Garnett LK, Waterhouse EJ, et al. The use of topiramate in refractory status epilepticus. Neurology 2003;60:332–4.

139. Tarulli A, Drislane FW. The use of topiramate in refractory status epilepticus. Neurology 2004;62:837.

140. Hottinger A, Sutter R, Marsch S, et al. Topiramate as an adjunctive treatment in patients with refractory status epilepticus: an observational cohort study. CNS Drugs 2012;26:761–72.

141. Yoshimura I, Kaneko S, Yoshimura N, et al. Long-term observations of two siblings with Lafora disease treated with zonisamide. Epilepsy Res 2001; 46:283–7.

142. Brodie MJ, Ben-Menachem E, Chouette I, et al. Zonisamide: its pharmacology, efficacy and safety in clinical trials. Acta Neurol Scand Suppl 2012;(194): 19–28.

143. Gaida-Hommernick B, Rieck K, Runge U. Oxcarbazepine in focal epilepsy and hepatic porphyria: a case report. Epilepsia 2001;42:793–5.

144. Zaatreh MM. Levetiracetam in porphyric status epilepticus: a case report. Clin Neuropharmacol 2005;28:243–4.

145. Misra UK, Kalita J, Maurya PK. Levetiracetam versus lorazepam in status epilepticus: a randomized, open labeled pilot study. J Neurol 2012;259:645–8.

146. Zelano J, Kumlien E. Levetiracetam as alternative stage two antiepileptic drug in status epilepticus: a systematic review. Seizure 2012;21:233–6.

147. Trinka E. What is the evidence to use new intravenous AEDs in status epilepticus? Epilepsia 2011; 52(Suppl 8):35–8.

148. Alvarez V, Januel JM, Burnand B, et al. Second-line status epilepticus treatment: comparison of phenytoin, valproate, and levetiracetam. Epilepsia 2011;52:1292–6.

149. Cherry S, Judd L, Muniz JC, et al. Safety and efficacy of lacosamide in the intensive care unit. Neurocrit Care 2012;16:294–8.

150. Hofler J, Trinka E. Lacosamide as a new treatment option in status epilepticus. Epilepsia 2013;54(3): 393–404.

151. Berger B, Vienenkoetter B, Korporal M, et al. Accidental intoxication with 60 mg intrathecal baclofen: survived. Neurocrit Care 2012;16:428–32.

152. Czuczwar P, Wojtak A, Cioczek-Czuczwar A, et al. Retigabine: the newer potential antiepileptic drug. Pharmacol Rep 2010;62:211–9.

Strategies for the Use of Mechanical Ventilation in the Neurologic Intensive Care Unit

Wan-Tsu W. Chang, MD[a,b,c],
Paul A. Nyquist, MD, MPH[a,b,c],*

KEYWORDS

- Mechanical ventilation • Brain injury • Intracranial pressure • Cerebral edema

KEY POINTS

- There are distinct patterns of respiration associated with brain injury reflecting different mechanisms of injury.
- Mechanical ventilation can help to control physiologic consequences of brain injury such as intracranial pressure.
- Strategies such as hyperoxia and positive end-expiratory pressure used to assist in oxygenation can affect brain physiology in a very direct fashion.

INTRODUCTION

Mechanical ventilation is used in the intensive care unit. It is estimated that among patients admitted to medical surgical intensive care units, the primary indication for mechanical ventilation is neurologic in 20% of cases.[1] This statistic is much higher in a dedicated Neurocritical Care Unit (NCCU), in which as many as 80% of patients are intubated for a primary neurologic injury.[2] Patients with acute neurologic injuries usually require mechanical ventilation for reasons other than direct injury to the lungs. Many patients with acute brain injury are intubated to protect the airway in the setting of altered mental status. Even after recovery from acute brain injury, there is a subset of neurologically injured patients who fail estuation from mechanical ventilation because of neurologic respiratory insufficiency without injury to the lungs or increased work of breathing.[2]

There are special considerations for the management of mechanical ventilation in patients with neurologic injuries. Clinicians must be aware of clinical issues surrounding ventilator management in these patients and must focus on strategies to enhance neurologic recovery and facilitate extubation. Included is a list of neurologic disorders seen in the NCCU commonly requiring intubation and ventilator support (**Box 1**).

Patients with brain injury who are comatose or obtunded often present with the concern of airway compromise caused by altered mental status. With decreased levels of consciousness, there is reduced tone of the oropharyngeal muscles leading to posterior displacement of the tongue often causing airway obstruction. Combined with impaired swallowing mechanisms and inhibition of the cough and gag reflexes, these patients are at risk for aspiration. If the state of their altered mental status is rapidly reversible, the patient may not require immediate intubation. However, the patient should be in a monitored setting where he or she can be easily intubated if necessary. If the patient will be neurologically impaired for a

Disclosures: None.
[a] Department of Neurology, The Johns Hopkins School of Medicine, Baltimore, MD, USA; [b] Department of Anesthesiology and Critical Care Medicine, The Johns Hopkins School of Medicine, Baltimore, MD, USA; [c] Department of Neurosurgery, The Johns Hopkins School of Medicine, Baltimore, MD, USA
* Corresponding author. 600 North Wolfe Street, Meyer 8-140, Baltimore, MD 21287.
E-mail address: pnyquis1@jhmi.edu

Neurosurg Clin N Am 24 (2013) 407–416
http://dx.doi.org/10.1016/j.nec.2013.02.004
1042-3680/13/$ – see front matter © 2013 Elsevier Inc. All rights reserved.

Box 1
Neurologic conditions requiring intubation and mechanical ventilation

- Primary neurologic processes often requiring intubation and mechanical ventilation:
  - Stroke of all types: ischemic strokes, intracerebral hemorrhages, and subarachnoid hemorrhages
  - Traumatic brain injury
  - Status epileptic us
  - Metabolic and septic encephalopathy
  - Meningitis/encephalitis
- Primary neurologic disorders often resulting in type II respiratory failure due to neuromuscular weakness:
  - Spinal cord injury
  - Myasthenia gravis
  - Guillain-Barre syndrome
  - Amyotrophic lateral sclerosis
  - Acute inflammatory myopathy
  - Genetic peripheral neuropathies such as spinal muscular atrophy
  - Intoxications/poisonings

long period of time, with absent cough and gag reflexes, intubation should be considered for airway protection.

In certain clinical circumstances, it may be prudent to institute mechanical ventilation based on the anticipation of neurologic deterioration during the progression of the underlying condition. In patients with aneurysmal subarachnoid hemorrhage with severe vasospasm, the best strategy may be to intubate and initiate mechanical ventilation, to insure adequate pulmonary gas exchange in the setting of hemodynamic augmentation and subsequent pulmonary edema and hypoxemia. Patients with hemispheric strokes and malignant cerebral edema may require early intubation in anticipation of the need for transient hyperventilation, hypoxemia, and surgical intervention.

Brain injury always causes dysregulation of the respiratory drive and/or altered pulmonary mechanical function. Neural control of respiration depends on both conscious and automatic inputs integrated in the pons and medulla. Automatic control of respiration is located in areas of the dorsolateral tegmentum of the pons as well as the medulla, specifically the nucleus tractus solitarus and retroambigualis. The descending pathways of the ventrolateral columns of the spinal cord allow for conscious input from the cortex.[3]

Automatic respiration is a homeostatic mechanism through which pulmonary function is controlled by regulatory centers in the brain stem. These centers act to regulate acid-base status and to meet oxygen demand. Central chemoreceptors in the medulla monitor the pH associated with CO_2 levels within the cerebrospinal fluid in the fourth ventricle. Peripheral chemoreceptors located in the carotid bodies and aortic bodies monitor the P_{CO_2}, pH, and P_{O_2} of arterial blood while relaying the information to the respiratory centers via the vagus and glossopharyngeal nerves. An increase in the P_{CO_2} in the blood decreases the pH, thereby stimulating the respiratory centers to increase ventilation and improve CO_2 elimination. The peripheral chemoreceptors also respond to a drop in arterial P_{O_2} less than 60 mm Hg, stimulating the respiratory centers to increase ventilation to achieve appropriate oxygenation. Hypercapnea is a more sensitive respiratory stimulus than hypoxemia in most people except those who have compensated for chronic CO_2 retention, such as in chronic obstructive pulmonary disease.

Human respiration is most strongly affected by conscious inputs originating from the cortex. These outputs represent most of the stimuli affecting respiration. In the healthy human these outputs often occur beyond awareness. In patients who are comatose with brain injury, conscious input from the cortex is eliminated. In this setting the architecture of respiration is controlled almost entirely by automatic input originating from the brain stem. It is in this setting that classical patterns of respiration associated with regional brain injury become apparent.

The most commonly observed patterns of breathing in patients with brain injury are tachypnea and hyperventilation. These patterns are frequently seen as a result of diffuse cortical and subcortical injury and can be seen even in patients who seem to be neurologically intact. This pattern is a consequence of inhibition of conscious input from the cortex and increased dependency on the Pa_{CO_2} as a trigger for respiratory drive from the automatic centers in the brain stem.[4] In patients with cortical injury a dysnchrony between the normal cortically initiated cues for respiration and the automatic regulation of respiration exists. Thus the coordination between conscious inputs and automatic inputs is disrupted with an increased dependence on automatic regulation and suppression of cortical output.

There are classic patterns of abnormal breathing associated with specific neurologic lesions in different locations in the brain. These patterns are seen in patients with intracranial mass lesions and elevated intracranial pressure. Cheynes-Stokes respiration is the most common pattern seen with brain injury. It is characterized by a regular cyclic crescendo-decrescendo pattern of variable respiratory rate and tidal volumes. It is associated with disruptions between the bilateral cortical hemispheres and dysfunction of the medial forebrain structures.[3,4] Apneustic breathing is characterized by prolonged inspiratory pause and is associated with lesions of the lower tegmentum of the pons.[3,4] Cluster breathing is irregular quick breaths regularly separated by long pauses. It is associated with lesions of the lower pons or upper medulla.[3,4] Ataxic breathing is similar to cluster breathing except that the there is a complete loss of rhythmicity of breathing with irregularly timed breaths with variable tidal volumes usually of smaller sizes. It is often called the atrial fibrillation of breathing and occurs lesions of the medulla.[4,5] Patients can be observed to have these abnormal breathing patterns in succession over minutes to hours with elevation of intracranial pressure and progressive downward herniation as brain function is compromised in a rostral to caudal fashion.

EFFECTS OF NEUROLOGIC INJURY ON THE PULMONARY SYSTEM

There is a subset of patients with neurologic disease who experience specific pulmonary complications caused by their neurologic illness. These associated pulmonary conditions are neurogenic pulmonary edema (NPE) and pulmonary edema from stunned myocardium. NPE has been reported extensively in the setting of acute neurologic injury, including seizures, traumatic brain injury (TBI), as well as cervical spinal cord injury associated with hanging.[3,6,7] This disorder can occur rapidly with onset of initial neurologic injury or it can occur at later stages of illness.[8] Reports suggest an incidence of 40% of neurogenic pulmonary edema for all head injury subtypes and a 90% incidence in the setting of intracranial hemorrhages.[8,9] The use of supportive measures, such as positive end-expiratory pressure (PEEP), to maintain sufficient blood and brain oxygenation are usually quite effective in this disorder.[10] Case reports also suggest that patients with this disorder may be particularly responsive to prone positioning, although such positioning is difficult in patients who have intraventricular drains or other monitors.[11,12]

NPE is strongly associated with lesions in specific regions of the brain. Several experimental models have demonstrated that focused damage to the nucleus of the tractus solitarus in the medulla of the human and experimentally in rodents causes NPE.[13] It has been studied extensively in

humans since the 1950s, at which time an association between high cervical cord injury and the immediate onset of pulmonary edema was observed.[8,12,14] Since then it has been studied in the setting of armed conflicts as well as in civilian emergency rooms.[14] It is caused by the extravasation of a proteinaceous fluid across the alveolar membrane of the lungs secondary to injury from the catecholamine storm associated with severe neurologic injury.[15] It is different from acute respiratory distress syndrome (ARDS), acute lung injury (ALI), and transfusion-associated lung injury (TRALI) in that the mechanism of injury in ARDS, ALI, and TRALI are the result of an inflammatory reaction to lung injury and the alveolar fluid is produced from the pneumocytes within the alveolar wall.[13,16]

The diagnosis of NPE is often difficult to separate from other forms of lung injury. Other causes of pulmonary edema commonly seen in the setting of acute neurologic injury include pulmonary edema from congestive heart failure and stunned myocardium, ARDs, ALI, and TRALI. In general, NPE is different from pulmonary edema from heart failure, ARDS, ALI, and TRALI in that the wedge pressure usually is not elevated and the echocardiogram is usually normal. It has a rapid onset at the time of neurologic injury and often involves only one lung field. NPE is usually temporary in duration and often exquisitely PEEP responsive. Treatment involves supportive measures including intubation, elevated PEEP, elevated Fio_2, and diuresis if necessary.

Acute neurologic injury has long been recognized as a primary cause of stunned myocardium. It has been used extensively in subarachnoid hemorrhage and has been associated with several neurologic diseases including brain tumors, seizures, ischemic stroke, hemorrhagic stroke of all types, and peripheral nerve injuries, such as Guillain-Barre syndrome. It has been documented to occur in up to 40% of all brain injuries and 90% of all ICHs. It is synonymous with Takotsubo's cardiomyopathy, typified as a syndrome of global hypokinesis associated with an increase in serum catecholamines with damage to the myocardium appearing as contraction band necrosis located in the fibers of the myocardium.[17-19] It is usually a reversible and temporary phenomenon lasting only a few days.

Myocardial stunning in the setting of acute neurologic injury often results in acute fulminant pulmonary edema. In subarachnoid hemorrhage patients with cardiogenic shock due to stunned myocardium, aggressive support with inotropic agents to maintain adequate brain perfusion to avoid focal ischemic from vasospasm is sometimes required.

Intraaortic balloon counterpulsation has also been used as a measure to facilitate cardiac output in this situation.[12,20] In the ventilated patient with severe neurologic injury, this entity can often be confused with other syndromes, such as NPE, ALI, ARDS, or TRALI. This issue is usually easily resolved with the use of echocardiography.

Diagnosis focuses on the detection of increased serum troponins and creatine kinase MB, with troponin levels disproportionately elevated in comparison to creatine kinase MB. However, overall the cardiac enzymes are only minimally elevated as compared with occlusive cardiac disease. Electrocardiogram changes are typified by nonspecific ST changes in an apical distribution. Global as opposed to segmental hypokinesis is observed on echocardiogram usually with an apical pattern. Early detection of this disorder and appropriate treatment with fluid management and inotropic support are essential to avoid potentially fatal outcomes. Intubation and appropriate ventilatory maneuvers to avoid hypoxia are often required to support the patient while the patient is treated for underlying myocardial dysfunction and neurologic injury.

ISSUES IN VENTILATION AFFECTING BRAIN OXYGENATION

No large studies have systematically examined the role of different mechanical ventilation strategies on brain oxygenation. Although most clinical strategies emphasize maximal oxygen support with an adequate fractional inspired oxygen (Fio_2) to maintain brain parenchymal oxygen levels, no study has demonstrated benefit from the prophylactic use of high Fio_2 in the setting of brain injury. There is a hypothetical consideration of lung injury from exposure to high Fio_2 in the setting of severe lung injury. In the past, study of brain oxygenation has been limited by the inability to measure parenchymal oxygenation directly. In recent years, jugular venous oxygen sensors and intraparenchymal oxygen sensors have been developed to provide direct measures of brain oxygenation through determination of vascular oxygenation and direct measurement of parenchymal oxygen levels ($PbtO_2$). Studies of jugular venous oximetry have demonstrated that hyperventilation can result in decreased global brain oxygenation.[21] A linear relationship between reduced oxygen availability and decreasing cerebral blood flow (CBF) with increasing hyperventilation in animals as well as humans has been observed.[22–24]

The use of brain parenchymal oxygen sensors has resulted in new recommendations for their use in TBI. The Brain Trauma Foundation guidelines suggest targets for brain $PbtO_2$ of greater than 15 mm Hg. The brain in general cannot tolerate levels less than 10 mm Hg for longer than 30 minutes, or at the lowest, 6 mm Hg, regardless of duration.[25] Direct $PbtO_2$ monitors measure $PbtO_2$ in units of tension (mm Hg). $PbtO_2$ reflects oxygen tension in the tissue bed not overall oxygen consumption and does not directly measure the metabolic state of the cell. Positron emission tomography studies suggest it may correlate inversely with the oxygen extraction fraction and reflect oxygen diffusion rather than total oxygen delivery or metabolism. In general a $PbtO_2$ of 1 mm Hg = 0.003 mL O_2/100 g brain.[26,27] When placed in approximation with injured tissue, the sensor can measure trends in tissue $PbtO_2$ concentrations that respond to interventions with mechanical ventilation. Normobaric hyperoxia administration has been demonstrated to restore mitochondrial oxygen levels in mice.[28] Maneuvers affecting ventilation, oxygen management, and ventilator strategies are now used with $PbtO_2$ as a guide. Interventions known to cause increases in $PbtO_2$ include increasing Fio_2 (eg, 50%–60%), increasing PEEP, limited periods of 100% normobaric oxygen, increasing minute ventilation, decreasing $Paco_2$ to lower intracranial pressure (ICP), paralysis, augmenting BP, sedation, and transfusion.[26,27]

ISSUES IN VENTILATION AFFECTING ICP

Mechanical ventilation is necessary in many patients with elevated ICP. Such patients almost invariably have an impaired level of consciousness and require intubation and mechanical ventilation to implement therapies aimed at lowering ICP.

HYPERVENTILATION

Hyperventilation reduces intracranial pressure through its effect on $Paco_2$. This process is mediated by arterial responses to changes in pH. Hypocapnia induces cerebral vasoconstriction and reduces CBF by causing a reduction in the volume occupied by the vascular component of the cranial vault, which is a rapidly effective measure to acutely reduce ICP. These changes can temporarily shift the autoregulatory curve to the right, resulting in lower ICP and lower CBF at higher mean arterial pressure (MAP) (**Fig. 1**). This change in the relationship of CBF to MAP will resolve with time as a new $Paco_2$ set point is created by the homeostatic pH regulatory mechanisms. This adaptation usually occurs within 6 to 12 hours after initiation of hypocapnia. As bicarbonate concentration shifts intracerebrally, this autoregulatory system adapts

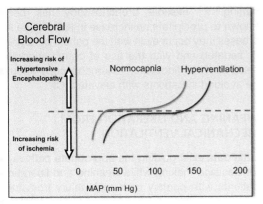

Fig. 1. The cerebral autoregulation curve in the setting of normocapnea and hyperventilation.

to higher $Paco_2$ set points and will shift back to the left with higher CBF at lower MAP. At this point, the effects of hypocapnia from hyperventilation will be lost.[29]

To most effectively induce hypocapnia for the management of elevated intracranial pressures, the patient must be intubated and sedated to allow for aggressive control of his or her ventilatory cycle. $Paco_2$ is reduced from its normal range of 40 to 60 mm Hg to a reduced range of 25 to 35 mm Hg. Acute ICP reduction through hyperventilation can be achieved in most patients by using bag breaths that result in doubling of the minute ventilation. A bag breath rate of 18 to 24 breaths per minute is often required. In healthy volunteers, a reduction of CBF to 40% lasts for 30 minutes after reduction of $Paco_2$ to 25 mm Hg.[30]

The end result of hypocapnia on most organ systems is a reduction in blood flow. Thus a consequence of reduced CBF on brain parenchyma is the development of hypoxia and cerebral ischemia. This effect can be amplified in the metabolically dynamic setting of severe brain injury. Hyperventilation is associated with increased rate of morbidity and early mortality if continued chronically.[31–33] The Brain Trauma Foundation guidelines on management of TBIs recommend against any strategy that uses prophylactic or chronic hyperventilation.[25]

ARDS AND PERMISSIVE HYPERCAPNEA

The ARDS Net protocol is the only known ventilatory strategy demonstrated to reduce mortality in the setting of ARDS.[34] It incorporates strategies that use elevated PEEP and permissive hypercapnea to reduce ventilator lung injury. ARDS and ALI are diagnoses frequently seen in the NCCU. Many patients with a neurologic injury are predisposed to ARDS and ALI, such as head trauma, sepsis,

neurologic surgery of the brain or spine, and stroke of all types. ARDS/ALI is found in 10% to 35% of patients who have severe TBI and aneurysmal subarachnoid hemorrhage and is a predictor of poor outcome in these settings.[35–41] Risk for ARDS/ALI in the neurologically injured patient population may be increased due to exposure to aspiration, transfusion, and sepsis. In a recent study the incidence of ALI and ARDs in 192 consecutive patients was 68% or 35%. It was found that the most significant predictors of ALI and ARDs were not neurologic markers but the coincidence of pneumonia and shock, with an absent gag reflex as the most predictive marker for the development of ALI and ARDs (odds ratio: 3.14, P .0097).[42]

Permissive hypercapnea has not been shown to induce brain injury and is frequently incorporated as a strategy to reduce ventilator lung injury in patients in the NCCU to allow lower tidal volumes and less PEEP. In neonates, permissive hypercapnea has been associated with more severe injury from intracranial hemorrhage. Permissive hypercapnea has not been observed in adults. The use of elevated PEEP is associated with increasing ICP. In the context of the ARDS Net protocol, the lower tidal volumes and reduced plateau pressures usually offset the effects of elevated PEEP on ICP and can be used safely. However, careful neurologic monitoring seems prudent.

PEEP AND ICP

Clinical studies have documented the relationship of elevated PEEP to ICP in brain injury. Some clinical studies have reported increases in ICP up to 14 mm Hg in response to as little as 10 cm H_2O of PEEP. These changes are reversible with the elimination of PEEP.[43,44] PEEP increases intrathoracic pressure, peak inspiratory pressure, and mean airway pressure. PEEP decreases venous return, mean arterial pressure, and cardiac output. Increased intrathoracic pressure reduces venous outflow from the cranium, thereby increasing jugular venous pressure. This increase in jugular venous pressure causes increased cerebral venous blood volume, which can be critical in situations where the ventricular compliance is already elevated by a space-occupying lesion or traumatic injury. In these settings, even small changes in intracranial volume result in steep increases in ICP. In patients with severe lung injury, the effects of PEEP on increases in intrathoracic pressure are often amplified due to a decline in lung compliance. In patients with both decreased ventricular compliance and decreased lung compliance, the effects of elevated PEEP on ICP seem greater.[45]

The decreased venous return and cardiac output associated with PEEP can also reduce cerebral perfusion pressure (CPP). If cerebral autoregulation is intact, decreases in CPP are compensated by cerebral vasodilation, which may also exacerbate ICP. If cerebral autoregulation is impaired, decreased CPP may lead to cerebral ischemia.

In patients with TBI and respiratory dysfunction, PEEP is often required to support the patient and improve oxygenation. Even though increased PEEP can lead to elevated ICP and some changes in hemodynamic parameters, PEEP should always be considered an option for patients with brain injury.[46] In general, PEEP seems well tolerated in the most brain-injured patients and it is unlikely to have deleterious intracranial effects if ICP is monitored and adequately controlled.[47]

HIGH-FREQUENCY VENTILATION AND ICP

High-frequency ventilation (HFV) incorporates high-frequency respiratory rates of more than 150 breaths per minute with low tidal volumes, usually 1 to 5 mL/kg. It allows for efficient ventilation and oxygenation with minimal induction of ventilator-induced lung injury. The effects of this ventilator mode are to reduce the mean peak airway pressure as well as the peak inspiratory pressure and therefore reduce intrathoracic pressure.[48] It thus has minimal effect on cerebral venous outflow and ICP, which is increased in situations with decreased cerebral venous outflow. This allows for a significant reduction of ICP when compared with conventional modes of ventilation. There are several variants of this technology: high-frequency oscillatory ventilation, high-frequency jet ventilation, high-frequency percussive ventilation, high-frequency flow interruption, and high-frequency positive pressure ventilation.

TBI with both severe lung injury as well as severe brain injury may benefit from HFV. These patients will have reduced pulmonary compliance and intracranial compliance and are likely to be sensitive to the effects of intrathoracic pressure on ICP caused by mechanical ventilation. Studies looking at patients with ARDS and elevated ICP who failed conventional mechanical ventilation and were placed on HFV showed reduction of peak inspiratory pressure and ICP without impairment of CO_2, oxygen delivery, or CPP.[49–51]

OTHER CONSIDERATIONS

The cycle time of inspiration I and expiration on changes in PEEP and ICP has been tested in humans and animals. There seems to be no direct effect of these inverted ratios on ICP at any PEEP setting.[52,53] Flexible bronchoscopy has been known to precipitate an increase in ICP. These increases may occur even with the patient paralyzed or sedated and with the use of cough suppressants such as lidocaine.[54] Bronchoscopy should be avoided in patients with elevated ICP.

WEANING AND LIBERATION FROM MECHANICAL VENTILATION

Little data exist guiding the appropriate pathways for decision-making while weaning and liberating patients with primary neurologic injury from mechanical ventilation. The Society of Critical Care Medicine has suggested that the best evidence supports using a standard spontaneous breathing trial with aggressive liberation of the patient from the ventilator if they pass this trial.[55] The use of weaning protocols incorporating slow weans through reduction of respiratory rate in the setting of SIMV or the use of CPAP as weaning modes without periods of rest are not supported by the present literature. However, in the neurologic patient, the primary injury is neurologic in nature and often does not involve pulmonary mechanical dysfunction and a concurrent increase in the work of breathing. These strategies are used until an autonomous respiratory rate is established and adequate peripheral strength is demonstrated.

Spinal or peripheral nerve injuries can cause a type II respiratory failure. In this setting, the standard daily breathing trial may be supplanted by early tracheostomy or extended CPAP trials designed to test for fatigue or neurologically impaired lungs with intact mechanical function. Many practitioners will use strategies incorporating slowly decreasing respiratory rate or a slow decrease in pressure support to obtain functional residual capacity and negative inspiratory force goals consistent with liberation from mechanical ventilation.

The transition from controlled ventilation to spontaneous ventilation can be performed safely if the patient's ICP is within the normal range. In any situation in which a patient has a markedly high ICP, a spontaneous breathing trial may be associated with significant and meaningful increases in ICP. A study on patients with severe TBI demonstrated that spontaneous breathing trials can increase ICP and that the most important factor predicting this increase is the ICP before beginning the trial.[56]

STRATEGIES FOR EXTUBATION OF THE NEUROLOGICALLY INJURED PATIENT

Liberating patients who are mechanically ventilated in the setting of neurologic injury can usually be performed safely and quickly. Coplin and colleagues[57] detected no differences in outcome when neurosurgical patients were extubated with Glasgow coma scores as low as 4, as long as the cough and gag reflexes were intact and there was a relatively short period of neurologic impairment.[58] In the authors' unit a very low rate of extubation failure was documented in patients 72 hours after liberation from mechanical ventilation. Of 1265 patients who were intubated because of primary neurologic injury of brain, spinal cord, or peripheral nerve, a total of 129 (10%) patients were reintubated. This rate is well below the extubation failure rates targeted in conventional units, usually around 15%. In addition, only 39% were reintubated because of increased work of breathing resulting from pneumonia or aspiration. Aspiration was reported in less than 5% of these patients. In 59% of these patients a syndrome of altered respiratory pattern associated with decrease tidal volume and irregular respiratory rates, atelectasis, and decreased Glasgow coma scores was the primary cause of reintubation.[2] It seems the combination of events involving reduced tidal volume and respiratory rate leading to atelectasis and shunting were the primary cause of reintubation in the patients.

The patient who is intubated for a primary neurologic disorder can be classified into 1 of 4 categories. The first type of patient is one who suffers from the effects of a central nervous system process and intubated solely for airway protection and has no signs of respiratory failure. These patients can usually be safely extubated if they have signs of airway protection, such as a cough and gag reflex. If the patient will be neurologically impaired for an indefinite period of time, the clinician may consider tracheostomy as an aid to liberation from mechanical ventilation. Tracheostomy allows for safe suctioning and immediate control of the airway in the event of acute respiratory failure.

The second type of patient is one that has a severe neurologic injury that inhibits the central respiratory drive who will experience acute respiratory arrest on cessation of mechanical ventilation. These patients cannot be safely extubated until they demonstrate an autonomous respiratory drive. Often these patients will require tracheostomy and prolonged mechanical ventilation.

The third type of patient is the one that is experiencing some kind of mechanical failure induced by their neurologic injury, including mechanical failure resulting from neurogenic pulmonary edema, pulmonary edema from stunned myocardium, and aspiration pneumonia. These patients cannot be safely liberated until they demonstrate both intact arousal and reversibility of their mechanical failure via standard spontaneous breathing trials. Early liberation and failure will result in dramatic setbacks, such as the acquisition of aspiration pneumonia or exacerbation of the cause of mechanical ventilatory failure.

Finally, the fourth type of patient one that has a primary peripheral nervous disorder resulting in type II respiratory failure. These patients are inherently different from all classes of ventilated patients with a primary neurologic injury. Care must be taken to identify the mechanical limits caused by their neurologic injury before liberation. These patients in general should not be liberated until they have demonstrated a prolonged period of independent ventilation such as a tolerance of prolonged CPAP trial or T-piece trial.

Weaning in type II respiratory failure is unique among patients who are ventilator dependent. Extubation of patients with severe peripheral nerve disease can be attempted when sufficient respiratory muscle recovery occurs, which is indicated by signs of improvement in overall muscle strength, vital capacity >15–20 mL/kg, and mean inspiratory pressure <−20 to −50 cm H_2O. The patient with a high cervical spinal cord injury presents a special case of type II respiratory failure. In general, the same rules apply. However, there are some special considerations. Respiratory failure usually involves a slow decline in which the patient progressively de-recruits alveoli, resulting in alveolar hypoventilation and atelectasis. The $Paco_2$ slowly increases with a concomitant decrease in oxygenation. Patients often exhibit paradoxic breathing whereby the intercostals muscles remain innervated while the diaphragm is flaccid, producing ineffective ventilation with chest expansion and abdominal contraction. The level of spinal injury may give insight into the severity of respiratory dysfunction. Injury of C1-C3 causes apnea. Injury of C3-C5 is often associated with a mixed presentation in which the patient is able to initiate ventilation but cannot do so with enough efficiency to ventilate independently or lacks the stamina to remain ventilator independent. Injury below C5 is usually associated with some form of recovery to ventilator independence. Special concerns for these patients revolve around 3 key clinical obstacles. The need to avoid atelectasis through maneuvers that promote alveolar recruitment with adequate inflation is required. The use of aggressive pulmonary toilet to avoid aspiration pneumonia is a key element. The education of the patient to use voluntary muscles of respiration and proper positioning to maximize pulmonary function is also important. A common pitfall is the rapid extubation of patients with a cervical spine injury within the first 72 hours. Often, these patients will perform well early in their injury but as the edema at the site of the injury expands and causes a more devastating neurologic injury, they will experience worsening respiratory failure.

SUMMARY

Patients who experience neurologic injury often do not have severe mechanical disruption of the pulmonary system. However, alterations of mental status, neurogenic respiratory failure, as well as mechanical pulmonary consequences of neurologic injury require special considerations. Critical care specialists need to address issues of elevated ICP and facilitate brain oxygenation in the management of the neurologically injured patient. Critical care specialists also need to determine the appropriate strategy in the weaning and liberation of the neurologically injured patient from mechanical ventilation.

REFERENCES

1. Esteban A, Anzueto A, Alia I, et al. How is mechanical ventilation employed in the intensive care unit? An international utilization review. Am J Respir Crit Care Med 2000;161(5):1450–8.
2. Karanjia N, Nordquist D, Stevens R, et al. A clinical description of extubation failure in patients with primary brain injury. Neurocrit Care 2011;15(1):4–12.
3. Simon RP. Pathophysiology of respiratory dysfunction. In: Diseases of the nervous system: clinical neurobiology. Philadelphia: WB Saunders; 1992.
4. Pulm F, Posner LB. The diagnosis of stupor and coma. Philadelphia: FA Davis; 1980.
5. Brazias PW, Masdeu JC, Biller J. Localization in clinical neurology. 4th edition. Philadelphia: Lipincott, Williams & Wilkins; 2001. p. 559–81.
6. Moutier F. Hypertension et mort par oedeme pulmonaire aigu, chez les blesses cranio-encephaliques. Presse Med 1918;26:108–9.
7. Shanahan WT. Pulmonary oedema in epilepsy. NY Med J 1908;37:54–6.
8. Paine R, Smith JR, Howard FA. Pulmonary edema in patients dying with disease of the central nervous system. J Am Med Assoc 1952;149(7):643–6.
9. Schievink WI, Wijdicks EF, Parisi JE, et al. Sudden death from aneurysmal subarachnoid hemorrhage. Neurology 1995;45:871–4.
10. Maron MB, Holcomb PH, Dawson CA, et al. Edema development and recovery in neurogenic pulmonary edema. J Appl Physiol 1994;77(3):1155–63.
11. Fletcher SJ, Atkinson JD. Use of prone ventilation in neurogenic pulmonary oedema. Br J Anaesth 2003; 90:238–40.

12. Lazaridis C, Pradilla G, Nyquist PA, et al. Intra-aortic balloon pump counterpulsation in the setting of subarachnoid hemorrhage, cerebral vasospasm, and neurogenic stress cardiomyopathy. Case report and review of the literature. Neurocrit Care 2010; 13(1):101–8.
13. Darragh TM, Simon RP. Nucleus tractus solitarius lesions elevate pulmonary arterial pressure and lymph flow. Ann Neurol 1985;17(6):565–9.
14. Simmons RL, Heisterkamp CA, Collins JA, et al. Acute pulmonary edema in battle casualties. J Trauma 1969;9:760–75.
15. Berthiaume Y, Broaddus VC, Gropper M, et al. Alveolar liquid and protein clearance from normal dog lungs. J Appl Physiol 1988;65(2):585–93.
16. Davison DL, Terek M, Chawla LS. Neurogenic pulmonary edema. Crit Care 2012;16(2):212.
17. Greenhoot JH, Reichenbach DD. Cardiac injury and subarachnoid hemorrhage. A clinical, pathological, and physiological correlation. J Neurosurg 1969; 30(5):521–31.
18. Kurisu S, Sato H, Kawagoe T, et al. Tako-tsubo-like left ventricular dysfunction with ST-segment elevation: a novel cardiac syndrome mimicking acute myocardial infarction. Am Heart J 2002;143(3): 448–55.
19. Samuels MA. The brain-heart connection. Circulation 2007;116:77–84.
20. Apostolides PJ, Greene KA, Zabramski JM, et al. Intra-aortic balloon pump counterpulsation in the management of concomitant cerebral vasospasm and cardiac failure after subarachnoid hemorrhage: technical case report. Neurosurgery 1996;38(5): 1056–60.
21. Unterberg AW, Kiening KL, Hartl R, et al. Multimodal monitoring in patients with head injury: evaluation of the effects of treatment on cerebral oxygenation. J Trauma 1997;42:S32–7.
22. Imberti R, Bellinzona G, Langer M. Cerebral tissue PO2 and SjvO2 changes during moderate hyperventilation in patients with severe traumatic brain injury. J Neurosurg 2002;96(1):97–102.
23. Manley GT, Pitts LH, Morabito D, et al. Brain tissue oxygenation during hemorrhagic shock, resuscitation, and alterations in ventilation. J Trauma 1999; 46(2):261–7.
24. van Hulst RA, Hasan D, Lachmann B. Intracranial pressure, brain PCO2, PO2, and pH during hypo- and hyperventilation at constant mean airway pressure in pigs. Intensive Care Med 2002;28(1):68–73.
25. The Brain Trauma Foundation, The American Association of Neurological Surgeons, The Joint Section on Neurotrauma and Critical Care. Guidelines for the management of severe traumatic brain injury. 3rd edition. J Neurotrauma 2007;24(Suppl):S1–106.
26. Maloney-Wilensky E, Gracias V, Itkin A, et al. Brain tissue oxygen and outcome after severe traumatic

brain injury: a systematic review. Crit Care Med 2009;37(6):2057–63.

27. Pascual JL, Georgoff P, Horan A, et al. Reduced brain tissue oxygen in traumatic brain injury: are most commonly used interventions successful? J Trauma 2011;70(3):535–46.

28. Zhou Z, Daugherty EP, Sun D, et al. Protection of mitochondrial function and improvement in cognitive recovery in rats treated with hyperbaric oxygen following lateral fluid-percussion injury. J Neurosurg 2007;106(4):687–94.

29. Diringer MN, Videen TO, Yundt K, et al. Regional cerebrovascular and metabolic effects of hyperventilation after severe traumatic brain injury. J Neurosurg 2002;96(1):103–8.

30. Raichle ME, Posner JB, Pulm F. Cerebral blood flow during and after hyperventilation. Arch Neurol 1970; 23:394–403.

31. Bouma GJ, Muizelaar JP, Choi SC, et al. Cerebral circulation and metabolism after severe traumatic brain injury: the elusive role of ischemia. J Neurosurg 1991;75:685–93.

32. Muizelaar JP, Marmarou A, Ward JD, et al. Adverse effects of prolonged hyperventilation in patients with severe head injury: a randomized clinical trial. J Neurosurg 1991;75:731–9.

33. Stocchetti N, Maas AI, Chieregato A, et al. Hyperventilation in head injury: a review. Chest 2005; 127(5):1812–27.

34. Ventilation with lower tidal volumes as compared with traditional tidal volumes for acute lung injury and the acute respiratory distress syndrome. The Acute Respiratory Distress Syndrome Network. N Engl J Med 2000;342(18):1301–8.

35. Bratton SL, Davis RL. Acute lung injury in isolated traumatic brain injury. Neurosurgery 1997;40:707–12 [discussion: 712].

36. Gruber A, Ungersbock K, Reinprecht A, et al. Evaluation of cerebral vasospasm after early surgical and endovascular treatment of ruptured intracranial aneurysms. Neurosurgery 1998;42(2):258–67 [discussion: 267–8].

37. Holland MC, Mackersie RC, Morabito D, et al. The development of acute lung injury is associated with worse neurologic outcome in patients with severe traumatic brain injury. J Trauma 2003;55(1):106–11.

38. Kahn JM, Caldwell EC, Deem S, et al. Acute lung injury in patients with subarachnoid hemorrhage: incidence, risk factors, and outcome. Crit Care Med 2006;34(1):196–202.

39. Mascia L, Mastromauro I, Viberti S. High tidal volume as a predictor of acute lung injury in neurotrauma patients. Minerva Anestesiol 2008;74(6): 325–7.

40. Robertson CS, Valadka AB, Hannay HJ, et al. Prevention of secondary ischemic insults after severe head injury. Crit Care Med 1999;27:2086–95.

41. Schirmer-Mikalsen K, Vik A, Gisvold SE, et al. Severe head injury: control of physiological variables, organ failure and complications in the intensive care unit. Acta Anaesthesiol Scand 2007;51:1194–201.

42. Hoesch RE, Lin E, Young M, et al. Acute lung injury in critical neurological illness. Crit Care Med 2012; 40(2):587–93.

43. Shapiro HM, Marshall LF. Intracranial pressure responses to PEEP in head-injured patients. J Trauma 1978;18(4):254–6.

44. Videtta W, Villarejo F, Cohen M, et al. Effects of positive end-expiratory pressure on intracranial pressure and cerebral perfusion pressure. Acta Neurochir Suppl 2002;81:93–7.

45. Burchiel KJ, Steege TD, Wyler AR. Intracranial pressure changes in brain-injured patients requiring positive end-expiratory pressure ventilation. Neurosurgery 1981;8(4):443–9.

46. Huynh T, Messer M, Sing RF, et al. Positive end-expiratory pressure alters intracranial and cerebral perfusion pressure in severe traumatic brain injury. J Trauma 2002;53(3):488–92 [discussion: 492–3].

47. Caricato A, Conti G, Della Corte F, et al. Effects of PEEP on the intracranial system of patients with head injury and subarachnoid hemorrhage: the role of respiratory system compliance. J Trauma 2005; 58(3):571–6.

48. Sjostrand U. High-frequency positive-pressure ventilation (HFPPV): a review. Crit Care Med 1980; 8(6):345–64.

49. Fuke N, Murakami Y, Tsutsumi H, et al. The effect of high frequency jet ventilation on intracranial pressure in the patients with severe head injury. No Shinkei Geka 1984;12(Suppl 3):297–302.

50. Hurst JM, Saul TG, DeHaven CB Jr, et al. Use of high frequency jet ventilation during mechanical hyperventilation to reduce intracranial pressure in patients with multiple organ system injury. Neurosurgery 1984;15(4):530–4.

51. Salim A, Miller K, Dangleben D, et al. High-frequency percussive ventilation: an alternative mode of ventilation for head-injured patients with adult respiratory distress syndrome. J Trauma 2004;57(3):542–6.

52. Georgiadis D, Schwarz S, Kollmar R, et al. Influence of inspiration:expiration ratio on intracranial and cerebral perfusion pressure in acute stroke patients. Intensive Care Med 2002;28(8):1089–93.

53. Taplu A, Gokmen N, Erbayraktar S, et al. Effects of pressure- and volume-controlled inverse ratio ventilation on haemodynamic variables, intracranial pressure and cerebral perfusion pressure in rabbits: a model of subarachnoid haemorrhage under isoflurane anaesthesia. Eur J Anaesthesiol 2003;20(9): 690–6.

54. Kerwin AJ, Croce MA, Timmons SD, et al. Effects of fiberoptic bronchoscopy on intracranial pressure in

patients with brain injury: a prospective clinical study. J Trauma 2000;48(5):878–82 [discussion: 882–3].

55. Ely EW, Meade MO, Haponik EF, et al. Mechanical ventilator weaning protocols driven by nonphysician health-care professionals: evidence-based clinical practice guidelines. Chest 2001;120(Suppl 6): 454S–63S.

56. Jaskulka R, Weinstabl C, Schedl R. The course of intracranial pressure during respiratory weaning after severe craniocerebral trauma. Unfallchirurg 1993;96(3):138–41 [in German].

57. Coplin WM, Pierson DJ, Cooley KD, et al. Implications of extubation delay in brain-injured patients meeting standard weaning criteria. Am J Respir Crit Care Med 2000;161:1530–6.

58. Namen AM, Ely EW, Tatter SB, et al. Predictors of successful extubation in neurosurgical patients. Am J Respir Crit Care Med 2001;163(3 Pt 1): 658–64.

Microdialysis in the Neurocritical Care Unit

Ryan Kitagawa, MD[a], Shoji Yokobori, MD, PhD[a,b],
Anna T. Mazzeo, MD[c], Ross Bullock, MD, PhD[a,*]

KEYWORDS

- Microdialysis • Neuromonitoring • Traumatic brain injury • Subarachnoid hemorrhage

KEY POINTS

- Microdialysis is a neuromonitoring technique for direct measurement of cerebral metabolism.
- Microdialysis has a role in traumatic brain injury and subarachnoid hemorrhage, and the clinical applications continue to expand.
- Microdialysis may be used as a research tool for studying the cerebral effects of medications, pathophysiologic mechanisms, or other cerebral metabolic processes.

INTRODUCTION/HISTORY

Monitoring the brain after acute injury is central to the practice of neurocritical care and is analogous to hemodynamic monitoring for the cardiovascular system. However, the most widely available clinical monitor, the physical examination, is unavailable in neurologically compromised or sedated patients. Current neuromonitoring techniques have evolved from the study of cerebral physiology and allow for the repeated or continuous measurement of multiple cerebral parameters. These measurements may detect evolving abnormalities and thus guide interventions designed to minimize secondary injury after neurosurgical interventions, traumatic brain injury (TBI), or subarachnoid hemorrhage (SAH).[1] However, no monitor alone can improve patient outcome. Only actions such as decompressive craniectomy for increased intracranial pressure (ICP), based on monitoring data, carry the prospect of improving outcome, and for

microdialysis (MD), this aspect requires further studies.

Many neuromonitoring devices attempt to assess changes in cerebral metabolism. This process may be indirectly estimated from global imaging modalities such as xenon computed tomography (CT) and through measuring cerebral oxygen content with jugular venous oxygen saturation (Sjvo$_2$) catheters and cerebral oxygenation (partial pressure of oxygen in brain tissue [Pbto$_2$]) probes. Direct metabolic substrate measurement in the living human brain currently can only be achieved with cerebral MD catheters or positron emission tomography (PET) scans, which can only be done at great cost and for 1 or 2 time points.

The use of small (approximately 1 mm) semipermiable coaxial and loop membrane tubes within the brain was first described by Bito and colleagues in 1960 and was later refined in 1972 with the advent of the coaxial MD catheter by Delgado

Disclosures: There are no financial disclosures or conflicts of interest for any of the authors.
[a] Department of Neurosurgery, Lois Pope LIFE Center, Miller School of Medicine, University of Miami, 1095 Northwest 14th Terrace, Miami, FL 33136, USA; [b] Department of Emergency and Critical Care Medicine, Nippon Medical School, 1-1-5 Sendagi Bunkyo-ku, Tokyo, Japan 113-0083; [c] Department of Anesthesia and Critical Care, Azienda Ospedaliera Città della Salute e della Scienza di Torino-Presidio Molinette, University of Turin, Corso Dogliotti 14, Torino 10126, Italy
* Corresponding author.
E-mail address: rbullock@med.miami.edu

and colleagues. In 1986, the first data on neurotransmitter concentrations in the rat brain were reported by Tossman and colleagues.[2]

The first human implantation occurred in 1987 in adipose tissue and was followed in 1990 with the first use in human cerebral tissues.[3] In 1992, the first clinical use of this device was reported, and the creation of commercially available catheters and bedside analysis systems followed shortly.[2,4–6] Over time, MD has gained popularity in trauma, stroke, and aneurysmal SAH, and, as more studies verify its usefulness, the indications for use will continue to expand. As of 2012, about 12 centers in North America and about 30 worldwide clinically use brain MD on a regular basis.

MD MEASUREMENT
The Device

The monitoring device consists of a double-lumen dialysis probe that is implanted within the cerebral tissue (**Fig. 1**). A physiologic fluid (artificial cerebrospinal fluid [CSF] or normal saline without lactate or glucose) is passed into the probe and over the dialysis membrane using a micropump injector. The concentration gradients between the probe fluid and the surrounding tissue cause various molecules to diffuse across the membrane and into the solution, which is collected and analyzed in sampling vials or passed over a

detector system such as a glucose oxidase–based electrochemical sensor.[7] This fluid analysis is not a direct measure of the extracellular concentrations because the concentration in the dialysate depends on the membrane (pore size and surface area), the rate of the fluid flow, the size of the extracellular space, and the individual solutes' rates of diffusion. It is therefore termed the relative recovery.[6]

There are commercially available 20-kD and 100-kD cutoff membrane probes; however, at the present time, only the 20-kD (CMA70, CMA Microdialysis AB, Solna, Sweden) probe has been approved by the US Food and Drug Administration for human use in the United States and Japan. In Europe, clinical trials with the 100-kD MD probe for the measurement of cerebral intercellular cytokines, neurotrophic factors, and biomarkers are ongoing.[8–11] A flow rate of 0.3 μL/min is used for 10 mm of membrane length using a 20-kD cutoff membrane. With these settings, the flow recovery rate of CMA70 is approximately 70% for small molecules such as glucose, lactate, pyruvate, glutamate, and glycerol.[12,13]

Once the device is assembled and secured, the system allows hourly sample collection with bedside, computerized analysis. The device consists of the MD probe, connection tubing, perfusion media, pump, and collection device (see **Fig. 1**).[2] Commercially available assays currently

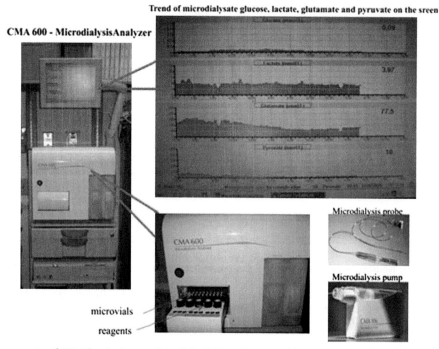

Fig. 1. Components of MD. The device consists of the MD probe, connection tubing, perfusion media, pump, and collection device. The MD analyzer then presents the data in a variety of formats including the trends over time.

include glucose, lactate, pyruvate, glycerol, and glutamate, in a 12-μL sample aliquot (**Table 1**). At present, the cost of the setup is approximately $120,000 ($60 per probe and $110,000 for the CMA 600 analyzer and pump). Thus, frequent use lowers the cost substantially per patient.

Reimbursement, and Cost Recovery

Several Swedish neurointensive care centers, such as Karolinska, Lund, and Uppsalla have shown that use of MD data can contribute to improved clinical decision making in the most severely injured patients with TBI and SAH. Nursing, critical care, and neurosurgical staff use data from MD to aid decisions, such as vasospasm management, ventilator weaning, choice of oxygen saturation, CSF drainage, and decompressive craniectomy. However, data to justify the cost of MD in terms of improved patient outcome are lacking. In European Union countries, costs have historically been amortized over general patient care and intensive care unit costs, but, in the countries of itemized billing, such as the United States, most centers have funded early MD experience from research grants.

Chen and colleagues[13] recently showed that MD costs can be successfully covered by using inpatient billing codes 99291, and 99292. The procedural code 61105 was introduced to cover twist-drill craniostomy and placement of monitoring catheters with devices such as MD.

Device Implantation

The probe tip is implanted through a twist-drill craniostomy or at the time of surgery. The dura is incised, and the catheter tip is passed to the appropriate depth. This insertion may be done freehand and then tunneled through a skin incision away from the skull defect, or the MD catheter may be a part of a bundled, bolt-based system. The freehand method allows for more precise anatomically selected positioning of the catheter tip but is more labor intensive because the bundle allows for the simultaneous placement of other monitoring devices such as ICP monitors and $Pbto_2$ probes.

Because the present system may only sample a small tissue zone, estimated to be about a 10-mm sphere around the catheter tip, several locations are potential targets for device implantation. For TBI, probes placed directly into contusions have been shown to yield severe derangements in metabolism consistent with tissue death and are unresponsive to any manipulations, and therefore this location is not recommended.

Egstrom and colleagues[14] investigated the placement of MD catheters within the penumbra zones as well as within the anatomically normal brain. They found a statistically significant difference in the glucose, lactate, lactate/pyruvate ratio (LPR), glutamate, and glycerol levels between the two catheter locations. Thus, placing the probe in structurally normal tissue may aid in assessing global cerebral metabolic condition, and placing the probe in pericontusional tissue may provide direct data on the microenvironment of the potentially salvageable tissue.[5] For aneurismal SAH, insertion of the device in the parent artery distribution aids in the detection of vasospasm and may be achieved at surgery for aneurysm clipping.[15]

STANDARD BIOMARKERS OF CLINICAL RELEVANCE (WITH 20-KD MD)

The range of investigational molecule analytes continues to expand, but glucose, lactate, pyruvate,

---

Table 1
Normal value of small molecule analytes that may be measured with commercially available reagents and analyzers such as the CMA 600 (collected with conventional 20-kD cutoff membrane)

Parameters	Clinical Significance	Normal Value (Mean ± SD)
Glucose	Decrease in hypoxia/ischemia	1.7 ± 0.9 mmol/L
Lactate	Increase in hypoxia/ischemia	2.9 ± 0.9 mmol/L
Pyruvate	Decrease in hypoxia/ischemia	166 ± 47 μmol/L
LPR	Best marker for anaerobic metabolism Increase in hypoxia/ischemia	23 ± 4
Glycerol	Increase with the destruction of cell membrane structure and free radical generation	82 ± 44 μmol/L
Glutamate	Increase in hypoxia/ischemia and excitotoxicity	16 ± 16 μmol/L

Abbreviations: LPR, lactate/pyruvate ratio; SD, standard deviation.
Data from Reinstrup P, Stahl N, Mellergard P, et al. Intracerebral microdialysis in clinical practice: baseline values for chemical markers during wakefulness, anesthesia, and neurosurgery. Neurosurgery 2000;47:701–10.

glycerol, and glutamate levels are the current standard for cerebral metabolism available from a 12-μL sample with the CMA analyzer device.[4] These data in combination with other monitoring tools such as ICP monitors, Pbto$_2$ probes, Sjvo$_2$ catheters, electroencephalography, and other modalities are commonly used in the intensive care unit.

Glucose, the primary energy substrate, is initially transported from the extracellular fluid into the cell cytoplasm and, through glycolysis, it is converted to pyruvate. Pyruvate is then aerobically metabolized in the mitochondria through the citric acid (TCA) cycle (**Fig. 2**). Under normal circumstances, 95% of the cerebral energy requirements come from the aerobic conversion of glucose to water (H$_2$O) and carbon dioxide (CO$_2$). Through this process, ATP synthesis is highly efficient and results in the generation of 38 molecules of ATP for each molecule of glucose:

$$1\ glucose + 6O_2 + 38ADP + 38Pi \rightarrow 6CO_2 + 6H_2O + 38ATP$$

Under hypoxic conditions such as TBI, conversion of glucose can only take place by anaerobic glycolysis because of mitochondrial dysfunction, and only 2 molecules of ATP and 2 molecules of lactate are generated for each molecule of glucose:

$$1\ glucose + 2ADP + 2Pi \rightarrow 2\ lactate + 2ATP$$

With normal aerobic states, pyruvate and the reduced form of nicotinamide adenine dinucleotide (NADH) are taken up by mitochondria, and their oxidation by the TCA cycle and respiratory chain provide most of the ATP production. With the anaerobic state, reoxidation of NADH through the respiratory chain is blocked and must instead occur by the reductive conversion of pyruvate to lactate by lactate dehydrogenase (LDH) (see **Fig. 2**). Thus, an increase of the LPR indicates failure of oxidative phosphorylation and may portend future or ongoing cerebral injury from ischemia or hypoxia.[5,15–19]

In general, the LPR normal range averages 23 $\pm$ 4 (mean $\pm$ standard deviation [SD]),[20] and the mean normal glucose values are 1.7 $\pm$ 0.9 mmol/L (see **Table 1**).[6] However, metabolic crisis may occur at a glucose less than 0.8 mmol/L with an LPR greater than 25, and thus several investigators have suggested the MD may indicate brain tissue at risk of delayed damage caused by high ICP or vasospasm.[20–22]

An additional target molecule, glycerol, is an integral component of cell membranes. The loss of

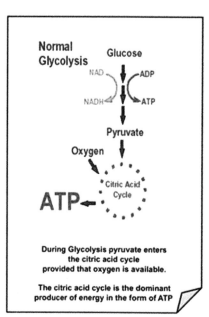
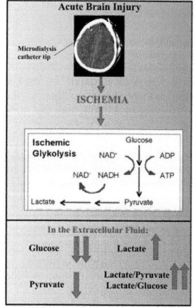

Fig. 2. Aerobic and anaerobic glycolytic cascade. Glucose is taken into the cytoplasm of neuronal cells and used as the main energy substrate. Under normal circumstance, 38 molecules of ATP are generated in the TCA cycle. Under hypoxic conditions, conversion of glucose takes place by anaerobic glycolysis, and 2 molecules of ATP and 2 molecules of lactate are generated. Under these conditions, reoxidation of the reduced form of nicotinamide adenine dinucleotide (NADH) through the respiratory chain is blocked and must instead occur by the reductive conversion of pyruvate to lactate by lactate dehydrogenase (LDH). NAD, nicotinamide adenine dinucleotide.

energy caused by ischemia causes an influx of calcium as well as a decomposition of cell membranes caused by free radical activation. When this breakdown occurs, glycerol is released into the interstitial fluid. This mechanism is supported by laboratory studies that show that glycerol generation occurs in proportion to free radical production in the tissues.[23] Thus, glycerol is an important marker of cell membrane damage. The glutamatergic system is also an important mediator for inducing excitotoxic damage in TBI. With brain injury, presynaptic glutamate secretion induces excitotoxicity and an increase in the influx of Ca2+ through N-methyl-D-aspartate (NMDA) receptors.[24] Thus, the glutamate measurements can aid in the evaluation of excitotoxicity after injury.[25]

CURRENT GUIDELINES FOR CLINICAL APPLICATION

As MD gained favor among intensive care doctors, a consensus meeting was held in 2002 to determine its use. The recommendations included[15] that:

1. This procedure is clinically indicated in aneurismal SAH and severe TBI.
2. The catheter should be placed in the tissue at risk (pericontusional tissues, right frontal in diffuse axonal injury, and within the distribution of vessels at risk for vasospasm) and an additional catheter should be place in CT normal-appearing tissue in patients with TBI.
3. All values are unreliable for the first hour after insertion.
4. Glutamate and the LPR are reliable markers of ischemia.
5. MD may assist with targeted therapy to prevent secondary ischemia.

MD IN TBI
Molecular Trends in TBI

MD has a multitude of research and clinical uses in TBI and, at present, the most common patient care indication is avoiding secondary injury. In TBI, ischemia after the primary injury is common and may lead to metabolic derangements that are reflected by changes in extracellular concentrations of key molecules. Thus, under anaerobic conditions, a decrease in glucose to zero or near zero, an increase in lactate, and an increase in the LPR to more than 20 to 30 is expected. If this ischemic pattern is detected before irreversible damage, interventions such as increasing inspired oxygen or decreasing ICP may help salvage vulnerable tissue and improve patient outcomes.

To test whether these alterations in glucose, lactate, and glutamate concentrations would accompany ischemia, Hlatky and colleagues[26] placed both Pbto2 probes and MD catheters in patients with severe TBI. They analyzed the MD findings when the Pbo2 probe indicated that ischemia was present (<10 mm Hg), and, as expected, the dialysate glucose significantly decreased, whereas the lactate, LPR, and glutamate increased under these hypoxic conditions. In addition, Belli and colleagues[27] explored the relationship between MD patterns and increases in ICP in 25 patients and showed that an LPR greater than 25 or a glycerol level greater than 100 μmol/L with a normal ICP strongly predicted an increase in ICP within 3 hours. Thus, if trends toward ischemia are noted, maneuvers to increase cerebral perfusion and decrease ICP may be instituted.

Several studies have attempted to identify critical substrate values that predict a poor outcome, and thus, if interventions could reverse the progression toward these critical values, the patient outcome may improve. Paraforou and colleagues[28] compared the MD results in 34 patients with severe TBI and found that all favorable outcome patients had LPRs less than 37 and glycerol levels less than 72 mmol/L. These findings raise the possibility of cutoff values similar to ICP, cerebral perfusion pressure (CPP), and Pbto2. However, at present, no study has found that interventions directly based on MD results improve patient outcomes. This may be because a single MD probe may only show changes in a small region of brain, whereas patient outcome depends on whole-brain changes. Thus, it is important to specify a detailed probe location when interpreting the literature concerning brain MD. Perhaps combining data sets from many of the centers that use MD worldwide could yield sufficient statistical power to achieve this aim.[15]

Outcome Prediction in TBI

After multiple animal and human studies verified the ability of MD to reliably detect ischemic and other putatively harmful neurochemical trends in TBI, investigators attempted to determine whether metabolic derangements recorded with MD could predict outcome. Goodman and colleagues[29] and other investigators reported that in severe patients with TBI, the median lactate level and the lactate-glucose ratio were statistically significantly higher in patients who died.[30] Chamoun and colleagues[31] studied glutamate levels in 165 patients with severe TBI and identified 2 distinct patterns. In pattern 1, the glutamate normalized over time (started low and remained low or started high and decreased over time), and, in pattern 2, the glutamate increased over time or remained increased. The pattern 2 patients had a statistically significant higher mortality and poorer outcome compared with pattern 1.[25]

Low and colleagues[32] attempted to predict patient outcomes based on parameters such as time of admission, mean arterial pressure, ICP, CPP, Pbto$_2$ data, and MD results. These investigators found that the addition of MD to this model improved its predictive value from 78% to 90%, and this variable was even shown to improve the predictive value more than Pbto$_2$ data.

Bullock and colleagues[25] initially developed an ischemia score based on hypoxemia, hypotension, cerebral blood flow, herniation, and low CPP, and this score was negatively correlated with the Glasgow Outcome Score (GOS) at 3 months and 6 months. With the addition of MD, a statistically significant relationship between lactate and pyruvate and the ischemic score was found. A correlation of the lactate/glucose ratio and the 3-month outcome was also found.[33]

Understanding TBI

MD can also play a major research role in understanding the pathophysiologic mechanisms that accompany TBI. We have explored neuronal vulnerability using MD with cerebral vascular autoregulation measurements in patients with severe TBI. In 3470 MD samples from 25 patients, the cerebral extracellular biomarkers (glucose, lactate, pyruvate, glycerol, and glutamate) were measured. The calculated pressure reactivity index (PRx), ICP, and mean arterial pressure were used to estimate cerebral vascular autoregulation.

After injury, the extracellular glucose concentration decreased, and the levels of glycerol, glutamate, and LPR, which indicate cerebral ischemia and neural cell damage, increased. On the fourth day after injury, the extracellular glucose concentration improved, and the value of LPR decreased. Along with these trends, the average PRx decreased daily and became negative on the fifth day after injury (**Fig. 3**). These results suggest that cerebral vascular autoregulation, and thus the cerebral vulnerability, may recover on the fourth day after TBI.[34]

MD IN SAH

The outcome of patients with aneurismal SAH is determined by the primary injury from the aneurysm rupture as well as by the secondary injury from events such as vasospasm, which can compromise the cerebral blood flow and significantly affect metabolism.[35] Similar to TBI, an increased concentration of brain tissue lactate and an increased LPR could reflect ischemia, and, with early intervention, a reduction in permanent neurologic deficits from vasospasm may be possible.[36,37]

These metabolic derangements were verified by Schulz and colleagues,[38] who found lower levels of energy substrates, higher levels of lactate, and higher levels of neuronal injury markers in patients with severe and complete ischemia. Unterberg and colleagues[39] also showed that, with ischemia, glucose decreased by 64%, lactate increased by 112%, and glutamate increased approximately 400% compared with a normal extracellular environment.[40]

One important SAH study found that this ischemic metabolic pattern preceded the occurrence of a delayed ischemic neurologic deficit (DIND). In this study, the mean delay from the peak in the LPR to the occurrence of a DIND was 23 hours (range 4–50 hours) and the mean delay from the ischemic metabolic pattern to a DIND was 11 hours. These results had a sensitivity for prediction of a DIND of 94%, a specificity of 88%, and a positive predictive value of 85%. Thus, in the proper clinical setting, MD may predict the occurrence of a DIND and cerebral infarction an average of 11 hours before its clinical appearance.[41] Although these data need more generalized validation in multiple centers, no other method of neuromonitoring offers the potential to preemptively detect harmful events and trends in patients with both SAH and severe TBI.

Glutamate has also been shown to be increased in the extracellular fluid of patients with SAH after secondary insults. This increase may be caused by an increased release from neurons or a decreased reuptake by astrocytes from the synaptic cleft,[42] and may lead to neuronal injury and poor outcome.[43]

Invasive metabolic monitoring may thus help to select those patients who may benefit from measures such as endovascular intervention or decompressive hemicraniectomy by the early detection of critical vulnerability. Studies on the effect of intracranial hypertension in patients with SAH showed that 83% of patients who developed increased ICP had cerebral metabolic derangements before the first increase in ICP (LPR >25, glycerol >80 μmol/L, and glutamate >10 μmol/L for >6 hours).[44] The sensitivity of MD for detecting cerebral compromise in patients with SAH may be better than that of ICP and CPP monitoring because the LPR or Pbto$_2$ were abnormal in many instances when the ICP was initially normal and then increased.

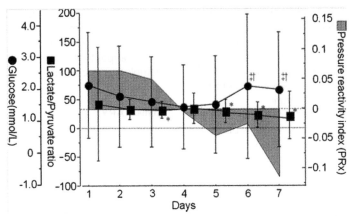

Fig. 3. The time course of biomarkers in 3470 microdialysates and PRx. The extracellular concentration of glucose decreased until day 4 and then increased until day 7. The daily average PRx decreased after day 1 and became negative after day 4. With improved cerebral pressure autoregulation, the extracellular glucose concentration increased, and LPR, which indicates tissue ischemia, decreased.

MOLECULES UNDER INVESTIGATION

In addition to the clinically available markers, many other molecules are currently being investigated for SAH and TBI. Mellergard and colleagues[45] reported the extracellular cerebral response of 2 of the most studied neurotrophic factors, fibroblast growth factor 2 (FGF2) and vascular endothelial growth factor (VEGF). The VEGF concentration was significantly higher in patients with TBI, whereas the FGF2 showed a tendency to be higher in patients with SAH. These data will assist in determining the inflammatory mechanism of injury and in identifying a potential threshold value for these chemokines for interventions as well as the possible timing of neural transplantation strategies.

Nitric oxide (NO) metabolite concentrations after SAH are another potential area of study. NO concentrations decreased on average by 21% in patients with SAH, which may lead to vasoconstriction and decreased local CBF.[46] Khaldi and colleagues[47] showed that brain tissue oxygen tension was strongly correlated with dialysate nitrate and nitrite, suggesting that substrate delivery and NO are linked in the pathophysiology of vasospasm after SAH.

Using 100-kDa MD probes, specific changes in certain protein concentrations occur approximately 4 days before the onset of symptomatic vasospasm. In particular, the protein concentrations of several isoforms of glyceraldehyde-3-phosphate dehydrogenase (GAPDH) were 1.79-fold higher in the patient group that later developed symptomatic vasospasm, whereas heat-shock cognate 71-kDa protein (HSP7C) isoforms were decreased to 0.50-fold. Thus, GAPDH and HSP7C may be used as early markers indicating the later development of symptomatic vasospasm after SAH.[48]

LIMITATIONS AND FUTURE DIRECTIONS

Although MD catheters have a multitude of uses, they have many drawbacks. The most limiting factor is the cost and labor-intensive nature of the collection and analytical systems despite the elegantly simple and robust pump and probes. This factor has restricted their widespread use throughout the neurointensive care community. Many samples are necessary for the acquisition of data and trends, and a qualified individual must spend time gathering and interpreting the results.[49] Also, many of the time-dependent changes in the 5 commonly used analytes are too complex for the current level of understanding, and thus cannot be translated into changes in patient care.

The limited volume of brain tissue sampled from the device is also a consideration. The current recommendation is to place the probe tip in pericontusional tissue in patients with TBI and the parent vessel territory in patients with SAH. Accurate placement can be difficult, and an aberrant probe position such as in the ventricle or outside the dura may render the data useless. In addition, the probes are delicate and cannot withstand pulling or head rotations unless carefully secured to the scalp, and inadvertent fracture of the membrane or disconnection from the pump preclude its use.[50]

In a series of 48 patients with MD probes, Stuart and colleagues[51] had 14 patients (29%) with catheter-related issues. These issues included catheter dislodgement, malfunction of the micro-pump collection system, and failure of sample analysis by the computer system. The limitations include the complications from the invasive procedure, and, although the risk is small, intracranial hemorrhage and infections are possible but have not been reported in the literature.

There are a multitude of studies attempting to expand the clinical indications for MD. In particular, quantifiable assays of antibiotics, anticonvulsants, neuroprotectants, and chemotherapeutic agents hold promise for more accurate and effective central nervous system dose determination.[52,53] In addition, catheters with higher membrane permeability may assist in studies of inflammatory markers and their effects on the brain.[50] Another area of interest is the use of MD to determine a drug's effect on cerebral metabolism. In a study by Mazzeo and colleagues,[54] cyclosporine A was administered to patients with severe TBI, and the brain energy metabolism was measured. This study showed that brain glucose, lactate, and pyruvate were higher in the cyclosporine group compared with the control group, and the LPR was decreased in the cyclosporine group.

Another active research area is novel biomarkers. Investigators are attempting to identify new molecules with prognostic value within the blood and CSF, but MD offers a unique opportunity for monitoring the extracellular fluid for potential targets.

From a clinical standpoint, nearly every area of cerebral dysfunction has the potential to benefit from these devices by determining prognosis, effectiveness of an intervention, and pathophysiologic mechanism. In the literature, multiple investigators have described its use in pediatric head trauma, stroke, intracerebral hematoma, and general comatose patients.

MD studies in epilepsy have shown a large increase in glutamate in the hippocampus of epileptic patients during the onset of a seizure. Extracellular glutamate has also been found to be increased in the epileptogenic focus as well as the pathway of propagation.[55] In studies with liver failure, extracellular glutamine correlated with the LPR as well as ICP. Thus, with the assistance of MD, the mechanism for cerebral edema may be elucidated and targeted therapies may be developed.[56]

Neuroanatomy and physiology also benefit from the use of MD. Fried and colleagues[57] placed MD catheters into epileptic patients in conjunction with depth electrodes and discovered that extracellular dopamine in the human amygdala increased with reading, memory, and learning. In patients who quickly mastered a task, the dopamine increased rapidly and slowly diminished, whereas the dopamine slowly increased in patients who required more time to gain experience. MD has a great potential impact on the study of both normal and pathologic processes.

SUMMARY

MD has yielded important results in neuromonitoring for neurologically compromised patients. This device allows the direct measurement of extracellular molecules in an attempt to characterize metabolic derangements before they become clinically relevant. Advancements in technology have allowed for the bedside assay of multiple markers of ischemia and dysfunction in energy production, and the applications for TBI and aneurismal SAH have been well established. As clinicians become more comfortable with these tools, their widespread use will increase and the potential for clinical impact will continue to increase. No other neuromonitoring technique has such potential at minimal cost in terms of invasiveness and risk to the patient.

Well-organized multicenter studies are needed to define new analyte biomarkers and to determine the threshold values of these analytes to suggest actions to be taken in the patient. Only on this basis can a rational study be designed to determine whether use of MD can improve patient outcome, which is the ultimate goal of the neurointensivist.

REFERENCES

1. Dunn IF, Ellegala DB, Kim DH, et al. Neuromonitoring in neurological critical care. Neurocrit Care 2006;4: 83–92.
2. Lee GJ, Park JH, Park HK. Microdialysis applications in neuroscience. Neurol Res 2008;30:661–8.
3. Hillered L, Persson L, Ponten U, et al. Neurometabolic monitoring of the ischaemic human brain using microdialysis. Acta Neurochir 1990;102:91–7.
4. Dhawan V, DeGeorgia M. Neurointensive care biophysiological monitoring. J Neurointerv Surg 2012; 4:407–13.
5. Goodman JC, Robertson CS. Microdialysis: is it ready for prime time? Curr Opin Crit Care 2009;15: 110–7.
6. Tisdall MM, Smith M. Cerebral microdialysis: research technique or clinical tool. Br J Anaesth 2006;97:18–25.
7. Jones DA, Ros J, Landolt H, et al. Dynamic changes in glucose and lactate in the cortex of the freely moving rat monitored using microdialysis. J Neurochem 2000;75:1703–8.

8. Helmy A, Carpenter KL, Skepper JN, et al. Microdialysis of cytokines: methodological considerations, scanning electron microscopy, and determination of relative recovery. J Neurotrauma 2009;26:549–61.

9. Hutchinson PJ, O'Connell MT, Nortje J, et al. Cerebral microdialysis methodology–evaluation of 20 kDa and 100 kDa catheters. Physiol Meas 2005;26: 423–8.

10. Magnoni S, Esparza TJ, Conte V, et al. Tau elevations in the brain extracellular space correlate with reduced amyloid-beta levels and predict adverse clinical outcomes after severe traumatic brain injury. Brain 2012;135:1268–80.

11. Petzold A, Tisdall MM, Girbes AR, et al. In vivo monitoring of neuronal loss in traumatic brain injury: a microdialysis study. Brain 2011;134:464–83.

12. Amberg G, Lindefors N. Intracerebral microdialysis: II. Mathematical studies of diffusion kinetics. J Pharmacol Methods 1989;22:157–83.

13. Chen JW, Rogers SL, Gombart ZJ, et al. Implementation of cerebral microdialysis at a community-based hospital: a 5-year retrospective analysis. Surg Neurol Int 2012;3:57.

14. Engstrom M, Polito A, Reinstrup P, et al. Intracerebral microdialysis in severe brain trauma: the importance of catheter location. J Neurosurg 2005;102: 460–9.

15. Bellander BM, Cantais E, Enblad P, et al. Consensus meeting on microdialysis in neurointensive care. Intensive Care Med 2004;30:2166–9.

16. Goodman JC, Valadka AB, Gopinath SP, et al. Lactate and excitatory amino acids measured by microdialysis are decreased by pentobarbital coma in head-injured patients. J Neurotrauma 1996;13:549–56.

17. Pellerin L, Magistretti PJ. Neuroenergetics: calling upon astrocytes to satisfy hungry neurons. Neuroscientist 2004;10:53–62.

18. Vespa P, Bergsneider M, Hattori N, et al. Metabolic crisis without brain ischemia is common after traumatic brain injury: a combined microdialysis and positron emission tomography study. J Cereb Blood Flow Metab 2005;25:763–74.

19. Yokobori S, Watanabe A, Matsumoto G, et al. Lower extracellular glucose level prolonged in elderly patients with severe traumatic brain injury: a microdialysis study. Neurol Med Chir (Tokyo) 2001;51: 265–71.

20. Reinstrup P, Stahl N, Mellergard P, et al. Intracerebral microdialysis in clinical practice: baseline values for chemical markers during wakefulness, anesthesia, and neurosurgery. Neurosurgery 2000; 47:701–10.

21. Stein NR, McArthur DL, Etchepare M, et al. Early cerebral metabolic crisis after TBI influences outcome despite adequate hemodynamic resuscitation. Neurocrit Care 2012;17:49–57.

22. Timofeev I, Carpenter KL, Nortje J, et al. Cerebral extracellular chemistry and outcome following traumatic brain injury: a microdialysis study of 223 patients. Brain 2011;134:484–94.

23. Merenda A, Gugliotta M, Holloway R, et al. Validation of brain extracellular glycerol as an indicator of cellular membrane damage due to free radical activity after traumatic brain injury. J Neurotrauma 2008; 25:527–37.

24. Choi DW. Glutamate neurotoxicity and diseases of the nervous system. Neuron 1988;1:623–34.

25. Bullock MR, Zauner A, Woodward JJ, et al. Factors affecting excitatory amino acid release following severe human head injury. J Neurosurg 1998;89: 507–18.

26. Hlatky R, Valadka AB, Goodman JC, et al. Patterns of energy substrates during ischemia measured in the brain by microdialysis. J Neurotrauma 2004;21: 894–906.

27. Belli A, Sen J, Petzold A, et al. Metabolic failure precedes intracranial pressure rises in traumatic brain injury: a microdialysis study. Acta Neurochir (Wien) 2008;150:461–70.

28. Paraforou T, Paterakis K, Fountas K, et al. Cerebral perfusion pressure, microdialysis biochemistry and clinical outcomes in patients with traumatic brain injury. BMC Res Notes 2011;4:540–6.

29. Goodman JC, Valadka AB, Gopinath SP, et al. Extracellular lactate and glucose alterations in the brain after head injury measured by microdialysis. Crit Care Med 1999;27:1965–73.

30. Hillered L, Persson L, Milsson P, et al. Continuous monitoring of cerebral metabolism in traumatic brain injury: a focus on cerebral microdialysis. Curr Opin Crit Care 2006;12:112–8.

31. Chamoun R, Suki D, Gopinath SP, et al. Role of extracellular glutamate measured by cerebral microdialysis in severe traumatic brain injury. J Neurosurg 2010;113:564–70.

32. Low D, Kuralmani V, Ng SK, et al. Prediction of outcome utilizing both physiological and biochemical parameters in severe head injury. J Neurotrauma 2009;26:1177–82.

33. Mazzeo AT, Kunene NK, Choi S, et al. Quantitation of ischemic events after severe traumatic brain injury in humans: a simple scoring system. J Neurosurg Anesthesiol 2006;18:170–8.

34. Yokobori S, Watanabe A, Matsumoto G, et al. Time course of recovery from cerebral vulnerability after severe traumatic brain injury: a microdialysis study. J Trauma 2001;71:1235–40.

35. Zetterling M, Hillered L, Samuelsson C, et al. Temporal patterns of interstitial pyruvate and amino acids after subarachnoid haemorrhage are related to the level of consciousness – a clinical microdialysis study. Acta Neurochir 2009;151: 771–80.

36. Kolias AG, Sen J, Belli A. Pathogenesis of cerebral vasospasm following aneurismal subarachnoid hemorrhage: putative mechanisms and novel approaches. J Neurosci Res 2009;87:1–11.

37. Noshe DP, Peerdeman SM, Comans EF, et al. Cerebral microdialysis and positron emission tomography after surgery for aneurysmal subarachnoid hemorrhage in grade I patients. Surg Neurol 2005; 64:109–15.

38. Schulz MK, Wang LP, Tange M, et al. Cerebral microdialysis monitoring: determination of normal and ischemic cerebral metabolisms in patients with aneurysmal subarachnoid hemorrhage. J Neurosurg 2000;93:808–14.

39. Unterberg AW, Sakowitz OW, Sarrafzadeh AS, et al. Role of bedside microdialysis in the diagnosis of cerebral vasospasm following aneurysmal subarachnoid hemorrhage. J Neurosurg 2001;94:740–9.

40. Sarrafzadeh A, Haux D, Sakowitz O, et al. Acute focal neurological deficits in aneurysmal subarachnoid hemorrhage: relation of clinical course, CT findings, and metabolite abnormalities monitored with bedside microdialysis. Stroke 2003;34:1382–8.

41. Skjoth-Rasmussen J, Schulz M, Kristensen SR, et al. Delayed neurological deficits detected by an ischemic pattern in the extracellular cerebral metabolites in patients with aneurysmal subarachnoid hemorrhage. J Neurosurg 2004;100:8–15.

42. Wu CT, Wen LL, Wong CS, et al. Temporal change in glutamate, glutamate transporters, basilar artery wall thickness, and neuronal variability in an experimental rat model of subarachnoid hemorrhage. Anesth Analg 2001;112:666–73.

43. Staub F, Graf R, Gabel P, et al. Multiple interstitial substances measured by microdialysis in patients with subarachnoid hemorrhage. Neurosurgery 2000;47:1106–16.

44. Nagel A, Graetz D, Vajkoczy P, et al. Decompressive craniectomy in aneurysmal subarachnoid hemorrhage: relation to cerebral perfusion pressure and metabolism. Neurocrit Care 2009;11:384–94.

45. Mellergard P, Sjogren F, Hillman J. Release of VEGF and FGF in the extracellular space following severe subarachnoid haemorrhage or traumatic head injury in humans. Br J Neurosurg 2010;24:261–7.

46. Sakowitz OW, Wolfrum S, Sarrafzadeh AS, et al. Relation of cerebral energy metabolism and extracellular nitrite and nitrate concentrations in patients after aneurysmal subarachnoid hemorrhage. J Cereb Blood Flow Metab 2001;21:1067–76.

47. Khaldi A, Zauner A, Reinert M, et al. Measurement of nitric oxide and brain tissue oxygen tension in patients after severe subarachnoid hemorrhage. Neurosurgery 2001;49:33–40.

48. Maurer MH, Haux D, Sakowitz OW, et al. Identification of early markers for symptomatic vasospasm in human cerebral microdialysate after subarachnoid hemorrhage: preliminary results of a proteome-wide screening. J Cereb Blood Flow Metab 2007;27 1675–83.

49. Wright W. Multimodal monitoring in the ICU: when could it be useful? J Neurol Sci 2007;261:10–5.

50. Oddo M, Villa F, Citerio G. Brain multimodality monitoring: an update. Curr Opin Crit Care 2012;18 111–8.

51. Stuart RM, Schmidt M, Kurtz P, et al. Intracranial multimodal monitoring for acute brain injury: a single institution review of current practices. Neurocrit Care 2010;12:188–98.

52. Alves OL, Doyle AJ, Clausen T, et al. Evaluation of topiramate neuroprotective effect in severe TBI using microdialysis. Ann N Y Acad Sci 2003;993: 25–53.

53. Miller CM. Update on multimodality monitoring. Curr Neurol Neurosci Rep 2012;12:474–80.

54. Mazzeo AT, Alves OL, Gilman CB, et al. Brain metabolic and hemodynamic effects of cyclosporin A after human severe traumatic brain injury: a microdialysis study. Acta Neurochir 2008;150: 1019–31.

55. Pan JW, Williamson A, Cavus I, et al. Neurometabolism in human epilepsy. Epilepsia 2008;49:31–41.

56. Bjerring PN, Hauerberg J, Frederiksken HJ, et al. Cerebral glutamine concentration and lactate-pyruvate ratio in patients with acute liver failure. Neurocrit Care 2008;9:3–7.

57. Fried I, Wilson CL, Morrow JW, et al. Increased dopamine release in the human amygdala during performance of cognitive tasks. Nat Neurosci 2001;4:201–6.

Parenchymal Brain Oxygen Monitoring in the Neurocritical Care Unit

Peter D. Le Roux, MD[a],*, Mauro Oddo, MD[b]

KEYWORDS

- Brain monitoring • Brain oxygen • Clark electrode • Hypoxia • Neurocritical care
- Optical fluorescence • Traumatic brain injury • Subarachnoid hemorrhage

KEY POINTS

- Parenchymal brain tissue oxygen ($PbtO_2$) monitoring is a safe and reliable technique for continuous bedside evaluation of patients with severe brain injury.
- Two techniques, a modified Clark electrode that uses the electrochemical properties of noble metals or optical fluorescence technology, can be used to measure $PbtO_2$.
- $PbtO_2$ indicates the balance between regional oxygen supply and cellular oxygen consumption and may be described by the equation $PbtO_2 = CBF \times AVTo_2$, where CBF is cerebral blood flow, Pvo_2 is partial oxygen pressure in mixed venous blood, and $AVTo_2$ is $Pao_2 - Pvo_2$.
- $PbtO_2$ values less than 20 mm Hg are considered worth treating and values less than 15 mm Hg are consistent with brain hypoxia or ischemia.
- Reduced $PbtO_2$ is associated with worse outcome in acute brain injury in adults and children, although the strength of this relationship may depend on probe location.
- When severe traumatic brain injury care is based on data from both a $PbtO_2$ and intracranial pressure (ICP) monitor, some (but not all) observational series suggest that outcome is better than when just ICP-based care is provided.

INTRODUCTION

Patients with a variety of severe, acute neurologic disorders such as traumatic brain injury (TBI), subarachnoid hemorrhage (SAH), acute ischemic stroke, and intracerebral hemorrhage (ICH) often are admitted to the neurocritical care unit (NCCU). Despite much research and success in animal models, effective drug therapies for these disorders have not been identified in clinical trials.[1] Instead, much of patient management in the NCCU is centered on the early identification and removal of mass lesions and on the detection, prevention, and management of secondary brain insults that exacerbate outcome (eg, hypotension, hypoxia, seizures, increased intracranial pressure [ICP]). Careful and repeated assessment and monitoring of clinical and laboratory findings, imaging studies, and bedside physiologic data are consequently what drive modern neurocritical care.

A variety of monitors are currently in clinical use (**Box 1**), although the ideal monitor to assess neurologic function in the NCCU does not yet exist. These monitors may be classified into 2 broad categories: (1) radiographic or tomographic techniques that provide information at a single point in time, and (2) bedside monitors that may

a The Brain and Spine Center, Lankenau Medical Center, 100 E. Lancaster Ave, Wynnewood, PA 19096, USA;
b Service de Médecine Intensive Adulte, Medico-Surgical ICU, Centre Hospitalier Universitaire Vaudois - CHUV, Rue du Bugnon 46, Lausanne 1011, Switzerland
* Corresponding author.
E-mail address: lerouxp@mlhs.org

Neurosurg Clin N Am 24 (2013) 427–439
http://dx.doi.org/10.1016/j.nec.2013.03.001
1042-3680/13/$ – see front matter © 2013 Elsevier Inc. All rights reserved.

- Clinical evaluation, serial assessment
- Laboratory analysis
- Systemic: electrocardiogram, heart rate, blood pressure, O_2 saturation, end tidal CO_2 ($Etco_2$), temperature
- Hydraulic: ICP/cerebral perfusion pressure (CPP)
- Electrophysiology: electroencephalogram, somatosensory evoked potentials, brain stem auditory evoked response
- Radiographic/tomographic: positron emission tomography (PET), single-photon emission computed tomography, CT-P, stable Xe-CT (^{133}XE), magnetic resonance imaging (MRI)
- Cerebral blood flow (CBF): transcranial Doppler, laser Doppler, thermal diffusion probe, transcranial cerebral oximetry
- Metabolic: microdialysis, jugular venous oximetry, direct brain oxygen, near infrared spectroscopy
- Biosamples (cerebrospinal fluid or serum): eg, S100B, GFAP, NSE

Abbreviations: CT-P, CT – perfusion scan (computed tomography); GFAP, Glial fibrillary acidic protein; NSE, neuron specific enolase.

be subdivided into monitors that are (1) invasive or noninvasive, or (2) continuous or noncontinuous. More than 1 monitor is ideally used because the brain is a complex organ and no single method can provide complete information about its health. Furthermore, monitoring by itself does not alter outcome. Instead, it is how the information provided by the monitor is used that contributes to patient wellbeing, particularly when targeted to patient-specific pathophysiology. This article reviews one type of continuous physiologic monitor: direct measurement of parenchymal brain oxygen.

THE IMPORTANCE OF BRAIN OXYGEN

Maintenance of adequate tissue oxygenation is a fundamental objective in critical care medicine in general, and the assessment of tissue oxygenation is indispensable to care of the critically ill patient. The adult brain represents about 2% of body weight, but consumes about 20% of the oxygen consumed by the body. Greater than 90% of this oxygen is used by the mitochondria to produce ATP, which is integral to cell function.[2] For this

energy metabolism, brain cells must be supplied with oxygen and glucose, the primary fuel for the brain (although, in some circumstances, lactate also may be used).[3] Only then, and with normal mitochondrial function, can sufficient energy (ATP) be produced to maintain neuronal integrity and function. The brain lacks fuel stores and requires a continuous supply of glucose and oxygen. Therefore, continuous CBF, cerebral oxygen tension and delivery, and normal mitochondrial function are of vital importance to maintain brain function and tissue viability.

DEFINITION

There are 4 basic methods to measure brain oxygen: jugular venous bulb oximetry, direct brain tissue (parenchymal) oxygen tension measurement, near infrared spectroscopy, and oxygen-15 PET. This article discusses parenchymal brain oxygen measurement, the commonest technique currently used in the NCCU to assess cerebral oxygenation. Brain tissue oxygen, or parenchymal brain oxygen, is defined as the partial pressure of oxygen in the brain interstitial space and reflects the availability of oxygen for oxidative energy production. There has been debate about whether the technique measures tissue oxygen pressure or tension, and, accordingly, several abbreviations have been used for brain tissue oxygen. A consensus conference at the 13th International Symposium on Intracranial Pressure and Brain Monitoring held in July 2007 in San Francisco, California, proposed that $PbtO_2$ be used as the standard abbreviation. Hence, this article uses $PbtO_2$ when referring to brain tissue oxygen or parenchymal brain oxygen. Consistent with this abbreviation, recent clinical studies suggest that $PbtO_2$ may be best defined by the equation: $PbtO_2 = CBF \times AVTo_2$, where $AVTo_2$ is $Pao_2 - Pvo_2$ (ie, $PbtO_2$ represents the interaction between plasma oxygen tension and CBF).[4]

TECHNOLOGY

Brain oxygen ($PbtO_2$) monitors were first used in the clinical environment in 1993 and included in the treatment guidelines for severe TBI in 2007.[5] Two techniques are available: (1) a modified Clark electrode that uses the electrochemical properties of noble metals (eg, Licox, Integra Lifesciences, Plainsboro, NJ; or Neurovent-P Temp, Raumedic AG, Munchberg, Germany), and (2) optical fluorescence technology (eg, Neurotrend, Diametrics Medical, St Paul, MN, and Codman, Johnson & Johnson, Raynham, MA; and OxyLab Po_2, Oxford Optronix Ltd, Oxford, UK).

The Licox probe has been most frequently used in the NCCU. It is based on the Clark principle, which is a temperature-dependent oxygen-consuming process, and so a temperature probe is supplied with the PbtO$_2$ probe. This temperature probe measures brain temperature and allows for automatic calibration. The new Licox PMO probe can measure PbtO$_2$ and brain temperature using a single probe.[6] The Clark principle uses the electrochemical properties of noble metals to measure tissue oxygen content.[7] The Clark electrode consists of a membrane that covers a layer of electrolyte and 2 metallic electrodes. Oxygen diffuses through the membrane and is electrochemically reduced at the cathode. The greater the oxygen partial pressure, the more oxygen diffuses through the membrane. The change in voltage between the reference electrode and the measuring electrode is proportional to the amount of oxygen being reduced on the cathode. The Neurovent-P Temp, which uses the same polagraphic technique as the Licox, can also measure PbtO$_2$ and brain temperature with 1 catheter. There are important differences in values obtained by the Neurovent and Licox, and so the values obtained by these devices cannot be used interchangeably.[8,9] The Licox system averages oxygen over a probe area of 14 to 18 mm^2 and has excellent long-term stability, even after 7 days. The Neurovent-P Temp has a greater surface area (24 mm^2).

The second technique used to measure PbtO$_2$ is based on fluorescence quenching in which a marker changes color according to the ambient amount of gas. Optode sensors are used to measure concentrations of substances by photochemical reactions that create changes in indicator compound optical properties.[7] Unlike the Licox, this process does not consume oxygen and does not affect the measured oxygen level. However, the probe measures a smaller area. The Neurotrend uses this technique but it is no longer commercially available for clinical use. The accuracy and clinical stability of the Neurotrend sensor also seems to be less than the Licox system.[10] There are several other important differences between the Clark principle (eg, the Licox) and optical techniques (eg, Neurotrend). First, Licox catheters are precalibrated and so can be inserted without any preuse calibration. However postinsertion stabilization (about 1 hour) is required before readings are reliable. By contrast, the Neurotrend monitor needs bedside calibration to a defined oxygen concentration. Second, the catheters are of different lengths; the Neurotrend is inserted at a greater depth than the Licox catheter. Third, the critical PbtO$_2$ threshold for hypoxia is different and so it is difficult to compare studies

that use the different techniques. In addition, the Neurotrend changed design in 1998, making it difficult to compare between old and more recent studies that describe this technology.[11]

Direct PbtO$_2$ monitors provide a measure of PbtO$_2$ in units of tension (mm Hg). A conversion factor of 1 mm Hg = 0.003 mL O$_2$/100 g brain can be used to convert PbtO$_2$ values to units of concentration (mL O$_2$/100 cm^3). A PbtO$_2$ monitor is not a blood flow monitor. Instead, it indicates the balance between regional oxygen supply and cellular oxygen consumption and may be described by the equation: PbtO$_2$ = CBF × AVTO$_2$ (ie, the interaction between plasma oxygen tension and CBF).[4] PbtO$_2$ is influenced by many factors (**Box 2**), including CBF and the factors that regulate it, such as CO$_2$ and mean arterial blood pressure (MAP) but also with changes in arterial oxygen tension (Pao$_2$) and so lung function and hemoglobin.[11–14] In addition, a PbtO$_2$ monitor is different from a jugular bulb catheter that measures the venous oxygen content in blood leaving the brain (ie, the balance between oxygen delivery and oxygen use). By contrast, PbtO$_2$ is consistent with the oxygen that accumulates in brain tissue and PET studies suggest it may correlate inversely with the oxygen extraction fraction[15] and reflect oxygen diffusion rather than total oxygen delivery or metabolism.[14,16,17]

MONITOR INSERTION

Parenchymal brain oxygen measurement involves the insertion of a fine catheter (about 0.5 mm in

---

Box 2
Factors that may influence brain oxygen

- Local factors of major influence on PbtO$_2$
  - Oxygen consumption of neurons and glia cells
  - Oxygen diffusion conditions/gradients in tissue
  - Number of perfused capillaries per tissue volume
  - Length and diameter of perfused capillaries
  - Capillary perfusion rate and microflow pattern
  - Hemoglobin oxygen release in microcirculation
- Systemic factors of major influence on PbtO$_2$
  - Arterial BP, ICP, Pao$_2$, Paco$_2$, pH, temperature
  - Blood hemoglobin content, P50, viscosity, and hematocrit

diameter) into the brain tissue, specifically the white matter. The PbtO$_2$ catheters or probes can be inserted through a single-lumen or multiple-lumen bolt secured in a burr hole or they may be tunneled under the scalp. The procedure to insert the monitor may be performed in the operating room or at the bedside in the NCCU. PbtO$_2$ monitors usually are placed by neurosurgeons but, in some institutions, neurointensivists may insert these devices with neurosurgical backup. In general, PbtO$_2$ monitors are placed for similar reasons as an ICP monitor (ie, Glasgow Coma Scale [GCS] ≤8). The Licox system includes a brain temperature probe (thermocouple) that is inserted through a triple-lumen bolt with the PbtO$_2$ and ICP monitor (eg, Camino, Integra Neuroscience). However, if brain temperature is not measured (eg, a microdialysis catheter is inserted through the lumen instead of the temperature probe), the monitor should be calibrated manually on a regular basis (eg, every 30 minutes) by using core body temperature. Hemorrhage is the most common procedural complication and is identified in less than 1% of parenchymal monitors. Most of these are identified on imaging and are not of clinical importance. An INR less than or equal to 1.6 and platelet count of more than 100,000 are necessary to safely place an ICP or PbtO$_2$ monitor. Infection is rare[18] but device malfunction, similar to other monitors, may require troubleshooting in up to 10% of devices.

NORMAL AND ABNORMAL PBTO$_2$ VALUES

Physiologic studies suggest that mitochondria need an oxygen concentration of 1.5 mm Hg to produce ATP.[19] This level corresponds with a PbtO$_2$ between 15 and 20 mm Hg. A similar PbtO$_2$ level is observed using 7-T MRI techniques and fluorescent quenching techniques. PbtO$_2$ threshold values depend on what type of monitor is used. In general, when using a Licox monitor, PbtO$_2$ greater than 2–30 mm Hg is considered normal; these values have been verified in awake patients undergoing elective functional neurosurgical procedures.[20,21] PbtO$_2$ values less than 20 mm Hg are considered worth treating and values less than 15 mm Hg are consistent with brain hypoxia or ischemia (**Table 1**).[11,21–24,48,49]

REGIONAL VERSUS GLOBAL MEASUREMENT

PbtO$_2$ probes sample approximately 15 mm^2 of tissue around the tip and the PbtO$_2$ value depends on oxygen diffusion from the vasculature to a small amount of tissue.[4,16] Therefore, it is a regional monitor, whose values depend on probe location

Table 1
Licox PbtO$_2$ values

Condition	PbtO$_2$ Values (mm Hg)
Increased	>50[a]
Normal	25–35
Compromised; begin treating	20[b]
Brain hypoxia	15
Severe brain hypoxia	10
Cell death	<5

[a] The meaning of supranormal PbtO$_2$ values is unclear.
[b] In a National Institutes of Health–sponsored phase II trial currently underway to study PbtO$_2$, treatment is initiated when PbtO$_2$ is less than 20 mm Hg. Other investigators suggest treatment be initiated when PbtO$_2$ is less than 15 mm Hg.
Data from Refs.[11,15,20,22–47]

(**Fig. 1**), which has led to debate about probe location and whether the value can be used to make decisions about global oxygenation. In most patients, PbtO$_2$ is measured in normal-appearing (ie, on admission computed tomography [CT] scan) frontal subcortical white matter; there is evidence that this local measurement is an indicator of global oxygenation.[11,22,25,26,42,43] Consistent with this, 2 clinical studies have shown good correlation between PbtO$_2$ and jugular bulb venous oxygen saturation (Sjo$_2$), used to assess global brain oxygenation, in areas without focal disorders after TBI.[22,25] In areas with focal disorders, this correlation between PbtO$_2$ and Sjo$_2$ was absent and the PbtO$_2$ values reflected regional brain oxygenation better than jugular bulb oximetry.[25] Other studies also show that, when the probe is in tissue immediately adjacent to a contusion or other disorder (eg, a subdural hematoma), values are often lower, even if CPP is higher.[27,50,51] In addition, when the monitor is placed adjacent to abnormal brain, regional hypoxia lasts longer than in normal-appearing tissue[50] and the relationship with outcome seems to be more robust.[27]

PRACTICAL USE IN THE NCCU

Once inserted, a run-in or equilibration time of up to 1 hour is required before readings are stable. Adjustment of insertion depth (when used through an access device) is not possible with the Licox system and, if the monitor is removed, the insertion bolt then should be replaced if a new monitor is inserted to avoid potential contamination. The position and function of the PbtO$_2$ monitor should ideally be confirmed with a head CT scan or oxygen challenge test, particularly if the initial PbtO$_2$ reading after 30 to 60 minutes of stabilization is

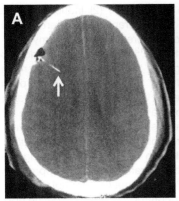
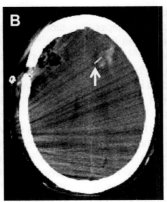
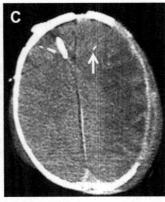

Fig. 1. A computed tomography (CT) head scan shows a Licox PbtO$_2$ probe (*arrow*) in (*A*) what appears to be normal white matter of the right frontal cortex, (*B*) in a contusion, and (*C*) adjacent to the penumbra. Brain oxygen levels may vary because of position. In particular, the probe in the contusion is unlikely to respond to an oxygen challenge and so would be considered nonfunctional.

abnormal. Transiently increasing the fraction of inspired oxygen (Fio$_2$) and observing the corresponding PbtO$_2$ increase can help confirm function or exclude the presence of surrounding microhemorrhages or sensor damage at insertion. An oxygen challenge is therefore performed when monitoring starts and, in some institutions, daily thereafter as part of regular clinical care to evaluate the function and responsiveness of the PbtO$_2$ probe or to determine oxygen reactivity. The oxygen challenge involves increasing the Fio$_2$ from baseline to 1.0 for approximately 5 minutes. This increase typically leads to a several-fold increase in the amount of oxygen dissolved in the plasma, translating into a mean 3-fold increase in PbtO$_2$.[4,13,14] However, the response to hyperoxia usually is less robust when the monitor is in an underperfused (CBF <20 mL/100 g/min) region.[52]

There are no specific recommendations on how long PbtO$_2$ should be monitored. In patients with TBI, we leave the monitor in place until ICP is normal for 24 hours without any specific treatment other than sedation for ventilation. On average, in patients with severe TBI this is 4 to 5 days. In patients with SAH, we tend to keep the monitor in place during the risk period for vasospasm. In addition, continuous PbtO$_2$ can be monitored twice as long as Sjo$_2$ and without needing recalibration. In studies that compare PbtO$_2$ with Sjo$_2$, good-quality data are acquired 95% of the time with PbtO$_2$, but only 43% of the time for Sjo$_2$.[22] Postinsertion noncontrast head CT confirmation of probe position in the brain parenchyma is important to interpret readings.[17,27,50] In some patients, a CT-perfusion study also may be useful. For example, if PbtO$_2$ readings are consistently low or poorly responsive to therapy, it is useful to know the monitor's proximity to a focal

abnormality or whether the region it is in is hypoperfused. In these cases, the PbtO$_2$ threshold for treatment may be lower than normally used.

THE PHYSIOLOGIC RATIONALE BEHIND PBTO$_2$ MONITORING

Monitoring in the NCCU has traditionally focused on ICP and its control. There is a large body of literature that shows a relationship between increased ICP, including even short episodes, and mortality.[53,54] The relationship between ICP and outcome among survivors is less clear[55] and, although ICP treatment benefits some patients, the results in large clinical series are less certain.[56–59] In part, this may stem from trial design, center variation, and prognostic heterogeneity. In addition, current management is largely a reactive model in which an abnormal value (threshold) from a single parameter triggers corrective action(s) to reverse the process largely in a phenomenological rather than mechanical manner. Hence treatment of the acutely injured brain based on an individual parameter (eg, ICP and CPP) may be an oversimplified approach to patient care,[60–63] and further treatment advances may depend on more rather than less information to better target and individualize care.

Several lines of clinical evidence using a variety of techniques suggest that PbtO$_2$ monitors, among other tools, may be an ideal complement to ICP monitors and hence targeted management of select patients in the NCCU. First, in cerebral microdialysis studies, decreases in PbtO$_2$ are associated with markers of cellular dysfunction[64]; hence PbtO$_2$ monitoring may be useful in clinical conditions in which cerebral ischemia or secondary brain injury may occur.[15] Second, pericontusional brain tissue exhibits persistent increase of lactate/pyruvate ratio (ie, cell energy dysfunction) independently of CPP.[65] Third, metabolic changes in the brain may occur before ICP increases.[66,67] Fourth, studies using jugular bulb catheters or $PbtO_2$ monitors show evidence for cellular hypoxia in the brain despite normal ICP and CPP in both adults and children, and that these events are common.[28–31,68–71] Fifth, PET studies show that cellular hypoxia after TBI is associated with abnormal oxygen diffusion rather than a perfusion deficit.[16] Together these findings suggest that a $PbtO_2$ monitor may provide unique, more, or earlier information about pathophysiologic changes occurring in the brain after acute injury that can supplement or complement information from other devices. An alternative is that $PbtO_2$ may be considered a novel target for resuscitation following brain injury and so expand potential therapeutic options.[31]

CLINICAL USE IN THE NCCU

A large body of observational clinical $PbtO_2$ data, primarily in patients with severe TBI and, less frequently, in SAH, has accrued since the early 1990s. In addition, use of $PbtO_2$ monitors has been described in several other conditions including brain tumors, intracerebral hemorrhage, stroke, cerebral edema associated with metabolic abnormalities, and meningitis. Recommendations about use are derived mainly from retrospective case-control and prospective observational studies. Based on these studies, $PbtO_2$ monitoring is recommended in patients with a GCS less than 9, particularly when there is an abnormal head CT scan or the patient is at risk for delayed ischemia (ie, when ICP monitoring is indicated).

   $PbtO_2$ monitoring is best used with other monitors (eg, an ICP monitor) and, like all other monitors, the information provided by a $PbtO_2$ monitor should be interpreted with data from the clinical examination, other monitors, and CT scan findings. The pathophysiologic changes that occur in the brain after injury, in the broad sense, are complex and different pathophysiologic processes may occur simultaneously or sequentially, and to varying degrees. Hence, use of a $PbtO_2$ and ICP (or other) monitor(s) together can improve insight about this complex pathophysiology (eg, provide information about autoregulation or help identify an optimal CPP target), and so allow intensive care unit staff to design strategies of care that are individualized and targeted.[72,73] Consistent with this, observational data suggest that $PbtO_2$ monitoring can potentially guide (eg, identify) potential deleterious effects of treatment or define responders and nonresponders of several therapies,

including (1) CPP[15,74–76]; (2) induced hypertension[74,77]; (3) osmotherapy and hypertonic saline use[78,79]; (4) decompressive craniectomy DC[80–82]; (5) hyperventilation[12,83–85]; (6) normobaric hyperoxia, although its role in resuscitation remains controversial[86–88]; (7) blood transfusion, particularly in patients with impaired cerebrovascular reserve who may be better transfused when oxygen delivery is compromised rather than a hemoglobin threshold reached[32,89–94]; (8) fluid balance[95]; (9) titration of sedatives, including use of propofol or barbiturates for burst suppression or ICP control[96–98]; (10) induced normothermia[99,100]; (11) ventilator control[101,102]; or (12) define optimal body position for nursing a patient.[103] Furthermore, information from a $PbtO_2$ monitor may help define a subset of patients who are at risk for patient transport.[104] In patients with SAH, $PbtO_2$ has also been used to help detect delayed cerebral ischemia (DCI) and to evaluate the effects of various therapies for DCI, angiography, or pharmacologic angioplasty.[74,105–107] In addition, studies in SAH have shown that, in some patients, nimodipine or intra-arterial papaverine can have unexpected adverse effects on $PbtO_2$.[108,109]

Use During Neurosurgical Procedures

$PbtO_2$ monitor use during neurosurgical procedures, in particular aneurysm or arteriovenous malformation (AVM) surgery is well described.[106,110,111] A correctly positioned $PbtO_2$ monitor allows the effects of temporary arterial occlusion to be examined; reduced $PbtO_2$ and especially brain hypoxia indicate low CBF and are associated with cerebral infarction.[110] $PbtO_2$ measurements have also been used during surgery to examine oxygenation of cerebral tissue during AVM or tumor surgery.[111,112] Reduced $PbtO_2$, before AVM resection suggests low perfusion and chronic hypoxia, whereas a marked $PbtO_2$ increase after AVM removal indicates hyperperfusion. The effects of inhalational agents[113] and propofol[98] on cerebral autoregulation and oxygenation during anesthesia have been examined using $PbtO_2$ monitoring. These studies show a dose-dependent loss of autoregulation but a corresponding increase in $PbtO_2$ provided CPP is maintained with inhalational agents, but not with propofol.

BRAIN OXYGEN INDICES
$PbtO_2$ Reactivity

The increase in $PbtO_2$ relative to an increase in arterial P_{O_2} is termed brain tissue oxygen reactivity. It is thought that this reactivity is controlled by an oxygen regulatory mechanism, and that this mechanism may be disturbed after brain injury. Van Santbrink and colleagues[114] examined the brain tissue oxygen response (ie, the change in $PbtO_2$ in response to changes in Pao_2) and showed that a greater response in the first 24 hours after injury was independently associated with an unfavorable outcome. The effect of $Paco_2$ on this mechanism has been studied in dogs[115] and in pigs[12]: $PbtO_2$ shows a linear correlation with CO_2 and MAP. A linear correlation with CBF during CO_2 reactivity testing was also found, which suggest that $PbtO_2$ is influenced by factors that regulate CBF, namely CO_2 and MAP.

Oxygen Reactivity Index

Soehle and colleagues[116] introduced the concept of $PbtO_2$ autoregulation, defined as the ability of the brain to maintain $PbtO_2$ despite CPP changes. This concept may facilitate identification of appropriate individual CPP targets. Additional studies by Lang and colleagues[73] showed a significant correlation between static cerebral autoregulation (determined using blood flow velocity in relation to changing CPP) and cerebral tissue oxygen reactivity (the rate of $PbtO_2$ change relative to changing CPP).[117] This finding suggests a close link between regulation of CBF and oxygenation. Impaired brain tissue oxygen pressure reactivity index is associated with worse outcome after TBI,[72] SAH,[118,119] and stroke.[72] These findings suggest that manipulation of Pbo_2 by altering Pao_2 or CPP can be used to optimize CPP management. In patients with acute ischemic stroke, impaired CPP brain tissue oxygen reactivity index predicts the development of

malignant edema after middle cerebral artery infarction.

BRAIN OXYGEN AND OUTCOME

Several observational studies suggest that reduced brain oxygen is associated with worse outcome in acute brain injury in adults[23,28,33–37,49,71,89] and children,[38,39,71] although the strength of this relationship may depend in part on probe location relative to other disorders, such as, in normal white matter, the penumbra or in a contusion.[27,51] Episodes of brain tissue hypoxia may occur when CPP and ICP are normal,[23,28,30,69,71] so emphasizing the value of using both monitors. The number, duration, and intensity of $PbtO_2$ episodes less than 15 mm Hg, and any $PbtO_2$ values less than or equal to 5 mm Hg are associated with poor outcome after TBI.[23,28,33–37,49] A $PbtO_2$ less than 10 mm Hg is associated with 2-fold to 4-fold increase in both mortality and unfavorable outcome,[37] including neuropsychological performance[40,41]; this is important because ICP generally is associated with mortality alone rather than outcome. Furthermore, the development of compromised $PbtO_2$ is an independent variable associated with outcome rather than simply an indicator of disease severity.[28] Reduced $PbtO_2$ is also associated with outcome in SAH, although the observed relationship is less robust than in TBI.[40,41]

MANAGEMENT OF BRAIN OXYGEN

The association between outcome and $PbtO_2$ in observational series has led to the concept of

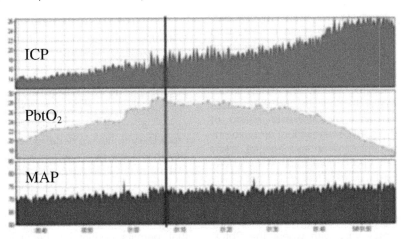

Fig. 2. Continuous monitoring of ICP, $PbtO_2$ and MAP, recorded over several hours, showing dynamic changes in ICP and its effect on $PbtO_2$. In particular, as ICP initially increases it is associated with an increase in $PbtO_2$. As ICP continues to increase, $PbtO_2$ eventually decreases (*vertical line*), which suggests the point at which ICP may be best treated in this individual (ie, targeted care), because it is at this point that the ICP increase is having an adverse effect on other measures of intracranial health. (*Adapted from* Rohlwink UK, Zwane E, Graham Fieggen A, et al. The relationship between intracranial pressure and brain oxygenation in children with severe traumatic brain injury. Neurosurgery 2012;70(5):1220–31; with permission.)

$PbtO_2$-based care. When severe TBI care is based on data from both a $PbtO_2$ and ICP monitor, some, but not all, observational series suggest that outcome is better than when just ICP-based care is provided[44–47]; this question is now being evaluated in a multicenter clinical trial. Oxygen delivery to the brain is the product of CBF and the arterial oxygen content and hence many variables can influence it (see **Box 2**). However, several physiologic factors suggest that even small changes in intracellular Po_2 can have a biological effect. First, neuronal mitochondria require an intracellular Po_2 as low as 1.5 mm Hg to maintain aerobic metabolism; this corresponds with a $PbtO_2$ between 15 and 20 mm Hg (ie, where treatment usually is initiated). Second, only oxygen dissolved in plasma can exchange between vascular and tissue compartments. However, oxygen is lipophilic and so can cross the endothelium (ie, influx through passive diffusion). Third, the apparent diffusion coefficient of oxygen is stable even with sustained ischemia. Fourth, cellular-mitochondrial gradients are small and, consistent with this, Zhou and colleagues[120] observed that normobaric hyperoxia administered after experimental TBI can restore mitochondrial ATP levels.

A $PbtO_2$ monitor does not influence outcome. Instead, information from a $PbtO_2$ monitor, like other monitors, should be interpreted and integrated with other data (eg, clinical examination, CT scan findings, ICP, CPP, pulmonary status, and hemoglobin). This approach allows patient-specific pathophysiology to be targeted and, in some circumstances, $PbtO_2$ to be used as a novel target or for otherwise unrecognized relationships to be defined, so moving away from empiric treatment alone. For example, in some patients who receive pressors to augment CPP in the presence of increased ICP, we have observed that induced hypotension (eg, nicardipine) instead has a better effect on physiology because it ameliorates an underlying hyperemia. In addition, the $PbtO_2$ data may permit avoidance of deleterious effects of other therapies (eg, hyperventilation) or avoid unnecessary treatment or overtreatment (eg, allow permissive intracranial hypertension in select patients who have a mild increase in ICP but otherwise normal cerebral physiology by defining when increased ICP adversely affects intracranial physiology) (**Fig. 2**). Although the relationship with outcome may vary with where the $PbtO_2$ probe is placed, treatment paradigms are largely based on the probe being in white matter that appears normal on head CT. In addition, the various techniques on how to manage $PbtO_2$ are still being elucidated. In large part, these therapies are based on understanding patient physiology (**Table 2**).

Table 2
Therapies to treat compromised brain oxygen

Frequently Used Therapy	Less Frequently Used Therapy
Adjust ventilator parameters to increase Pao_2 Increase Fio_2 (eg, 50%–60%) Increase PEEP	Ventriculostomy Continuous or intermittent CSF drainage
Transient hyperoxia 100% Fio_2	Blood transfusion
Augment CPP Colloid bolus Neosynephrine, dopamine	Neuromuscular paralysis Pancuronium, vecuronium
Pharmacologic analgesia and sedation Propofol, versed, ativan Fentanyl, morphine	Adjust ventilator rate Increase to lower $Paco_2$ (ICP) Decrease to increase $Etco_2$, $Paco_2$
Head position or avoid turning, certain positions	Pulmonary toilet and suction
ICP control Sedation, mannitol, IV lidocaine	Pentothal
Ensure temperature <38°C	DCH (or other cranial surgery)
	Labetalol, nicardipine

Abbreviations: DCH, decompressive hemicraniectomy; IV, intravenous; PEEP, positive end-expiratory pressure.
Data from Refs.[11,121,122]

Common therapies include changing head position, ventilator manipulation, transient increases in inspired oxygen, CPP augmentation, transfusion, and sedation, and these therapies are successful in correcting the abnormality in about 70% of episodes of reduced $PbtO_2$. Those patients who respond to a corrective therapy are more likely to have a better outcome[44,121,122] and treatments are best used in a cause-specific tier fashion rather than a stepwise linear fashion.

SUMMARY

$PbtO_2$ monitoring is a safe and reliable technique that permits continuous bedside evaluation of cellular function in patients with severe brain injury. Several variables including CBF, blood pressure, hemoglobin concentration, and systemic oxygenation influence $PbtO_2$. Reduced $PbtO_2$ (<20 mm Hg), often independent of ICP and CPP, is frequent after acute brain injury and can result from several pathologic mechanisms (eg, increased ICP, ischemia, impaired oxygen extraction, anemia, or altered lung function). Information from a $PbtO_2$ monitor can guide the care of patients in the NCCU and help optimize CPP, $Paco_2$, Pao_2, and hemoglobin targets in individual patients, particularly when used in an integrated fashion with other monitors. Furthermore, observational data show an independent association between $PbtO_2$ and outcome. This finding has led to the concept of $PbtO_2$-based care to supplement and complement management based on ICP and CPP; whether this benefits outcome is still to be fully elucidated but early clinical series have produced promising results.

REFERENCES

1. Maas AI, Menon DK, Lingsma HF, et al. Re-orientation of clinical research in traumatic brain injury: report of an international workshop on comparative effectiveness research. J Neurotrauma 2011;29: 32–46.

2. Astrup J, Sorensen PM, Sorensen HR. Oxygen and glucose consumption related to Na+-K+ transport in canine brain. Stroke 1981;12:726–30.

3. Oddo M, Levine JM, Frangos S, et al. Brain lactate metabolism in humans with subarachnoid hemorrhage. Stroke 2012;43(5):1418–21.

4. Rosenthal G, Hemphill JC 3rd, Sorani M, et al. Brain tissue oxygen tension is more indicative of oxygen diffusion than oxygen delivery and metabolism in patients with traumatic brain injury. Crit Care Med 2008;36:1917–24.

5. Brain Trauma Foundation, American Association of Neurological Surgeons; Congress of Neurological Surgeons, Joint Section on Neurotrauma and Critical Care, AANS/CNS. Guidelines for the management of severe traumatic brain injury. X. Brain oxygen monitoring and thresholds. J Neurotrauma 2007;24(Suppl 1):S65–70.

6. Stewart C, Haitsma I, Zador Z, et al. The new Licox combined brain tissue oxygen and brain temperature monitor: assessment of in vitro accuracy and clinical experience in severe traumatic brain injury. Neurosurgery 2008;63:1159–64 [discussion: 64–5].

7. Siegemund M, van Bommel J, Ince C. Assessment of regional tissue oxygenation. Intensive Care Med 1999;25:1044–60.

8. Dengler J, Frenzel C, Vajkoczy P, et al. Cerebral tissue oxygenation measured by two different probes: challenges and interpretation. Intensive Care Med 2011;37:1809–15.

9. Orakcioglu B, Sakowitz OW, Neumann JO, et al. Evaluation of a novel brain tissue oxygenation probe in an experimental swine model. Neurosurgery 2010;67(6):1716–22 [discussion: 1722–3].

10. Jaeger M, Soehle M, Meixensberger J. Brain tissue oxygen ($Ptio_2$): a clinical comparison of two monitoring devices. Acta Neurochir Suppl 2005; 95:79–81.

11. Maloney-Wilensky E, Le Roux P. The physiology behind direct brain oxygen monitors and practical aspects of their use. Childs Nerv Syst 2010;26(4): 419–30.

12. Hemphill JC 3rd, Knudson MM, Derugin N, et al. Carbon dioxide reactivity and pressure autoregulation of brain tissue oxygen. Neurosurgery 2001;48: 377–83.

13. Scheufler KM, Lehnert A, Rohrborn HJ, et al. Individual values of brain tissue oxygen pressure, microvascular oxygen saturation, cytochrome redox level and energy metabolites in detecting critically reduced cerebral energy state during acute changes in global cerebral perfusion. J Neurosurg Anesthesiol 2004;16:210–9.

14. Scheufler KM, Rohrborn HJ, Zentner J. Does tissue oxygen-tension reliably reflect cerebral oxygen delivery and consumption? Anesth Analg 2002;95: 1042–8.

15. Johnston AJ, Steiner LA, Coles JP, et al. Effect of cerebral perfusion pressure augmentation on regional oxygenation and metabolism after head injury. Crit Care Med 2005;33(1):189–95.

16. Menon DK, Coles JP, Gupta AK, et al. Diffusion limited oxygen delivery following head injury. Crit Care Med 2004;32:1384–90.

17. Longhi L, Valeriani V, Rossi S, et al. Effects of hyperoxia on brain tissue oxygen tension in cerebral focal lesions. Acta Neurochir Suppl 2002; 81:315–7.

18. Bailey RL, Quattrone F, Curtain C, et al. In: Proceedings of Neurocritical Care Society Annual meeting. The safety of multimodal monitoring in severe brain injury. Neurocritical Care Society Meeting. Montreal, 2011.

19. Siesjo BK, Siesjo P. Mechanisms of secondary brain injury. Eur J Anaesthesiol 1996;13:247–68.

20. Pennings FA, Schuurman PR, van den Munckhof P, et al. Brain tissue oxygen pressure monitoring in awake patients during functional neurosurgery: the assessment of normal values. J Neurotrauma 2008;25:1173–7.

21. Hoffman WE, Charbel FT, Edelman G. Brain tissue oxygen, carbon dioxide, and pH in neurosurgical patients at risk for ischemia. Anesth Analg 1996; 82(3):582–6.

22. Kiening KL, Unterberg AW, Bardt TF, et al. Monitoring of cerebral oxygenation in patients with severe head injuries: brain tissue Po_2 versus jugular vein oxygen saturation. J Neurosurg 1996;85(5): 751–7.

23. Chang JJ, Youn TS, Benson D, et al. Physiologic and functional outcome correlates of brain tissue

hypoxia in traumatic brain injury. Crit Care Med 2009;37(1):283–90.

24. Gopinath SP, Valadka AB, Uzura M, et al. Comparison of jugular venous oxygen saturation and brain tissue Po_2 as monitors of cerebral ischemia after head injury. Crit Care Med 1999;27:2337–45.

25. Gupta AK, Hutchinson PJ, Al-Rawi P, et al. Measuring brain tissue oxygenation compared with jugular venous oxygen saturation for monitoring cerebral oxygenation after traumatic brain injury. Anesth Analg 1999;88:549–53.

26. Gopinath SP, Valadka A, Contant CF, et al. Relationship between global and cortical cerebral blood flow in patients with head injuries. Neurosurgery 1999;44:1273–8.

27. Ponce LL, Pillai S, Cruz J, et al. Position of probe determines prognostic information of brain tissue Po_2 in severe traumatic brain injury. Neurosurgery 2012;70(6):1492–502.

28. Oddo M, Levine JM, Mackenzie L, et al. Brain hypoxia is associated with short-term outcome after severe traumatic brain injury independently of intracranial hypertension and low cerebral perfusion pressure. Neurosurgery 2011;69(5):1037–45 [discussion: 1045].

29. Figaji AA, Zwane E, Thompson C, et al. Brain tissue oxygen tension monitoring in pediatric severe traumatic brain injury. Part 2: relationship with clinical, physiological and treatment factors. Childs Nerv Syst 2009;25(10):1335–43.

30. Chen HI, Stiefel MF, Oddo M, et al. Detection of cerebral compromise with multimodality monitoring in patients with subarachnoid hemorrhage. Neurosurgery 2011;69(1):53–63 [discussion: 63].

31. Eriksson EA, Barletta JF, Figueroa BE, et al. Cerebral perfusion pressure and intracranial pressure are not surrogates for brain tissue oxygenation in traumatic brain injury. Clin Neurophysiol 2012; 123(6):1255–60.

32. Oddo M, Milby A, Chen I, et al. Hemoglobin concentration and cerebral metabolism in patients with aneurysmal subarachnoid hemorrhage: a microdialysis study. Stroke 2009;40(4):1275–81.

33. Valadka AB, Gopinath SP, Contant CF, et al. Relationship of brain tissue Po_2 to outcome after severe head injury. Crit Care Med 1998;26: 1576–81.

34. van den Brink WA, van Santbrink H, Steyerberg EW, et al. Brain oxygen tension in severe head injury. Neurosurgery 2000;46:868–76 [discussion: 76–8].

35. van Santbrink H, Maas AI, Avezaat CJ. Continuous monitoring of partial pressure of brain tissue oxygen in patients with severe head injury. Neurosurgery 1996;38:21–31.

36. Sarrafzadeh AS, Kiening KL, Callsen TA, et al. Metabolic changes during impending and manifest cerebral hypoxia in traumatic brain injury. Br J Neurosurg 2003;17:340–6.

37. Maloney-Wilensky E, Gracias V, Itkin A, et al. Brain tissue oxygen and outcome after severe traumatic brain injury: a systematic review. Crit Care Med 2009;37(6):2057–63.

38. Figaji AA, Zwane E, Thompson C, et al. Brain tissue oxygen tension monitoring in pediatric severe traumatic brain injury. Part 1: relationship with outcome Childs Nerv Syst 2009;25(10):1325–33.

39. Narotam PK, Burjonrappa SC, Raynor SC, et al. Cerebral oxygenation in major pediatric trauma its relevance to trauma severity and outcome. J Pediatr Surg 2006;41:505–13.

40. Meixensberger J, Renner C, Simanowski R, et al. Influence of cerebral oxygenation following severe head injury on neuropsychological testing. Neurol Res 2004;26:414–7.

41. O'Brien D, Frangos S, Watson E, et al. Brain oxygen and long-term functional and neurocognitive outcome after severe traumatic brain injury and subarachnoid hemorrhage. National Neurotrauma Annual Meeting, Las Vegas, 2010.

42. Meixensberger J, Vath A, Jaeger M, et al. Monitoring of brain tissue oxygenation following severe subarachnoid hemorrhage. Neurol Res 2003;25: 445–50.

43. Ramakrishna R, Stiefel M, Udoteuk J, et al. Brain oxygen and outcome in patients with aneurysmal subarachnoid hemorrhage. J Neurosurg 2008; 109(6):1075–82.

44. Spiotta AM, Stiefel MF, Gracias VH, et al. Brain tissue oxygen-directed management and outcome in patients with severe traumatic brain injury. J Neurosurg 2010;113:571–80.

45. Narotam PK, Morrison JF, Nathoo N. Brain tissue oxygen monitoring in traumatic brain injury and major trauma: outcome analysis of a brain tissue oxygen-directed therapy. J Neurosurg 2009;111: 672–82.

46. Martini RP, Deem S, Yanez ND, et al. Management guided by brain tissue oxygen monitoring and outcome following severe traumatic brain injury. J Neurosurg 2009;111(4):644–9.

47. Nangunoori R, Maloney-Wilensky E, Stiefel M, et al. Brain tissue oxygen-based therapy and outcome after severe traumatic brain injury: a systematic literature review. Neurocrit Care 2012; 17(1):131–8.

48. Doppenberg EM, Zauner A, Watson JC, et al. Determination of the ischemic threshold for brain oxygen tension. Acta Neurochir Suppl 1998;71: 166–9.

49. Bardt TF, Unterberg AW, Hartl R, et al. Monitoring of brain tissue Po_2 in traumatic brain injury: effect of cerebral hypoxia on outcome. Acta Neurochir Suppl 1998;71:153–6.

50. Longhi L, Pagan F, Valeriani V, et al. Monitoring brain tissue oxygen tension in brain-injured patients reveals hypoxic episodes in normal-appearing and in peri-focal tissue. Intensive Care Med 2007;33:2136–42.

51. Sarrafzadeh AS, Kiening KL, Bardt TF, et al. Cerebral oxygenation in contusioned vs. nonlesioned brain tissue: monitoring of Ptio$_2$ with Licox and Paratrend. Acta Neurochir Suppl 1998;71: 186–9.

52. Hlatky R, Valadka AB, Gopinath SP, et al. Brain tissue oxygen tension response to induced hyperoxia reduced in hypoperfused brain. J Neurosurg 2008; 108(1):53–8.

53. Vik A, Nag T, Fredriksli OA, et al. Relationship of "dose" of intracranial hypertension to outcome in severe traumatic brain injury. J Neurosurg 2008; 109(4):678–84.

54. Stein DM, Hu PF, Brenner M, et al. Brief episodes of intracranial hypertension and cerebral hypoperfusion are associated with poor functional outcome after severe traumatic brain injury. J Trauma 2011; 71(2):364–74.

55. Badri S, Chen J, Barber J, et al. Mortality and long-term functional outcome associated with intracranial pressure after traumatic brain injury. Intensive Care Med 2012;38(11):1800–9.

56. Stein SC, Georgoff P, Meghan S, et al. Relationship of aggressive monitoring and treatment to improved outcomes in severe traumatic brain injury. J Neurosurg 2010;112:1105–12.

57. Cremer OL, van Dijk GW, van Wensen E, et al. Effect of intracranial pressure monitoring and targeted intensive care on functional outcome after severe head injury. Crit Care Med 2005;33(10): 2207–13.

58. Shafi S, Diaz-Arrastia R, Madden C, et al. Intracranial pressure monitoring in brain-injured patients is associated with worsening of survival. J Trauma 2008;64(2):335–40.

59. Chesnut RM, Temkin N, Carney N, et al. A trial of intracranial-pressure monitoring in traumatic brain injury. N Engl J Med 2012;367(26):2471–81.

60. Oddo M, Le Roux P. What is the etiology, pathogenesis and pathophysiology of elevated intracranial pressure?. In: Neligan P, Deutschman CS, editors. The evidenced based practice of critical care. Philadelphia: Elsevier Science; 2009. p. 399–405.

61. Aries MJ, Czosnyka M, Budohoski KP, et al. Continuous determination of optimal cerebral perfusion pressure in traumatic brain injury. Crit Care Med 2012;40(8):2456–63.

62. Steiner LA, Czosnyka M, Piechnik SK, et al. Continuous monitoring of cerebrovascular pressure reactivity allows determination of optimal cerebral perfusion pressure in patients with traumatic brain injury. Crit Care Med 2002;30:733–8.

63. Jaeger M, Dengl M, Meixensberger J, et al. Effects of cerebrovascular pressure reactivity-guided optimization of cerebral perfusion pressure on brain tissue oxygenation after traumatic brain injury. Crit Care Med 2010;38:1343–7.

64. Hlatky R, Valadka AB, Goodman JC, et al. Patterns of energy substrates during ischemia measured in the brain by microdialysis. J Neurotrauma 2004; 21(7):894–906.

65. Vespa PM, O'Phelan K, McArthur D, et al. Pericontusional brain tissue exhibits persistent elevation of lactate/pyruvate ratio independent of cerebral perfusion pressure. Crit Care Med 2007;35(4): 1153–60.

66. Adamides AA, Rosenfeldt FL, Winter CD, et al. Brain tissue lactate elevations predict episodes of intracranial hypertension in patients with traumatic brain injury. J Am Coll Surg 2009;209:531–9.

67. Belli A, Sen J, Petzold A, et al. Metabolic failure precedes intracranial pressure rises in traumatic brain injury: a microdialysis study. Acta Neurochir (Wien) 2008;150:461–9.

68. Le Roux P, Lam AM, Newell DW, et al. Cerebral arteriovenous difference of oxygen: a predictor of cerebral infarction and outcome in severe head injury. J Neurosurg 1997;87:1–8.

69. Stiefel MF, Udoetek J, Spiotta A, et al. Conventional neurocritical care and cerebral oxygenation after traumatic brain injury. J Neurosurg 2006;105: 568–75.

70. Gracias VH, Guillamondegui OD, Stiefel MF, et al. Cerebral cortical oxygenation: a pilot study. J Trauma 2004;56:469–74.

71. Rohlwink UK, Zwane E, Graham Fieggen A, et al. The relationship between intracranial pressure and brain oxygenation in children with severe traumatic brain injury. Neurosurgery 2012;70(5): 1220–31.

72. Jaeger M, Schuhmann MU, Soehle M, et al. Continuous assessment of cerebrovascular autoregulation after traumatic brain injury using brain tissue oxygen pressure reactivity. Crit Care Med 2006; 34:1783–8.

73. Lang EW, Czosnyka M, Mehdorn HM. Tissue oxygen reactivity and cerebral autoregulation after severe traumatic brain injury. Crit Care Med 2003;31: 267–71.

74. Muench E, Horn P, Bauhuf C, et al. Effects of hypervolemia and hypertension on regional cerebral blood flow, intracranial pressure, and brain tissue oxygenation after subarachnoid hemorrhage. Crit Care Med 2007;35:1844–51.

75. Stocchetti N, Chieregato A, De Marchi M, et al. High cerebral perfusion pressure improves low values of local brain tissue O$_2$ tension (Ptio$_2$) in focal lesions. Acta Neurochir Suppl 1998;71: 162–5.

76. Marin-Caballos AJ, Murillo-Cabezas F, Cayuela-Dominguez A, et al. Cerebral perfusion pressure and risk of brain hypoxia in severe head injury: a prospective observational study. Crit Care 2005;9: R670–6.

77. Johnston AJ, Steiner LA, Chatfield DA, et al. Effect of cerebral perfusion pressure augmentation with dopamine and norepinephrine on global and focal brain oxygenation after traumatic brain injury. Intensive Care Med 2004;30:791–7.

78. Oddo M, Levine JM, Frangos S, et al. Effect of mannitol and hypertonic saline on cerebral oxygenation in patients with severe traumatic brain injury and refractory intracranial hypertension. J Neurol Neurosurg Psychiatry 2009;80(8):916–20.

79. Sakowitz OW, Stover JF, Sarrafzadeh AS, et al. Effects of mannitol bolus administration on intracranial pressure, cerebral extracellular metabolites, and tissue oxygenation in severely head-injured patients. J Trauma 2007;62:292–8.

80. Stiefel MF, Heuer GG, Smith MJ, et al. Cerebral oxygenation following decompressive hemicraniectomy for the treatment of refractory intracranial hypertension. J Neurosurg 2004;101:241–7.

81. Weiner GM, Lacey MR, Mackenzie L, et al. Decompressive craniectomy for elevated intracranial pressure and its effect on the cumulative ischemic burden and therapeutic intensity levels after severe traumatic brain injury. Neurosurgery 2010;66: 1111–9.

82. Ho CL, Wang CM, Lee KK, et al. Cerebral oxygenation, vascular reactivity, and neurochemistry following decompressive craniectomy for severe traumatic brain injury. J Neurosurg 2008;108: 943–9.

83. Carmona Suazo JA, Maas AI, van den Brink WA, et al. CO_2 reactivity and brain oxygen pressure monitoring in severe head injury. Crit Care Med 2000;28:3268–74.

84. Coles JP, Minhas PS, Fryer TD, et al. Effect of hyperventilation on cerebral blood flow in traumatic head injury: clinical relevance and monitoring correlates. Crit Care Med 2002;30:1950–9.

85. Clausen T, Scharf A, Menzel M, et al. Influence of moderate and profound hyperventilation on cerebral blood flow, oxygenation and metabolism. Brain Res 2004;1019:113–23.

86. Tolias CM, Reinert M, Seiler R, et al. Normobaric hyperoxia–induced improvement in cerebral metabolism and reduction in intracranial pressure in patients with severe head injury: a prospective historical cohort-matched study. J Neurosurg 2004;101:435–44.

87. Nortje J, Coles JP, Timofeev I, et al. Effect of hyperoxia on regional oxygenation and metabolism after severe traumatic brain injury: preliminary findings. Crit Care Med 2008;36:273–81.

88. Diringer MN. Hyperoxia: good or bad for the injured brain? Curr Opin Crit Care 2008;14:167–71.

89. Oddo M, Levine JM, Kumar M, et al. Anemia and brain oxygen after severe traumatic brain injury. Intensive Care Med 2012;38(9):1497–504.

90. Smith MJ, Stiefel MF, Magge S, et al. Packed red blood cell transfusion increases local cerebral oxygenation. Crit Care Med 2005;33:1104–8.

91. Figaji AA, Zwane E, Kogels M, et al. The effect of blood transfusion on brain oxygenation in children with severe traumatic brain injury. Pediatr Crit Care Med 2010;11(3):325–31.

92. Leal-Noval SR, Munoz-Gomez M, Aerllano-Orden V, et al. Impact of age of transfused blood on cerebral oxygenation in male patients with severe traumatic brain injury. Crit Care Med 2008; 36:1290–6.

93. Le Roux P. Haemoglobin management in acute brain injury. Curr Opin Crit Care 2013;19(2):83–91.

94. Le Roux PD. Participants in the International Multidisciplinary Consensus Conference on the Critical Care Management of Subarachnoid Hemorrhage. Anemia and transfusion after subarachnoid hemorrhage. Neurocrit Care 2011;15(2):342–53.

95. Fletcher JJ, Bergman K, Blostein PA, et al. Fluid balance, complications, and brain tissue oxygen tension monitoring following severe traumatic brain injury. Neurocrit Care 2010;13(1):47–56.

96. Chen HI, Malhotra NR, Oddo M, et al. Barbiturate infusion for intractable intracranial hypertension and its effect on brain oxygenation. Neurosurgery 2008;63:880–6 [discussion: 6–7].

97. Thorat JD, Wang EC, Lee KK, et al. Barbiturate therapy for patients with refractory intracranial hypertension following severe traumatic brain injury: its effects on tissue oxygenation, brain temperature and autoregulation. J Clin Neurosci 2008; 15:143–8.

98. Johnston AJ, Steiner LA, Chatfield DA, et al. Effects of propofol on cerebral oxygenation and metabolism after head injury. Br J Anaesth 2003;91: 781–6.

99. Oddo M, Frangos S, Milby A, et al. Induced normothermia attenuates cerebral metabolic distress in patients with aneurysmal subarachnoid hemorrhage and refractory Fever. Stroke 2009;40(5): 1913–6.

100. Oddo M, Frangos S, Maloney-Wilensky E, et al. Effect of shivering on brain tissue oxygenation during induced normothermia in patients with severe brain injury. Neurocrit Care 2010;12(1):10–6.

101. Oddo M, Nduom E, Frangos S, et al. Acute lung injury is an independent risk factor for brain hypoxia after severe traumatic brain injury. Neurosurgery 2010;67(2):338–44.

102. Rosenthal G, Hemphill JC, Sorani M, et al. The role of lung function in brain tissue oxygenation

following traumatic brain injury. J Neurosurg 2008; 108(1):59–65.

103. Ledwith MB, Bloom S, Maloney-Wilensky E, et al. Effect of body position on cerebral oxygenation and physiologic parameters in patients with acute neurological conditions. J Neurosci Nurs 2010; 42(5):280–7.

104. Swanson E, Mascitelli J, Stiefel M, et al. The effect of patient transport on brain oxygen in comatose patients. Neurosurgery 2010;66:925–32.

105. Ekelund A, Reinstrup P, Ryding E, et al. Effects of iso- and hypervolemic hemodilution on regional cerebral blood flow and oxygen delivery for patients with vasospasm after aneurysmal subarachnoid hemorrhage. Acta Neurochir (Wien) 2002;144: 703–12 [discussion: 12–3].

106. Kett-White R, Hutchinson PJ, Al-Rawi PG, et al. Cerebral oxygen and microdialysis monitoring during aneurysm surgery: effects of blood pressure, cerebrospinal fluid drainage, and temporary clipping on infarction. J Neurosurg 2002;96: 1013–9.

107. Dudkiewicz M, Proctor KG. Tissue oxygenation during management of cerebral perfusion pressure with phenylephrine or vasopressin. Crit Care Med 2008;36:2641–50.

108. Stiefel MF, Heuer GG, Abrahams JM, et al. The effect of nimodipine on cerebral oxygenation in patients with poor-grade subarachnoid hemorrhage. J Neurosurg 2004;101:594–9.

109. Stiefel MF, Spiotta A, Udoetek J, et al. Intra-arterial papaverine used to treat cerebral vasospasm reduces brain oxygen. Neurocrit Care 2006;4:113–8.

110. Gelabert-Gonzalez M, Fernandez-Villa JM, Ginesta-Galan V. Intra-operative monitoring of brain tissue O$_2$ (Ptio$_2$) during aneurysm surgery. Acta Neurochir (Wien) 2002;144:863–6 [discussion: 6–7].

111. Hoffman WE, Charbel FT, Edelman G, et al. Brain tissue oxygenation in patients with cerebral occlusive disease and arteriovenous malformations. Br J Anaesth 1997;78:169–71.

112. Pennings FA, Bouma GJ, Kedaria M, et al. Intraoperative monitoring of brain tissue oxygen and carbon dioxide pressures reveals low oxygenation in peritumoral brain edema. J Neurosurg Anesthesiol 2003;15:1–5.

113. Hoffman WE, Edelman G. Isoflurane increases brain oxygen reactivity in dogs. Anesth Analg 2000;91:637–41.

114. van Santbrink H, vd Brink WA, Steyerberg EW, et al. Brain tissue oxygen response in severe traumatic brain injury. Acta Neurochir (Wien) 2003;145: 429–38 [discussion: 38].

115. Hoffman WE, Edelman G, Wheeler P. Cerebral oxygen reactivity in the dog. Neurol Res 2000;22: 620–2.

116. Soehle M, Jaeger M, Meixensberger J. Online assessment of brain tissue oxygen autoregulation in traumatic brain injury and subarachnoid hemorrhage. Neurol Res 2003;25:411–7.

117. Ang BT, Wong J, Lee KK, et al. Temporal changes in cerebral tissue oxygenation with cerebrovascular pressure reactivity in severe traumatic brain injury. J Neurol Neurosurg Psychiatry 2007;78: 298–302.

118. Jaeger M, Schuhmann MU, Soehle M, et al. Continuous monitoring of cerebrovascular autoregulation after subarachnoid hemorrhage by brain tissue oxygen pressure reactivity and its relation to delayed cerebral infarction. Stroke 2007;38: 981–6.

119. Dohmen C, Bosche B, Graf R, et al. Identification and clinical impact of impaired cerebrovascular autoregulation in patients with malignant middle cerebral artery infarction. Stroke 2007;38:56–61.

120. Zhou Z, Daugherty WP, Sun D, et al. Protection of mitochondrial function and improvement in cognitive recovery in rats treated with hyperbaric oxygen following lateral fluid-percussion injury. J Neurosurg 2007;106(4):687–94.

121. Pascual JL, Georgoff P, Horan A, et al. Brain tissue hypoxia in traumatic brain injury: are most commonly used interventions successful at correcting brain tissue oxygen deficits? J Trauma 2011;70(3):535–46.

122. Bohman LE, Heuer GG, Macyszyn L, et al. Medical management of compromised brain oxygen in patients with severe traumatic brain injury. Neurocrit Care 2011;14:361–9.

Use of Transcranial Doppler (TCD) Ultrasound in the Neurocritical Care Unit

Atul Kalanuria, MD[a], Paul A. Nyquist, MD[a],
Rocco A. Armonda, MD[b],
Alexander Razumovsky, PhD, FAHA[c],*

KEYWORDS

- Transcranial Doppler • Neurocritical care unit • Vasospasm • Stroke • Intracranial hypertension

KEY POINTS

- Transcranial Doppler (TCD) is a bedside procedure that measures linear cerebral blood flow velocity (CBFV) through the intracranial circulation and pulsatility index (PI).
- Several different disease processes can lead to intracerebral vasospasm, for example after subarachnoid hemorrhage, and traumatic brain injury. Intracerebral vasospasm will be represented by abnormally high CBFV.
- The PI's changes can be used for evaluation of high intracranial pressure (ICP). The PI is the reflection of downstream resistance and will be affected by abnormally high ICP.
- TCD can be used for detection of cerebral vessel occlusion and estimation of cerebrovascular reactivity. Contrast TCD is used for the diagnosis of right to left cardiac shunts, for patients with cryptogenic stroke.
- TCD is the unique standard for the detection of microembolic signals in real-time.
- TCD has high accuracy to confirm total cerebral circulatory arrest and has been used as an ancillary test to support clinical diagnosis of brain death.

INTRODUCTION

Transcranial Doppler ultrasonography (TCD) was introduced into the practice of medicine in 1986 and has been used extensively in a variety of inpatient and outpatient settings. TCD ultrasonography uses a handheld 2-MHz transducer that is placed on the surface of the scalp to measure the cerebral blood flow velocity (CBFV) and pulsatility index (PI) within the intracranial arteries. Because of its noninvasiveness and easy applications, TCD examinations have gained an important role in the very early phase, as well during the repetitive assessment of patients with cerebrovascular diseases (CVDs). This has led to a broad application of TCD in outpatients and inpatients, and emergency and intraoperative settings. This article describes specific clinical applications of TCD to diagnose and monitor vasospasm (VSP) for patients after subarachnoid hemorrhage (SAH) of different etiologies (aneurysm rupture, traumatic brain injury [TBI]) and cerebral hemodynamic changes in patients after stroke (including cryptogenic stroke). Other important clinical applications of TCD discussed are emboli monitoring, management of patients with sickle-cell disease, and so-called functional TCD. Advanced TCD application for

[a] Division of Neurocritical care, Department of Anesthesiology and Critical Care Medicine, The Johns Hopkins Hospital, 600 N. Wolfe Street, Baltimore, MD 21287, USA; [b] Walter Reed National Military Medical Center, 8901 Wisconsin Avenue, Bethesda, MD 20889, USA; [c] Sentient NeuroCare Services, 11011 McCormick Rd, Suite 200, Hunt Valley, MD 21031, USA
* Corresponding author.
E-mail address: arazumovsky@sentientmedical.com

Neurosurg Clin N Am 24 (2013) 441–456
http://dx.doi.org/10.1016/j.nec.2013.02.005

diagnosis and monitoring of patients with intracranial hypertension and confirmation of clinical diagnosis of brain death are also presented.

It should be noted that TCD has also been frequently used for the clinical evaluation of cerebral autoregulatory reserve, and to monitor cerebral circulation and emboli during cardiopulmonary bypass, carotid endarterectomies, and carotid artery stenting. Over the past decade, Power M mode, color Doppler imaging, and use of ultrasound contrast agents have extended the scope of TCD clinical applications. In addition, TCD is being increasingly used as a research tool.

Basic Concepts

TCD examination involves placement of the probe of a range-gated ultrasound Doppler instrument, allowing the velocities in the arteries to be determined from the Doppler signals.[1] At 2-MHz frequency, the attenuation in bone and soft tissues is considerably less as compared with higher frequencies and provides satisfactory recordings of intracranial CBFVs.[1] An ultrasonic beam transmitted by the probe crosses the skull at prespecified locations and is reflected back from the flowing erythrocytes in the blood vessels. These erythrocytes move at different speeds and the resultant Doppler signal obtained is a mixture of different frequency components. The Doppler shift is the difference between the transmitted signal and the received signal and the time interval from pulse emission to reception determines the depth from which any Doppler frequency shift is detected.[1,2] Spectral analysis then presents 3-dimensional Doppler data in a 2-dimensional format. The time vector is represented on the horizontal scale while velocity (frequency shift) is displayed on the vertical scale. The brightness of color represents the signal intensity. Mean CBFV is calculated using a spectral envelope (also known as Fast Fourier transformation [FFT]), which corresponds to the time averaged flow velocity

throughout a cardiac cycle[3]: Mean CBFV = [PSV + (EDV × 2)]/3, where PSV is peak systolic CBFV and EDV is end-diastolic CBFV.[4]

The relationship between the velocity and pressure exerted by blood flowing through the cerebral arteries is described by the Bernoulli principle, which states that as the velocity of flow increases, the pressure exerted by that fluid decreases. TCD ultrasonography is based on the principle that the CBFV in a given artery is inversely related to the cross-sectional area of that artery.[5] Thus, TCD ultrasonography provides an indirect evaluation of the vessel diameter by calculating the Doppler shift.[4] TCD also allows measurement of PSV and EDV. Using these values, the mean CBFV, PI, and resistance index (RI) can be calculated.[6]

There are several physiologic factors affecting CBFV, among them age, hematocrit, vessel diameter, gender, fever, metabolic factors, exercise, and brain activity.[6–9] **Table 1** outlines mean CBFV based on different age groups in anterior and posterior circulation. Other variables measured with TCD examination are a PI (Gosling Index) and/or RI (Pourcelot Index): PI = (PSV − EDV)/mean CBFV and RI = (PSV − EDV)/PSV.[4] The physiologic meaning of these indices is the reflection of downstream resistance. **Table 2** outlines Mean CBFVs and associated conditions.[4–6,14,15]

PI It is a calculated index of the TCD waveform. The pulsatility of the waveform reflects the amount of resistance in the more distal cerebral blood vessels.[4,16] With the intracranial pressure (ICP) higher than 20 mm Hg, the PI has been evaluated as an alternative to direct ICP measurement.[15,17,18] There is also a significant correlation between the cerebral perfusion pressure (CPP) and PI.[4,18] Similarly, it has been observed that that RI also has good correlation with elevated ICP in various intracranial processes. However, as compared with the PI, the RI is less sensitive to ICP changes.[17] The PI and RI have been observed to be influenced by factors such as arterial blood pressure, cerebral vascular resistance, partial pressure of carbon

Table 1
Mean cerebral blood flow velocities (cm/s) based on age groups

Artery	Age 20–40 y	Age 40–60 y	Age >60 y
Anterior cerebral artery	56–60	53–61	44–51
Middle cerebral artery	74–81	72–73	58–59
Posterior cerebral artery (PCA) (P1)	48–57	41–56	37–47
PCA (P2)	43–51	40–57	37–47
Vertebral artery	37–51	29–50	30–37
Basilar artery	39–58	27–56	29–47

Data from Refs.[10–13]

Table 2
Clinical scenarios associated with changes in CBFV

Elevated CBFV	Decreased CBFV
Vasospasm/Hyperemia	Elevated intracranial
Elevated $Paco_2$	pressure
Loss of autoregulatory	Hypothermia
mechanism	Low blood
Stenosed arterial tree	pressure (BP)
Increasing age	Reduced cerebral
Volatile anesthetic	blood flow
agents	Reduced cardiac
Sickle cell anemia	output (below 35%
AV malformation	ejection fraction)
Meningitis (especially	Reduced $Paco_2$
bacterial)	Pregnancy
Preeclampsia	Anesthetics except
Fever	ketamine
Sepsis	Fulminant hepatic
	failure
	Brain death

Abbreviations: AV, arteriovenous; CBFV, cerebral blood flow velocity.

dioxide, and presence of arteriovenous malformation.[4,19] Agewise distribution of normal PIs are outlined in **Table 3** and variations in PI and RI values with disease states are given in **Table 4**. Insonation of cerebral arteries is done using 4 windows: (1) Temporal, (2) Orbital (3) Foraminal, and (4) Submandibular. Power M-mode (PMD) simplifies operator dependence by simultaneously displaying the power and direction of the blood flow over a wide range of depth, without sound or spectral clues.[20]

Variations

Few studies have discussed side-to-side as well as day-to-day variations in TCD CBFV.[6,11,21] These studies suggest that side-to-side variation of more than 14% should be considered abnormal.

Most individuals (95%) should have day-to-day variation less than 10 cm per second. Same day interobserver variability has been reported to be approximately 7.5%, and approximately 13% on different days.[6,21] Variation in middle cerebral artery (MCA) CBFV has also been observed with age, pregnancy, menstruation, and arousal of individuals.[6,11,22,23]

NEUROINTENSIVE CARE UNIT TCD APPLICATIONS
Vasospasm after SAH, TBI, and Tumor Resection

Symptomatic VSP after aneurysm rupture (aSAH) is associated with a high incidence of permanent disability and death.[24,25] TCD ultrasonography is a noninvasive and relatively inexpensive investigative modality and is being used increasingly after aSAH for the surveillance and monitoring of VSP.[2,26,27] VSP detected on TCD may precede neurologic deficits, prompting earlier intervention.[28] Hemodynamic changes seen in intracerebral vasculature after aSAH can be diagnosed and monitored using TCD; therefore, the primary application of TCD in aSAH is in the surveillance of VSP.[10,29]

Symptomatic VSP is a clinical diagnosis and its pathophysiology defined as decrease in blood flow through the regions of the brain after aSAH due to the constriction of cerebral arteries and it contributes to significant morbidity and mortality (up to 20%) after aSAH.[4,10,30,31] Angiographic VSP, as seen on digital subtraction angiography (DSA) and computed tomography angiography (CTA) occurs in up to 50% to 70% of patients of aSAH with about half of them suffering from clinical symptoms.[31,32] The exact reason for the occurrence of delayed cerebral ischemia is not clearly understood, and several theories exist.[33] Clinically, terms of delayed ischemic neurologic deficit

Table 3
Normal pulsatility index (mean ± SD) based on age groups

Artery	Age 20–40 y	Age 40–60 y	Age >60 y
Anterior cerebral artery	0.80 ± 0.14	0.85 ± 0.16	1.02 ± 0.18
Middle cerebral artery	0.83 ± 0.14	0.82 ± 0.13	0.96 ± 0.17
Posterior cerebral artery	0.76 ± 0.12	0.79 ± 0.12	0.94 ± 0.16
Vertebral artery	0.82 ± 0.03	0.78 ± 0.04	0.94 ± 0.05
Basilar artery	0.81 ± 0.05	0.78 ± 0.05	0.95 ± 0.09

Data from Marshall SA, Nyquist P, Ziai WC. The role of transcranial Doppler ultrasonography in the diagnosis and management of vasospasm after aneurysmal subarachnoid hemorrhage. Neurosurg Clin N Am 2010;21(2):291–303; and Martin PJ, Evans DH, Naylor AR. Transcranial color-coded sonography of the basal cerebral circulation. Reference data from 115 volunteers. Stroke 1994;25(2):390–6.

Table 4	
PI and RI indices and associated conditions	
Elevated PI/RI	**Decreased PI/RI**
Elevated ICP (due to TBI, ICH, SAH, stroke)	Vasospasm/Hyperemia AV malformation
Hydrocephalus	
Fulminant hepatic failure	
Meningitis (especially bacterial)	
Encephalopathy	
Brain death	

Abbreviations: AV, arteriovenous; ICH, intracranial hemorrhage; ICP, intracranial pressure; PI, pulsatility index; RI, resistance index; SAH, subarachnoid hemorrhage; TBI, traumatic brain injury.
    Insonation of cerebral arteries is done using 4 windows: (1) Temporal, (2) Orbital (3) Foraminal, and (4) Submandibular.
    Data from Refs.[4–6,14,15]

(DIND) and delayed cerebral ischemia (DCI) have been used to describe symptomatic VSP. Although VSP has been classically reported to occur between days 4 and 14 after aSAH, variations to this do occur and VSP has been reported as early as within 48 hours (in up to 13% of patients), and as late as 17 days[10,34–38] but could be also evident up to day 20 by TCD.[51,52]

Vasospasm on TCD ultrasound
Mild VSP Mean CBFV (cm/s): Terminal internal carotid artery (ICA) 120–130, MCA 120–130, basilar artery (BA) 60–80, vertebral artery (VA) 60–80.[10,39–49]

Moderate VSP Mean CBFV (cm/s): Anterior cerebral artery (ACA) >50% increase in 24 hours, terminal ICA >130, MCA 130–200, posterior cerebral artery (PCA) >110, BA 80–115, VA >80.[10,39–49]

Severe VSP Mean CBFV (cm/s): ACA >50% increase in 24 hours, MCA >200, PCA >110, BA >115, VA >80.[10,39–49]

In the intensive care unit (ICU), patients after aSAH often will be treated with triple-H therapy (hypertension, hypervolemia, hemodilution) that would cause increased cerebral blood flow (CBF) to the brain.[27,50] Therefore, it is very important to compliment full TCD examination with the measurement of so-called Lindegaard Index (LI), defined as the ratio of the mean CBFV of the MCA to that of extracranial portion of the ipsilateral ICA. This ratio increases with the severity of VSP. Normal values for this index ranges from 1.1 to

2.3 (median 1.7 at days 1–2) and in the absence of vasospasm is less than 3.[14] If the CBFV is found to elevated but the ratio is less that 3, then the elevation is thought to be due to hyperemia Also, a ratio more than 6 is consistent with severe VSP.[3,5,12]

Lindegaard index
Mild to moderate VSP: >3, as measured by MCA CBFV/extracranial ICA CBFV.
    Severe VSP: >6, as measured by MCA CBFV/extracranial CBFV.
    VSP and its consequences represents significant events in a high proportion of patients after aSAH, therefore by our opinion daily TCD monitoring when a patient is in the ICU is warranted for the management of this subpopulation. Therefore, knowledge of the time course of the development and resolution of VSP after aSAH using TCD may help the clinician predict which patients are at higher risk of developing DCI, thereby guiding medical treatment or endovascular intervention.[52]
    TCD has long been used for diagnosis and monitoring of VSP in patients with SAH, but studies of diagnostic accuracy for detection of VSP vary widely with regard to sensitivity and specificity of TCD. The sensitivity and specificity of TCD in prediction of VSP vary according to the vessel, diagnostic criteria, and timing of correlative angiography (**Table 5**).[29] In addition, CBFV's on TCD can be influenced by technical issues (absence of temporal bone windows), vessel anatomy, and skills of neurosonographers. For the MCA, TCD is not likely to indicate a spasm when angiography does not show one (high specificity), and TCD may be used to identify patients with a spasm (high positive predictive value [PPV]).[53] Earlier work indicates relatively low sensitivity of TCD for detecting ACA VSP, therefore caution should be exercised in using negative TCD results to make treatment decisions based on the assumed absence of VSP.[54] TCD appears to be highly predictive of an angiographically demonstrated VSP in the MCA; however, its diagnostic accuracy is lower with regard to VSP in the BA.[55,56] In this regard, the combination of predictive factors (clinical, CT and TCD) to detect VSP after aSAH may be superior in accuracy compared with the single independent tests.[57]
    In general, increased mean CBFV on TCD predicts VSP of large intracranial arteries after aSAH. However, Rajajee and colleagues[58] retrospectively studied 81 patients with aSAH who underwent TCD between days 2 and 14 and reported that low PI (mean 0.71 ± 0.19) was found to be an independent predictor of large vessel VSP ($P = .03$, odds ratio [OR] 0.04, 95% confidence

Table 5
Ranges of sensitivity, specificity, PPV, and NPV of transcranial Doppler ultrasonography to detect vasospasm in different arteries

Vessels	Sensitivity (%)	Specificity (%)	PPV (%)	NPV (%)
Internal carotid artery C1 segment	100	91	73	56
Anterior cerebral artery A1 segment	13–82	65–100	41–100	37–80
Middle cerebral artery M1 segment	38–91	94–100	83–100	29–98
Posterior cerebral artery P1 segment	48	69	37	78
Vertebral artery	43.8	88	54	82
Basilar artery	73–76.9	79	63	88

Abbreviations: NPV, negative predictive value; PPV, positive predictive value.
Data from Refs.[29,37,44,45,48,49,53,55]

interval [CI] 0.001–0.54). In this large study, the investigators analyzed 1877 TCD examinations in 441 patients with aSAH within 14 days of onset.[52] After controlling for variables, all TCD CBFV between 120 and 180 cm/s implied an incremental risk of DCI after SAH, with maximal sensitivity by day 8.

TCD criteria for BA VSP are still poorly defined. However, Sviri and colleagues[55] showed that the CBFV ratio between the BA and the extracranial VAs strongly correlated with the degree of BA narrowing ($r^2 = 0.648$; $P<.0001$). A ratio higher than 2.5 with BA velocity greater than 85 cm/s was associated with 86% sensitivity and 97% specificity for BA narrowing of more than 25%. A BA/VA ratio higher than 3.0 with BA velocities higher than 85 cm/s was associated with 92% sensitivity and 97% specificity for BA narrowing of more than 50%. The investigators argued that the BA/VA ratio improves the sensitivity and specificity of TCD detection of BA VSP. Grading criteria for BA VSP still needed to be validated in a prospective trial.

It is clear that quest for "fine tuning" of this TCD application is still not over. By our opinion, trending of the CBFVs and day-to-day comparison of the changes are critical and has good predictive value. In addition, CBFV increase of 50 cm/s or more during a 24-hour period indicates high risk for DCI.[59]

Monitoring Cerebral Vasospasm

Early studies on angiographic VSP revealed maximal spasm at the site of lesion, which extended several centimeters to adjacent arteries to a lesser degree.[60] The time course of VSP as evaluated by TCD ultrasonography has been found to be similar to that reported in angiographic studies.[61] One such review of 26 studies comparing TCD and angiography showed 99% specificity for absence of elevated CBFV by TCD

in the MCA when angiography is also negative, and, thus, TCD had a high PPV to identify patients with VSP.[53]

Although digital subtraction angiography is the gold standard for diagnosis of cerebral VSP, TCD ultrasonography is relatively inexpensive and noninvasive, and can be repeatedly done at the bedside.[62] Moreover, a relationship between TCD-measured CBFVs and intracerebral vessel diameter (as observed on DSA) has been demonstrated.[14,40] TCD is typically performed from the day of SAH and can be repeated either twice daily or every other day, until there is absence of elevated CBFVs.[5,25,29]

To examine the predictive value of a rapid rise (>50 cm/s/24 h) in TCD CBFV in diagnosis of progressive VSP, Grosset and colleagues[59] correlated TCD-measured CBFV with increases to regional CBF changes (on single-photon emission computed tomography) and clinical course in 20 patients. Almost all the patients' perfusion patterns were abnormal and correlated with sites of increased CBFV on TCD. The investigators proposed that patients could be selected for prophylactic anti-ischemic therapy using TCD.

To test the predictive reliability of TCD to monitor cerebral VSP after aSAH, Nakae and colleagues[63] retrospectively measured increases in CBFV ratio of the ipsilateral to contralateral MCA and compared that to conventional absolute CBFV in 142 patients with aSAH, who underwent 1262 TCD studies. Their results showed that the receiver operating characteristic curve for delayed cerebral ischemia had an area under the curve of 0.86 (95% CI: 0.76–0.96) when the 2 sides were compared versus 0.80 (95% CI 0.71–0.88) when the absolute CBFV was used. The threshold value that best discriminated between patients with and without DCI was 1.5.

TBI represents the leading cause of morbidity and mortality in individuals younger than 45 years.

Outcome from TBI is determined by 2 substantially different factors: (1) the primary insult occurring at the moment of impact and (2) the secondary insult represents consecutive pathologic processes initiated at the moment of injury with delayed clinical presentation. Cerebral ischemia due to the onset of posttraumatic VSP and intracranial hypertension are major contributing factors for secondary injury. In addition, parenchymal contusions and fever are defined as independent risk factors for development of posttraumatic VSP.[9] The extent and timing of posttraumatic cerebral hemodynamic disturbances have significant implications for the monitoring and treatment of patients with TBI. Martin and colleagues[64] have described a triphasic pattern in CBF after TBI. Immediately after TBI, global CBF is reduced leading to hypoperfusion. This may be ensued by hyperperfusion over the next 24 to 72 hours, following which VSP may be seen.[64,65] After TBI, elevated CBFV not due to hyperemia can be captured on TCD as a waveform notch during diastole, which is absent in patients with hyperemia.[66]

In the past decade, it was also seen that TBI is associated with the severest casualties from Operation Iraqi Freedom and Operation Enduring Freedom. Armonda and colleagues[30] indicated that VSP occurred in a substantial number of patients with war-time TBI and clinical outcomes were worse in such patients. Their recent work indicates that TCD signs of mild, moderate, and severe VSP were observed in 37%, 22%, and 12% of patients, respectively.[67] These findings demonstrate that cerebral arterial VSP is a frequent and significant complication of combat TBI; therefore, daily TCD monitoring is recommended for their recognition and subsequent management (**Fig. 1**).

Post TBI, brain swelling is a frequent cause of intracranial hypertension and herniation syndromes.[68] Recently, decompressive craniectomy has experienced a revival, although its actual benefit on neurologic outcome remains debateable.[68] A better understanding of ICP dynamics, as well as of the metabolic and cerebral hemodynamic processes, may be useful in assessing the effect of this surgery on the pathophysiology of the swollen brain. Few studies have addressed the effect of decompressive craniectomy on intracranial hemodynamics. Nineteen patients with swelling and herniation after TBI had TCD CBFV's measurements of bilateral MCA and distal ICA before and after surgery, in one prospective study.[68] The investigators reported a significant elevation of ipsilateral CBFV and decrease in PI in most patients with swelling and transtentorial herniation syndrome. This elevation in CBFV was also seen on the contralateral side. In patients with post-

hemicraniectomy, cerebral vessels may shift and the distance from the scalp to the intracranial vessel may be increased. Therefore, this factor must be considered while performing TCD ultrasonography for this group of patients. Further studies will be needed to advocate the routine use of TCD to monitor effect of decompressive craniectomy on cerebral hemodynamics.

The occurrence of VSP and DCI after resection of intracranial tumor has not received extensive attention clinically, and is often misdiagnosed and improperly treated as surgical brain damage or brain swelling. Reports are sparse and mainly as case series.[69] VSP is an infrequent but definite complication of surgery for tumors. Some of the factors that appear to correlate with a higher incidence of postoperative VSP include a larger tumor size, the need for preoperative embolization indicating increased tumor vascularity, vessel encasement, displacement, and narrowing and increased intraoperative blood loss.[70,71] However, DCI from VSP after tumor resection is a complication that is being reported in increasing numbers. It is suggested that accumulation of blood in the basal cisterns may have been responsible for this unusual condition, and it is therefore important to consider VSP as a probable etiologic cause of clinical deterioration in patients undergoing the surgical removal of a cerebral tumor.[70] For this reason, whenever any neurologic deterioration occurs in such patients, it is advisable to perform TCD to verify the presence of any VSP and promptly commence suitable treatment.

One of the limitations of TCD is that it is unknown if TCD has the ability to predict clinical deterioration and infarction after aSAH, TBI, and tumor resection due to DCI. In spite of this, TCD examination is noninvasive, inexpensive, and the pattern of CBFVs observed in patients after aSAH is very distinctive, enabling immediate detection of abnormally high CBFVs and appears to be predictive of VSP and DCI.[11,24,46,48,51,52,55,59,68–74] TCD is useful in monitoring the temporal course of VSP after SAH. Even though repeat angiography is unavoidable in most aSAH patients, TCD can guide the timing of this procedure and the tailoring of aggressive treatment regimens. The key is not to predict compromised perfusion by TCD, but to identify patients going into VSP and to quickly confirm VSP when subtle signs are present, before apparent neurologic deterioration. It is useful to perform TCD test on admission (or as soon as possible after surgery) and perform daily TCD studies when the patient is in the ICU. The frequency with which TCD should be performed may be guided by patient clinical presentation, knowledge of risk factors for VSP, and early clinical course. Infrequently,

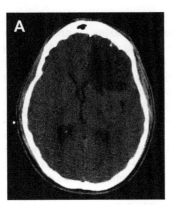

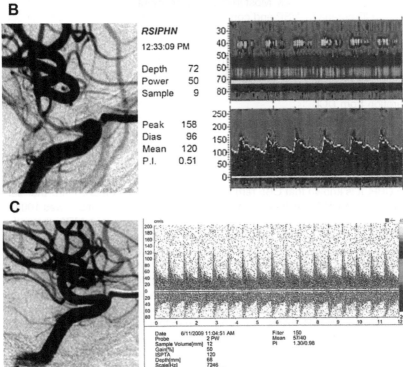

Fig. 1. Patient with right side contusion, base skull Fx, L1–L5–Fx. (*A*) CT scan demonstrating contusion. (*B*) Right common carotid artery injection showing severe vasospasm affecting right carotid siphon before angioplasty and corresponding TCD measured CBFV in the right carotid siphon. (*C*) Resolution of vasospasm after transluminal angioplasty and TCD showed CBFV normalization after angioplasty.

clinical VSP occurs earlier than natural history would suggest; daily TCD can be the least expensive option to identify patients at risk for deterioration. The presence and temporal profile of CBFVs in all available vessels must be detected and serially monitored. TCD studies should be performed after endovascular treatment to identify patients with recurrent VSP. The high sensitivity of TCD to identify abnormally high CBFVs due to the onset of VSP demonstrates that TCD is an excellent first-line examination to identify those patients who may need urgent aggressive treatment.

However, prior endovascular treatment presence of VSP must be confirmed by cerebral angiography, which still is the gold standard for cerebral vessel visualization. In addition, a dedicated and experienced team of neurointensivists, neurologists, neurosurgeons, and neuroradiologists are required to provide the best available care and better outcome for those patients suffering SAH and TBI.

To conclude, VSP continues to adversely affect a significant proportion of aSAH and TBI population and remains a challenge for all clinicians interested in reducing the adverse outcomes associated with aSAH and TBI. Today, if the question were to be asked if TCD can be used for evaluation of the presence or absence of abnormally elevated CBFV that is most likely due to the VSP; the unequivocal answer will be yes. TCD is a noninvasive ultrasound modality capable of identifying patients who are progressing to or suffering VSP. Several features of TCD assessment of VSP are similar to cerebral angiography. High CBFV measured by TCD, like severe angiographic VSP, are associated with DCI and infarction, although some patients can remain asymptomatic despite these changes. Most likely, validation of new TCD criteria for VSP and combination of different physiologic monitoring modalities that includes TCD, electroencephalography, brain tissue oxygen monitoring, cerebral microdialysis, and near-infrared spectroscopy will improve TCD accuracy to predict clinical deterioration and infarction from DCI.

Cerebral Autoregulation

Cerebral autoregulation (CA) is a homeostatic mechanism which reduces changes in CBF due to variations in CPP. It is known that CBF remains relatively constant when CPP is within 50 to 150 mm Hg[3].

In patients with TBI, TCD may be useful as a noninvasive means of calculating CPP. Czosnyka and colleagues[72] studied the reliability of CPP using TCD-measured CBFV in MCA (mean and diastolic) in 96 patients with TBI (Glasgow Coma Scale <13). The CPP measured by TCD and the calculated CPP (MAP minus ICP, measured using an intraparenchymal sensor) were compared. The results showed that in 71% of the studies, the estimation error was less than 10 mm Hg and in 84% of the examinations, the error was less than 15 mm Hg. The TCD method had a high positive predictive power (94%) for detecting low CPP (<60 mm Hg). Day-by-day variability in 41 patients was reasonable ($r = 0.71$). In addition, continuous waveform analysis of MCA CBFV and CPP correlates with coma score after resuscitation and outcome and hence may be considered reliable for assessment of autoregulation in ventilated TBI patients.[73]

Lang and colleagues[74] recorded CBFV and continuous arterial BP at a controlled ventilatory frequency in 12 patients with severe aSAH and compared it with 40 controls. Cerebral autoregulation was significantly impaired in patients with SAH when compared with normal subjects ($P<.01$ for days 1–6, and $P<.001$ for days 7–13). The investigators concluded that autoregulation can be assessed in a graded fashion in patients with SAH and impairment in autoregulation precedes VSP. Also, ongoing VSP worsened autoregulation and in the early phase (days 1–6) after SAH, autoregulation impairment is predictive of outcome.

Stroke Diagnosis and Management

The American Academy of Neurology Report of the Therapeutics and Technology Assessment Subcommittee mentions that TCD can detect acute MCA occlusions with greater than 90% sensitivity, specificity, PPV and NPV.[62] This report also mentions that TCD has 70% to 90% sensitivity and PPV and excellent specificity and NPV for occlusion of ICA siphon, VA, and BA.[62] A few studies have evaluated the prognostic value of TCD in acute ischemic stroke. TCD has been compared with magnetic resonance angiography (MRA) and CTA in acute stroke.[75–77] It can be used to evaluate intracranial steno-occlusive disease, particularly in the terminal ICA, ICA siphon, and MCA. In a prospective study including 30 patients, TCD showed a sensitivity of 96% and specificity of 33% for recognizing abnormal CBFV (anterior and posterior circulation vessels were evaluated together).[76] In the same study, for MCA lesions, specificity was 100% and sensitivity was 93%, whereas MRA showed a sensitivity of 46% and a specificity of 74% for assessing intracranial vascular anatomy. In the emergency room, bedside TCD is in agreement with urgent CT angiogram of the brain in the evaluation of patients with acute cerebral ischemia. TCD may provide real-time flow findings that are complementary to information provided by CTA.[77]

In a study involving 705 patients, Wong and colleagues[78] observed that in patients with predominantly intracranial large-artery occlusive disease, the presence and the total number of occlusive arteries in the cranio-cervical circulation (based on TCD measurements) can predict further vascular events or death within 6 months after stroke (adjusted OR 1.25 per occlusive artery, 95% CI 1.12–1.39). Molina and colleagues[79] studied the effect of delayed spontaneous recanalization on hemorrhagic conversions of MCA strokes in 53 patients. In their study, TCD detected delayed recanalization (>6 hours) after acute cardio-embolic stroke of MCA, and was found to be an independent predictor of hemorrhagic transformation (OR 8.9; 95% CI 2.1–33.3).

TCD detections of complete intracranial arterial occlusions were associated with poor neurologic recovery, disability, or death after 90 days in 2 separate studies.[80,81] Normal TCD results may be predictive of early improvement from stroke.[62,82] In patients with acute ICA occlusion, TCD finding of arterial occlusion along with stroke severity at 24 hours and CT lesion size were independent predictors of outcome after 30 days.[80] In one study, the investigators determined TCD accuracy for occlusion of intracranial arteries in patients with cerebral ischemia.[75] In this study, sensitivity for occlusion site was as follows: proximal ICA 94%, distal ICA 81%, MCA 93% terminal VA 56%, BA 60%, and specificity ranged from 96% to 98%. This study also demonstrated that TCD had specificity of 94.4 and NPV of 94.4% in the diagnosis of anterior or posterior circulatory occlusion.[75] TCD had the highest accuracy for ICA and MCA occlusions and if the results of TCD were normal, there was a 94% chance that angiographic studies were negative. Another study performed CT scan, DSA and TCD on 48 patients within 4 hours of the onset of acute hemispheric ischemic stroke.[83] In this study, the most significant TCD findings were absence of flow in the occluded carotid siphon or MCA origin (correlated by angiography) and reduced CBFV and asymmetry (symptomatic <asymptomatic) when the occlusion was located in the terminal MCA. TCD was used to assess collateral circulation by demonstrating higher CBFV in ACA and PCA.

To test the utility of TCD in demonstration of arterial occlusion and subsequent recanalization in patients with acute ischemic stroke treated with intravenous tissue plasminogen activator (tPA), Burgin and colleagues[84] compared posttreatment TCD with angiography (DSA or MRA) in 25 patients. TCD was performed at 12 ± 16 hours and angiography at 41 ± 57 hours after stroke onset. Accuracy of TCD to recognize recanalization was as follows: sensitivity 91%, specificity 93%, PPV 91%, and NPV 93%. TCD predicted the presence of complete occlusion on angiography with sensitivity of 50%, specificity of 100%, PPV of 100%, and NPV of 75%. TCD flow signals correlated with angiographic patency ($\chi^2 = 24.2$, $P<.001$).

Emergency TCD findings over the first 48 hours are related to early neurologic changes in patients with acute ischemic stroke. In a study with 93 patients, Toni and colleagues[85] performed serial TCDs at 6, 24, and 48 hours after stroke onset. On logistic regression, normal TCD was found to be an independent predictor of early improvement (OR 0.17; 95% CI 0.06–0.46). Abnormal TCD (asymmetry or no-flow) was an independent predictor of early deterioration (OR 5.02; 95% CI, 1.31–19.3). Abnormal TCD has been found to be predictive of larger chronic CT lesions and more extensive ischemic change within the MCA territory. This was demonstrated by Kushner and colleagues,[82] who compared TCD findings at 6 hours or less after acute proximal MCA occlusion with CT scan findings at 1 to 3 months ($P<.005$). Abnormal TCD was predictive of chronic cortical infarct in MCA territory and correlated with angiographic findings as well ($P<.001$).

Ischemic stroke occurs in an estimated 11% of patients with homozygous sickle cell disease (Hb SS) by the age of 20 years and is a major cause of morbidity.[86] The Stroke Prevention Trial in Sickle Cell Anemia (STOP Trial) demonstrated a significant benefit of chronic red-cell transfusion in reducing the risk of a first stroke by 90% and it used TCD to screen and identify children at greatest risk of ischemic stroke.[86] The STOP study is the most successful stroke prevention trial to date and the data provide the strongest evidence for effective clinical application of TCD to prevent ischemic stroke in children with sickle cell anemia; therefore, TCD screening is recommended as practice standard. Adams and colleagues[87] followed 315 patients with sickle cell disease for more than 5 years and found that elevated maximal CBFV (especially >200 cm/s) in the intracranial ICA and MCA were independently predictive of ischemic stroke ($P<.0001$). In another study including 130 patients, transfusion greatly reduced the risk of a first stroke in children with sickle cell anemia who had abnormal results on TCD examination.[88]

TCD examination performed within 24 hours of stroke symptom onset greatly improves the accuracy of early stroke subtype diagnosis in patients with acute cerebral ischemia.[89] Early and accurate detection of occluded arteries affects therapeutic strategies in patients with acute cerebral ischemia. It is well known that clinical course of stroke may include either spontaneous improvements or deterioration related to dynamic changes in cerebral perfusion. Serial daily TCD examinations may reveal dynamic changes in cerebral circulation that may be missed on a single neuroimaging study.[90] These serial rapid measurements of cerebral hemodynamics in patients with acute cerebral ischemia with TCD offers new insight into the process of diagnosis of acute stroke and provides guidance for and monitoring of therapeutic interventions.[90]

Patent Foramen Ovale Screening for Cryptogenic Stroke and Risk Assessment

Approximately 30% of adults have a patent foramen ovale (PFO) in the heart, but the frequency is even higher (approximately 50%) in patients with cerebral infarct of unknown etiology (cryptogenic infarct), especially in the younger age group.[91–94]

Although transesophageal echocardiogram (TEE) is better than contrast TCD (cTCD) because it provides direct anatomic information on the nature of the shunt or atrial septal aneurysm presence, cTCD is comparable with contrast TEE for detecting right-to-left shunts due to PFO.[62] However, cTCD is noninvasive, provides direct evidence of emboli passage through the cerebral vessels, and an optimal Valsalva maneuver performance because it does not require sedation and is easy to perform at the bedside. Almost perfect concordance between simultaneous contrast TCD and TEE in the quantification of right-to-left shunts was shown by Belvís and colleagues.[95] Recently, in a prospective study with 134 patients, it was shown that among patients diagnosed with PFO, the shunt was detected at baseline by cTCD in 69% of cases, by transthoracic echocardiography (TTE) in 74%, and by TEE in 58%. TTE and cTCD showed higher sensitivity (100% vs 97%; nonsignificant difference) than TEE in the diagnosis of PFO (86%; $P<.001$).[96]

In a study involving 69 patients, Albert and colleagues[97] concluded that observation of more than 10 microbubbles of agitated saline at less than 10 seconds on cTCD (with Valsalva maneuver), is highly sensitive and specific for the diagnosis of right-to-left cardiac shunts. Similarly, Droste,[98] in a study with 81 patients, showed that cTCD performed with Echovist-300 (D-galactose microparticulate) yielded a 100% sensitivity to identify TEE-proven cardiac right-to-left shunts. Also, Schwarze and colleagues[99] described the optimal methodology for performance of cTCD. Their findings suggested that 10 mL of contrast medium should be injected with the patient in the supine position and Valsalva maneuver must be performed 5 seconds after the start of the injection.

Emboli Monitoring

TCD ultrasonography currently represents only one available standard of detecting microembolic material in gaseous and solid state in real-time, within the intracranial cerebral arteries. Various disease states in which microembolic signals can be found are listed in **Table 6**.

These microembolic signals, also called MES or high-intensity transient signals (HITS) have distinct acoustic impedance properties when compared with erythrocytes that flow simultaneously.[62,100] The ultrasound signals reflect off emboli before flowing erythrocytes in blood and because of this phenomenon, the reflected Doppler signal has a higher intensity signal.[62] Asymptomatic embolic signals detected using TCD are frequent in

Table 6
Microembolic signals
Microembolic signals have been detected in patients with the following:
Asymptomatic high-grade ICA
Symptomatic high-grade ICA
Prosthetic cardiac valves
Myocardial infarction
Atrial fibrillation
Aortic arch atheroma
Fat embolization syndrome
Cerebral vascular disease
Coronary artery catheterization
Coronary angioplasty
Direct current cardioversion
Cerebral angiography
Carotid endarterectomy (CEA)
Carotid angioplasty
Cardiopulmonary bypass
Brain aneurysm
Hughes-Stovin syndrome
Marantic endocarditis
Deep vein thrombosis
Mitral valve prolapse
Polyarteritis nodosa
Pelvic vein thrombosis
Intravenous catheter infection
Renal vein thrombosis
Idiopathic dilated cardiomyopathy
Renal vein thrombosis
Dilated cardiomyopathy
Aortic aneurysm, abdominal
Idiopathic dilated cardiomyopathy
Endocarditis
Atrial myxoma
Ventricular aneurysm
Surgery complication
Cholesterol embolism

patients with carotid artery disease and detection of embolic signals by TCD can identify groups of patients with asymptomatic carotid stenosis who are at low or high risk of future stroke.[101]

In a study involving 81 patients, Goertler and colleagues[102] used TCD ultrasonography to localize an embolic source and to monitor the effects of antithrombotic treatment in patients with atherosclerotic cerebrovascular disease. Stork[103] hypothesized that smaller platelet aggregates and fibrin clots, which are not detected macroscopically, are the most likely sources of TCD-detected microembolic signals. Molloy and Markus observed that TCD-based identification of asymptomatic embolization in patients with carotid artery stenosis may be an independent predictor of future stroke risk in patients with both symptomatic and asymptomatic carotid stenosis.[104]

Patients with ischemic strokes, transient ischemic attacks, or asymptomatic high-grade ICA stenosis can also undergo TCD monitoring to detect, localize, and quantify cerebral embolization.[105] This information is helpful to establish the diagnosis and change management strategy. Asymptomatic embolic signals on TCD helps predict stroke risk in symptomatic carotid stenosis and postoperatively after carotid endarterectomy.[106] Sometimes the presence of emboli can be the only sign of a proximal arterial dissection, partially occlusive thrombus, or unrecognized cardiac source of embolism.[105,107]

Carotid Endarterectomy/Carotid Artery Stenting Treatment Effect Evaluation

TCD monitoring of the ipsilateral MCA during carotid endarterectomy (CEA) provides surgeons with constant status of flow velocities, which correlate with stump pressure during cross-clamping.[62,108] Large reductions in CBFV on TCD during CEA may be an indication for procedures that maintain blood flow to the brain (including shunt placement and augmentation of blood pressure).[62]

During CEA, microembolic signals are most commonly encountered intraoperatively during dissection and while shunting or unclamping. The presence of microembolic signals during dissection correlates best with new ischemic lesions seen on magnetic resonance imaging.[62] These signals are also noticed on TCD during wound closure and in the immediate postoperative phase.[103,108–113]

Jansen and colleagues[114] used combined electroencephalogram (EEG) and TCD intraoperative monitoring of thromboembolic phenomena to focus on the additional value of TCD to detect ischemia during surgery. They concluded that during CEA, information from intraoperative TCD directly influenced surgical technique and provided information about thromboembolism and hemodynamic changes that are not detected by EEG alone.

In a study involving 65 patients, Levi and colleagues[110] observed TCD signals for microembolisms within 24 hours after CEA. They concluded that more than 50 microembolic signals occurred in about 10% of cases and are predictive of ipsilateral focal cerebral ischemia (PPV = 0.71). Gaunt and colleagues[109] studied 100 consecutive patients undergoing CEA with intraoperative TCD. They found that more than 10 particulate emboli during initial carotid dissection correlated with a significant deterioration in postoperative cognitive function. They concluded that immediate

intervention, based on TCD evidence of embolization, has the potential to avert neurologic deficits during CEA. Also, Ackerstaff and colleagues,[112] in their study of 31 patients undergoing CEA, concluded that factors associated with operative stroke were TCD-detected microemboli during dissection and wound closure, 90% or higher MCA velocity decrease at cross-clamping, and 100% or more PI increase at clamp release.

In one study, 500 patients underwent CEA with TCD monitoring of the ipsilateral MCA during various phases of CEA to determine hemodynamic changes and incidence of microembolic signals. This study concluded that embolism (54%) is the primary cause of cerebrovascular complications from CEA. Hypoperfusion (17%) and hyperperfusion (29%) were also identified by TCD. By responding to information provided by TCD, the incidence of permanent deficits in these patients decreased from 7% in the first 100 operations to 2% in the last 400 ($P \leq .01$).[108]

In conclusion, TCD monitoring during CEA and CAS provides information about embolic phenomena and flow patterns in cerebral vasculature that may prompt appropriate measures at several stages of CEA to reduce the risk of perioperative stroke. However, TCD monitoring is still considered an investigational technique for application and clinical use during different cardiovascular surgeries.[62]

Diagnosis and Monitoring of Intracranial Hypertension and Brain Death Evaluation

Brain death is a medical, social, and legal issue and brain death is accepted as a legal and medical criterion for death. Brain death is confirmed with the help of physical examination and ancillary diagnostic modalities, such as EEG, radionuclide scans, and angiography. TCD ultrasonography can also be used for supporting diagnosis of brain death. TCD may be of value in this indication, as it is portable, less time consuming, and can be performed at bedside.

TCD provides information on the flow velocity, direction of flow, shape of the Doppler waveform, and also differences in pulsatility amplitudes between systolic and diastolic CBFV, which can be used to support diagnosis of brain death.[115]

Increased ICP initially leads to increased PIs, followed by progressive reduction in mean and diastolic CBFVs. Changes in PI are also known to occur when CPP is lower than 70 mm Hg. With severe elevation of ICP exceeding end-diastolic BP, diastolic CBFV approaches nil. With further elevations in ICP, there is observation of retrograde diastolic flow, appearance of small systolic spikes, and finally absence of flow. With prolonged presence of these lethal flow patterns, brain death is likely.[62,116–120]

Classically described waveform patterns in brain death diagnosis are an oscillating "to-and-fro" movement of blood flow (attributed to reversal of flow in diastole), as well as small early systolic spikes.[115,121] These waveform abnormalities represent arrest of intracerebral circulation and occur as a result of elevated ICP.

Zurynski and colleagues[116] studied 111 patients who were brain dead (vs 29 comatose patients in the control group) with TCDs performed before formal clinical brain death testing. They described short, sharp systolic patterns on TCD followed by diastolic reversal of flow or systolic peaks with absence of flow in either direction in all (100%) patients. In comparison, none of the patients in the control group showed reversal of flow. Another study explored the diagnostic accuracy of TCD in 184 patients who were brain dead. The investigators of this study concluded that TCD was able to diagnose brain death with a specificity of 100% and sensitivity (on serial testing) of 95.6%. No false-positives were observed.[122] Hadani and colleagues[123] had similar results when they studied TCD readings in 137 patients.

The consensus opinion on diagnosis of cerebral circulatory arrest using Doppler-sonography Task Force Group confirms that extracranial and intracranial Doppler sonography is useful as a confirmatory test to establish irreversibility of cerebral circulatory arrest. Although optional, TCD is of special value when the therapeutic use of sedative drugs renders EEG unreliable.[124] This statement also mentions that the absence of flow in MCA precedes complete loss of brain stem functions. The AAN Practice Parameters for Determining Brain Death in Adults considers TCD a confirmatory test of brain death along with clinical testing and other allied tests.[125]

SUMMARY

In the contemporary neurointensive care of patients with CVD, SAH, TBI, and other illnesses in which cerebral hemodynamics can be disturbed or impaired, basic neurologic monitoring should be expanded by extended neuromonitoring, including TCD. Growing evidence clearly supports the integration of extended neuromonitoring to unmask otherwise occult alterations and to differentially adapt the type, extent, and duration of therapeutic interventions. By expanding our knowledge and experience, the integration of extended neuromonitoring in daily clinical routine will provide us with the means to improve outcome, which has not been possible by relying only on neurologic examination alone, as practiced in the past.

REFERENCES

1. Aaslid R, Markwalder TM, Nornes H. Noninvasive transcranial Doppler ultrasound recording of flow velocity in basal cerebral arteries. J Neurosurg 1982;57(6):769–74.
2. Aaslid R, Huber P, Nornes H. Evaluation of cerebrovascular spasm with transcranial Doppler ultrasound. J Neurosurg 1984;60(1):37–41.
3. Rasulo FA, De Peri E, Lavinio A. Transcranial Doppler ultrasonography in intensive care. Eur J Anaesthesiol Suppl 2008;42(Suppl 42): 167–73.
4. White H, Venkatesh B. Applications of transcranial Doppler in the ICU: a review. Intensive Care Med 2006;32(7):981–94.
5. Rigamonti A. Transcranial Doppler monitoring in subarachnoid hemorrhage: a critical tool in critical care. Can J Anaesth 2008;55:112–24.
6. Moppett IK, Mahajan RP. Transcranial Doppler ultrasonography in anaesthesia and intensive care. Br J Anaesth 2004;93(5):710–24.
7. Droste DW, Harders AG, Rastogi E. A transcranial Doppler study of blood flow velocity in the middle cerebral arteries performed at rest and during mental activities. Stroke 1989;20(8):1005–11.
8. Patel PM, Drummond JC. Cerebral physiology and the effects of anesthetic drugs. 7th edition. Elsevier Inc; p. 305–39.
9. Shahlaie K, Keachie K, Hutchins IM, et al. Risk factors for posttraumatic vasospasm. J Neurosurg 2011;115(3):602–11.
10. Marshall SA, Nyquist P, Ziai WC. The role of transcranial Doppler ultrasonography in the diagnosis and management of vasospasm after aneurysmal subarachnoid hemorrhage. Neurosurg Clin N Am 2010;21(2):291–303.
11. Transcranial color Doppler sonography of basal cerebral arteries in 182 healthy subjects: age and sex variability and normal reference values for blood flow parameters. AJR Am J Roentgenol 1999; 172(1):213–8.
12. Martin PJ, Evans DH, Naylor AR. Transcranial color-coded sonography of the basal cerebral circulation. Reference data from 115 volunteers. Stroke 1994;25(2):390–6.
13. Tegeler CH, Crutchfield K, Katsnelson M, et al. Transcranial Doppler velocities in a large, healthy population. J Neuroimaging 2012;1–7.
14. Lindegaard KF, Nornes H, Bakke SJ, et al. Cerebral vasospasm after subarachnoid haemorrhage investigated by means of transcranial Doppler ultrasound. Acta Neurochir Suppl 1988;42:81–4.

15. Bellner J, Romner B, Reinstrup P, et al. Transcranial Doppler sonography pulsatility index (PI) reflects intracranial pressure (ICP). Surg Neurol 2004; 62(1):45–51.

16. Gosling RG, King DH. Arterial assessment by Doppler-shift ultra-sound. Proc R Soc Med 1974; 67:447–9.

17. Ursino M, Giulioni M, Lodi CA. Relationships among cerebral perfusion pressure, autoregulation, and transcranial Doppler waveform: a modeling study. J Neurosurg 1998;89(2):255–66.

18. Zweifel C, Czosnyka M, Carrera E, et al. Reliability of the blood flow velocity pulsatility index for assessment of intracranial and cerebral perfusion pressures in head-injured patients. Neurosurgery 2012;71(4):853–61.

19. Jo KI, Kim JS, Hong SC, et al. Hemodynamic changes in arteriovenous malformations after radiosurgery: transcranial Doppler evaluation. World Neurosurg 2012;77(2):316–21.

20. Moehring MA, Spencer MP. Power M-mode Doppler (PMD) for observing cerebral blood flow and tracking emboli. Ultrasound Med Biol 2002; 28(1):49–57.

21. Maeda H, Matsumoto M, Handa N, et al. Reactivity of cerebral blood flow to carbon dioxide in various types of ischemic cerebrovascular disease: evaluation by the transcranial Doppler method. Stroke 1993;24(5):670–5.

22. Brass LM, Pavlakis SG, DeVivo D, et al. Transcranial Doppler measurements of the middle cerebral artery. Effect of hematocrit. Stroke 1988;19(12): 1466–9.

23. Mattle H, Grolimund P, Huber P, et al. Transcranial Doppler sonographic findings in middle cerebral artery disease. Arch Neurol 1988;45(3):289–95.

24. Velat GJ, Kimball MM, Mocco JD, et al. Vasospasm after aneurysmal subarachnoid hemorrhage: review of randomized controlled trials and meta-analyses in the literature. World Neurosurg 2011; 76(5):446–54.

25. Dorsch N. A clinical review of cerebral vasospasm and delayed ischaemia following aneurysm rupture. Acta Neurochir Suppl 2011;110(Pt 1):5–6.

26. Saqqur M, Zygun D, Demchuk A. Role of transcranial Doppler in neurocritical care. Crit Care Med 2007;35(Suppl 5):S216–23.

27. Bederson JB, Connolly ES, Batjer HH, et al. Guidelines for the management of aneurysmal subarachnoid hemorrhage: a statement for healthcare professionals from a special writing group of the Stroke Council, American Heart Association. Stroke 2009;40(3):994–1025.

28. McGirt MJ, Blessing RP, Goldstein LB. Transcranial Doppler monitoring and clinical decision-making after subarachnoid hemorrhage. J Stroke Cerebrovasc Dis 2003;12(2):88–92.

29. Washington CW, Zipfel GJ. Detection and monitoring of vasospasm and delayed cerebral ischemia: a review and assessment of the literature. Neurocrit Care 2011;15(2):312–7.

30. Armonda RA, Bell RS, Vo AH, et al. Wartime traumatic cerebral vasospasm: recent review of combat casualties. Neurosurgery 2006;59(6):1215–25 [discussion: 1225].

31. Keyrouz SG, Diringer MN. Clinical review: prevention and therapy of vasospasm in subarachnoid hemorrhage. Crit Care 2007;11(4):220.

32. Höllerhage HG. Nimodipine treatment in poorgrade aneurysm patients. J Neurosurg 1988; 69(5):803–5.

33. Rowland MJ, Hadjipavlou G, Kelly M, et al. Delayed cerebral ischaemia after subarachnoid haemorrhage: looking beyond. Br J Anaesth 2012;22879655.

34. Zubkov AY, Rabinstein AA. Medical management of cerebral vasospasm: present and future. Neurol Res 2009;31(6):626–31.

35. Smith M. Intensive care management of patients with subarachnoid haemorrhage. Curr Opin Anaesthesiol 2007;20(5):400–7.

36. Dorsch NW, King MT. A review of cerebral vasospasm in aneurysmal subarachnoid haemorrhage Part I: incidence and effects. J Clin Neurosci 1994;1(1):19–26.

37. Mascia L, Fedorko L, terBrugge K, et al. The accuracy of transcranial Doppler to detect vasospasm in patients with aneurysmal subarachnoid hemorrhage. Intensive Care Med 2003;29(7):1088–94.

38. Otten ML, Mocco J, Connolly ES, et al. A review of medical treatments of cerebral vasospasm. Neurol Res 2008;30(5):444–9.

39. Ionita CC, Graffagnino C, Alexander MJ, et al. The value of CT angiography and transcranial Doppler sonography in triaging suspected cerebral vasospasm in SAH prior to endovascular therapy. Neurocrit Care 2008;9(1):8–12.

40. Sloan MA, Burch CM, Wozniak MA, et al. Transcranial Doppler detection of vertebrobasilar vasospasm following subarachnoid hemorrhage. Stroke 1994;25(11):2187–97.

41. Aaslid R. Transcranial Doppler assessment of cerebral vasospasm. Eur J Ultrasound 2002;16(1–2): 3–10.

42. Grolimund P, Seiler RW, Aaslid R, et al. Evaluation of cerebrovascular disease by combined extracranial and transcranial Doppler sonography. Experience in 1,039 patients. Stroke 1987;18(6):1018–24.

43. Soustiel JF, Bruk B, Shik B, et al. Transcranial Doppler in vertebrobasilar vasospasm after subarachnoid hemorrhage. Neurosurgery 1998;43(2): 282–91 [discussion: 291–3].

44. Langlois O, Rabehenoina C, Proust F, et al. Diagnosis of vasospasm: comparison between

arteriography and transcranial Doppler. A series of 112 comparative tests. Neurochirurgie 1992;38(3): 138–40 [in French].

45. Burch CM, Wozniak MA, Sloan MA, et al. Detection of intracranial internal carotid artery and middle cerebral artery vasospasm following subarachnoid hemorrhage. J Neuroimaging 1996;6(1):8–15.

46. Vora Y, Suarez-Almazor M, Steinke D, et al. Role of transcranial Doppler monitoring in the diagnosis of cerebral vasospasm after subarachnoid hemorrhage. Neurosurgery 1999;44(6):1237–47 [discussion: 1247–8].

47. Sviri GE, Lewis DH, Correa R, et al. Basilar artery vasospasm and delayed posterior circulation ischemia after aneurysmal subarachnoid hemorrhage. Stroke 2004;35(8):1867–72.

48. Soustiel JF, Shik V, Shreiber R, et al. Basilar vasospasm diagnosis: investigation of a modified "Lindegaard Index" based on imaging studies and blood velocity measurements of the basilar artery. Stroke 2002;33(1):72–7.

49. Wozniak MA, Sloan MA, Rothman MI, et al. Detection of vasospasm by transcranial Doppler sonography. The challenges of the anterior and posterior cerebral arteries. J Neuroimaging 1996; 6(2):87–93.

50. Diringer MN, Bleck TP, Claude Hemphill J, et al. Critical care management of patients following aneurysmal subarachnoid hemorrhage: recommendations from the Neurocritical Care Society's Multidisciplinary Consensus Conference. Neurocrit Care 2011;15(2):211–40.

51. Harders AG, Gilsbach JM. Time course of blood velocity changes related to vasospasm in the circle of Willis measured by transcranial Doppler ultrasound. J Neurosurg 1987;66(5):718–28.

52. Carrera E, Schmidt JM, Oddo M, et al. Transcranial Doppler for predicting delayed cerebral ischemia after subarachnoid hemorrhage. Neurosurgery 2009;65(2):316–23 [discussion: 323–4].

53. Lysakowski C, Walder B, Costanza MC, et al. Transcranial Doppler versus angiography in patients with vasospasm due to a ruptured cerebral aneurysm: a systematic review. Stroke 2001; 32(10):2292–8.

54. Lennihan L, Petty GW, Fink ME, et al. Transcranial Doppler detection of anterior cerebral artery vasospasm. J Neurol Neurosurg Psychiatr 1993;56(8): 906–9.

55. Sviri GE, Ghodke B, Britz GW, et al. Transcranial Doppler grading criteria for basilar artery vasospasm. Neurosurgery 2006;59(2):360–6 [discussion: 360–6].

56. Wardlaw JM, Offin R, Teasdale GM, et al. Is routine transcranial Doppler ultrasound monitoring useful in the management of subarachnoid hemorrhage? J Neurosurg 1998;88(2):272–6.

57. Gonzalez NR, Boscardin WJ, Glenn T, et al. Vasospasm probability index: a combination of transcranial Doppler velocities, cerebral blood flow and clinical risk factors to predict cerebral vasospasm after aneurysmal subarachnoid hemorrhage. J Neurosurg 2007;107(6):1101–12.

58. Rajajee V, Fletcher JJ, Pandey AS, et al. Low pulsatility index on transcranial Doppler predicts symptomatic large-vessel vasospasm after aneurysmal subarachnoid hemorrhage. Neurosurgery 2012; 70(5):1195–206 [discussion: 1206].

59. Grosset DG, Straiton J, Du Trevou M, et al. Prediction of symptomatic vasospasm after subarachnoid hemorrhage by rapidly increasing transcranial Doppler velocity and cerebral blood flow changes. Stroke 1992;23(5):674–9.

60. Ecker A, Riemenschneider PA. Arteriographic demonstration of spasm of the intracranial arteries. With special reference to saccular arterial aneurisms. J Neurosurg 1951;8:660–7.

61. Aaslid R, Huber R, Nornes H. A transcranial Doppler method in the evaluation of cerebrovascular spasm. Neuroradiology 1986;28:11–6.

62. Sloan MA, Alexandrov AV, Tegeler CH, et al. Assessment: transcranial Doppler ultrasonography: report of the Therapeutics and Technology Assessment Subcommittee of the American Academy of Neurology. Neurology 2004;62(9):1468–81.

63. Nakae R, Yokota H, Yoshida D, et al. Transcranial Doppler ultrasonography for diagnosis of cerebral vasospasm after aneurysmal subarachnoid hemorrhage: mean blood flow velocity ratio of the ipsilateral and contralateral middle cerebral arteries. Neurosurgery 2011;69(4):876–83.

64. Martin NA, Patwardhan RV, Alexander MJ, et al. Characterization of cerebral hemodynamic phases following severe head trauma: hypoperfusion, hyperemia, and vasospasm. J Neurosurg 1997; 87(1):9–19.

65. Werner C, Engelhard K. Pathophysiology of traumatic brain injury. Br J Anaesth 2007;99(1):4–9.

66. Chan KH, Dearden NM, Miller JD, et al. Transcranial Doppler waveform differences in hyperemic and nonhyperemic patients after severe head injury. Surg Neurol 1992;38(6):433–6.

67. Razumovsky A, Tigno T, Hochheimer SM, et al. Cerebral hemodynamic changes after wartime traumatic brain injury. Acta Neurochir Suppl 2013; 115:87–90.

68. Bor-Seng-Shu E, Hirsch R, Teixeira MJ, et al. Cerebral hemodynamic changes gauged by transcranial Doppler ultrasonography in patients with posttraumatic brain swelling treated by surgical decompression. J Neurosurg 2006;104(1):93–100.

69. Cervoni L, Salvati M, Santoro A. Vasospasm following tumor removal: report of 5 cases. Ital J Neurol Sci 1996;17(4):291–4.

70. Alotaibi NM, Lanzino G. Cerebral vasospasm following tumor resection. J Neurointerv Surg 2012;1–6.

71. Bejjani GK, Sekhar LN, Yost AM. Vasospasm after cranial base tumor resection: pathogenesis, diagnosis, and therapy. Surg Neurol 1999;52(6): 577–83.

72. Czosnyka M, Matta BF, Smielewski P, et al. Cerebral perfusion pressure in head-injured patients: a noninvasive assessment using transcranial Doppler ultrasonography. J Neurosurg 1998; 88(5):802–8.

73. Czosnyka M, Kirkpatrick PJ, Pickard JD. Multimodal monitoring and assessment of cerebral haemodynamic reserve after severe head injury. Cerebrovasc Brain Metab Rev 1996;8(4):273–95.

74. Lang EW, Diehl RR, Mehdorn HM. Cerebral autoregulation testing after aneurysmal subarachnoid hemorrhage: the phase relationship between arterial blood pressure and cerebral blood flow velocity. Crit Care Med 2001;29(1):158–63.

75. Demchuk AM, Christou I, Wein TH, et al. Accuracy and criteria for localizing arterial occlusion with transcranial Doppler. J Neuroimaging 2000;10(1): 1–12.

76. Razumovsky AY, Gillard JH, Bryan RN, et al. TCD, MRA and MRI in acute cerebral ischemia. Acta Neurol Scand 1999;99(1):65–76.

77. Tsivgoulis G, Sharma VK, Lao AY, et al. Validation of transcranial Doppler with computed tomography angiography in acute cerebral ischemia. Stroke 2007;38(4):1245–9.

78. Wong KS, Li H, Chan YL, et al. Use of transcranial Doppler ultrasound to predict outcome in patients with intracranial large-artery occlusive disease. Stroke 2000;31(11):2641–7.

79. Molina CA, Montaner J, Abilleira S, et al. Timing of spontaneous recanalization and risk of hemorrhagic transformation in acute cardioembolic stroke. Stroke 2001;32(5):1079–84.

80. Camerlingo M, Casto L, Censori B, et al. Prognostic use of ultrasonography in acute non-hemorrhagic carotid stroke. Ital J Neurol Sci 1996;17(3):215–8.

81. Baracchini C, Manara R, Ermani M, et al. The quest for early predictors of stroke evolution: can TCD be a guiding light? Stroke 2000;31(12):2942–7.

82. Kushner MJ, Zanette EM, Bastianello S, et al. Transcranial Doppler in acute hemispheric brain infarction. Neurology 1991;41(1):109–13.

83. Zanette EM, Fieschi C, Bozzao L, et al. Comparison of cerebral angiography and transcranial Doppler sonography in acute stroke. Stroke 1989;20(7): 899–903.

84. Burgin WS, Malkoff M, Felberg RA, et al. Transcranial Doppler ultrasound criteria for recanalization after thrombolysis for middle cerebral artery stroke. Stroke 2000;31(5):1128–32.

85. Toni D, Fiorelli M, Zanette EM, et al. Early spontaneous improvement and deterioration of ischemic stroke patients: a serial study with transcranial Doppler ultrasonography. Stroke 1998;29(6):1144–8.

86. Lee MT, Piomelli S, Granger S, et al. Stroke Prevention Trial in Sickle Cell Anemia (STOP): extended follow-up and final results. Blood 2006;108(3): 847–52.

87. Adams RJ, McKie VC, Carl EM, et al. Long-term stroke risk in children with sickle cell disease screened with transcranial Doppler. Ann Neurol 1997;42(5):699–704.

88. Adams RJ, McKie VC, Hsu L, et al. Prevention of a first stroke by transfusions in children with sickle cell anemia and abnormal results on transcranial Doppler. N Engl J Med 1998;339:5–11.

89. Wijman CA, McBee NA, Keyl PM, et al. Diagnostic impact of early transcranial Doppler ultrasonography on the TOAST classification subtype in acute cerebral ischemia. Cerebrovasc Dis 2001;11(4): 317–23.

90. Akopov S. Hemodynamic studies in early ischemic stroke: serial transcranial Doppler and magnetic resonance angiography evaluation. Stroke 2002; 33(5):1274–9.

91. Hagen PT, Scholz DG, Edwards WD. Incidence and size of patent foramen ovale during the first 10 decades of life: an autopsy study of 965 normal hearts. Mayo Clin Proc 1984;59(1):17–20.

92. Adams HP, Bendixen BH, Kappelle LJ, et al. Classification of subtype of acute ischemic stroke. Definitions for use in a multicenter clinical trial. TOAST. Trial of Org 10172 in Acute Stroke Treatment. Stroke 1993;24(1):35–41.

93. Job FP, Ringelstein EB, Grafen Y, et al. Comparison of transcranial contrast Doppler sonography and transesophageal contrast echocardiography for the detection of patent foramen ovale in young stroke patients. Am J Cardiol 1994;74(4):381–4.

94. Serena J, Segura T, Perez-Ayuso MJ, et al. The need to quantify right-to-left shunt in acute ischemic stroke: a case-control study. Stroke 1998;29(7): 1322–8.

95. Belvís R, Leta RG, Martí-Fàbregas J, et al. Almost perfect concordance between simultaneous transcranial Doppler and transesophageal echocardiography in the quantification of right-to-left shunts. J Neuroimaging 2006;16(2):133–8.

96. Cardiol RE. Diagnosis and quantification of patent foramen ovale. Which is the reference technique? Simultaneous study with transcranial Doppler, transthoracic and transesophageal echocardiography. Rev Esp Cardiol 2011;64(2):12–3.

97. Albert A, Müller HR, Hetzel A. Optimized transcranial Doppler technique for the diagnosis of cardiac right-to-left shunts. J Neuroimaging 1997;7(3): 159–63.

98. Droste DW. Optimizing the technique of contrast transcranial Doppler ultrasound in the detection of right-to-left shunts. Stroke 2002; 33(9):2211–6.

99. Schwarze JJ, Sander D, Kukla C, et al. Methodological parameters influence the detection of right-to-left shunts by contrast transcranial Doppler ultrasonography. Stroke 1999;30(6):1234–9.

100. Bernd Ringelstein E, Droste DW, Babikian VL, et al. Consensus on microembolus detection by TCD. Stroke 1998;29(3):725–9.

101. Markus HS, King A, Shipley M, et al. Asymptomatic embolisation for prediction of stroke in the Asymptomatic Carotid Emboli Study (ACES): a prospective observational study. Lancet Neurol 2010;9(7): 663–71.

102. Goertler M, Blaser T, Krueger S, et al. Cessation of embolic signals after antithrombotic prevention is related to reduced risk of recurrent arterioembolic transient ischaemic attack and stroke. J Neurol Neurosurg Psychiatr 2002;72(3):338–42.

103. Stork JL. Source of microembolic signals in patients with high-grade carotid stenosis. Stroke 2002;33(8):2014–8.

104. Molloy J, Markus HS. Asymptomatic embolization predicts stroke and TIA risk in patients with carotid artery stenosis. Stroke 1999;30(7):1440–3.

105. Alexandrov AV, Sloan MA, Tegeler CH, et al. Practice standards for transcranial Doppler (TCD) ultrasound. Part II. Clinical indications and expected outcomes. J Neuroimaging 2012;22(3):215–24.

106. King A, Markus HS. Doppler embolic signals in cerebrovascular disease and prediction of stroke risk: a systematic review and meta-analysis. Stroke 2009;40(12):3711–7.

107. Alexandrov AV, Demchuk AM, Felberg RA, et al. Intracranial clot dissolution is associated with embolic signals on transcranial Doppler. J Neuroimaging 2000;10(1):27–32.

108. Spencer MP. Transcranial Doppler monitoring and causes of stroke from carotid endarterectomy. Stroke 1997;28(4):685–91.

109. Gaunt ME, Martin PJ, Smith JL, et al. Clinical relevance of intraoperative embolization detected by transcranial Doppler ultrasonography during carotid endarterectomy: a prospective study of 100 patients. Br J Surg 1994;81(10):1435–9.

110. Levi CR, O'Malley HM, Fell G, et al. Transcranial Doppler detected cerebral microembolism following carotid endarterectomy. High microembolic signal loads predict postoperative cerebral ischaemia. Brain 1997;120(Pt 4):621–9.

111. Jansen C, Ramos LM, Van Heesewijk JP, et al. Impact of microembolism and hemodynamic changes in the brain during carotid endarterectomy. Stroke 1994;25(5):992–7.

112. Ackerstaff RG, Moons KG, Van de Vlasakker CJ, et al. Association of intraoperative transcranial Doppler monitoring variables with stroke from carotid endarterectomy. Stroke 2000;31(8):1817–23.

113. Lennard N, Smith J, Dumville J, et al. Prevention of postoperative thrombotic stroke after carotid endarterectomy: the role of transcranial Doppler ultrasound. J Vasc Surg 1997;26(4):579–84.

114. Jansen C, Vriens EM, Eikelboom BC, et al. Carotid endarterectomy with transcranial Doppler and electroencephalographic monitoring. A prospective study in 130 operations. Stroke 1993;24(5): 665–9.

115. Feri M, Ralli L, Felici M, et al. Transcranial Doppler and brain death diagnosis. Crit Care Med 1994; 22(7):1120–6.

116. Zurynski Y, Dorsch N, Pearson I, et al. Transcranial Doppler ultrasound in brain death: experience in 140 patients. Neurol Res 1991;13(4):248–52.

117. Babikian VL, Feldmann E, Wechsler LR, et al. Transcranial Doppler ultrasonography: year 2000 update. J Neuroimaging 2000;10(2):101–15.

118. Hassler W, Steinmetz H, Pirschel J. Transcranial Doppler study of intracranial circulatory arrest. J Neurosurg 1989;71(2):195–201.

119. Hassler W, Steinmetz H, Gawlowski J. Transcranial Doppler ultrasonography in raised intracranial pressure and in intracranial circulatory arrest. J Neurosurg 1988;68(5):745–51.

120. Petty GW, Mohr JP, Pedley TA, et al. The role of transcranial Doppler in confirming brain death: sensitivity, specificity, and suggestions for performance and interpretation. Neurology 1990;40(2): 300–3.

121. Yoneda S, Nishimoto A, Nukada T, et al. To-and-fro movement and external escape of carotid arterial blood in brain death cases. A Doppler Ultrasonic Study. Stroke 1974;5(6):707–13.

122. Conti A, Iacopino DG, Spada A, et al. Transcranial Doppler ultrasonography in the assessment of cerebral circulation arrest: improving sensitivity by transcervical and transorbital carotid insonation and serial examinations. Neurocrit Care 2009; 10(3):326–35.

123. Hadani M, Bruk B, Ram Z, et al. Application of transcranial Doppler ultrasonography for the diagnosis of brain death. Intensive Care Med 1999; 25(8):822–8.

124. Ducrocq X, Hassler W, Moritake K, et al. Consensus opinion on diagnosis of cerebral circulatory arrest using Doppler-sonography: task Force Group on cerebral death of the Neurosonology Research Group of the World Federation of Neurology. J Neurol Sci 1998;159(2):145–50.

125. Wijdicks EF. Determining brain death in adults. Neurology 1995;45(5):1003–11.

Hypothermia in Neurocritical Care

Neeraj Badjatia, MD, MS

KEYWORDS

- Therapeutic hypothermia • Traumatic brain injury • Cardiac arrest • Shivering • Spinal cord injury

KEY POINTS

- The ability of hypothermia to protect tissue from ischemic damage is primarily related to its effects on metabolism, with oxygen use decreasing linearly by 5% to 9% per degree centigrade.
- Therapeutic hypothermia applied within hours of injury designed as a neuroprotective strategy and delayed TH designed to mitigate the effect of increased intracranial pressure (ICP).
- At present, hypothermia has only been shown to be an effective therapy for cardiac arrest and reducing ICP.
- Shivering and immune suppression are the most significant concerns during the maintenance phase of cooling.
- Rewarming is the most dangerous phase of cooling because of the increased risk for rebound cerebral edema and increased ICP.

INTRODUCTION

Although use of hypothermia has only recently become commonplace, the neuroprotective properties of cooling have been studied for decades. Beneficial effects of hypothermia during cardiac arrest were first described in case reports during the 1940s, and the findings were reproduced in animal studies in the 1950s.[1–5] Findings from animal studies later suggested that induction of mild hypothermia (32–35°C) could achieve neuroprotective benefits while avoiding serious adverse effects caused by deep hypothermia.[6] Two randomized clinical trials in 2002 showed that hypothermia improved neurologic outcomes in patients following cardiac arrest.[7,8] Since these landmark trials the use of therapeutic hypothermia (TH) has gained momentum and its clinical use has increased substantially over the past decade.

Effective clinical use of TH requires a firm understanding of the mechanisms by which cooling induces neuroprotection, the physiologic consequences of hypothermia, and the potential for serious complications following temperature reduction. Given the complexity of the application of TH and the physiologic changes caused by mild hypothermia, standardized clinical management protocols are essential for optimal patient care, regardless of the indication.

MECHANISM OF ACTION

Preclinical trials have shown that hypothermia exerts multiple neuroprotective effects in models of both global and focal injury. The ability of hypothermia to protect tissue from ischemic damage is primarily related to its effects on metabolism, with oxygen use decreasing linearly by 5% to 9% per degree centigrade,[9] resulting in decreased oxygen requirements and tolerance of lower tissue perfusion.[10] When oxygen and glucose delivery is limited there is a reduced risk of energy failure, which causes failure of sodium pumps, calcium influx, and cell death.[11]

A broad range of beneficial effects of hypothermia have been well described, including effects

Section of Neurocritical Care, R Adams Cowley Shock Trauma Center, University of Maryland Medical Center, 22 South Greene Street, Baltimore, MD 21201, USA
E-mail address: nbadjatia@umm.edu

Neurosurg Clin N Am 24 (2013) 457–467
http://dx.doi.org/10.1016/j.nec.2013.02.001
1042-3680/13/$ – see front matter © 2013 Elsevier Inc. All rights reserved.

neurosurgery.theclinics.com

on many cellular and molecular processes from microRNA responses to differential gene expression.[12,13] The response to hypothermia causes an overall reduction in excitotoxic neurotransmitter release, free radical formation, sustained electrical depolarizations, and inhibition of proinflammatory and apoptotic pathways.[14–19] These mechanisms stabilize the blood-brain barrier, decrease edema, and reduce intracranial pressure (ICP).[20]

The effect of TH on these mechanisms depends on the timing of the therapy (**Fig. 1**). Hypothermia applied within hours of the injury is designed to optimize the potential for neuroprotection, working primarily at a cellular level to arrest pathologic processes that play a significant role in secondary injury. As injury progresses, TH is administered to reduce the impact of cerebral edema and mass effect that the primary injury has on uninjured areas of the brain. The distinction between neuroprotective and ICP-reducing mechanisms is important when administering hypothermia in the neurocritical care unit (NCCU).

INDICATIONS
Cardiac Arrest

During no-flow states such as observed in cardiac arrest, there is membrane depolarization, calcium influx, glutamate release, acidosis, and activation of lipases, proteases, and nucleases. This process allows for reoxygenation injury involving iron, free radicals, nitric oxide, catecholamines, excitatory amino acid release, and renewed calcium shifts.[21] During postischemic reperfusion, even after prolonged ischemic periods, the high-energy ATP

load recovers rapidly and approaches normal levels quickly after return of spontaneous circulation (ROSC); however, tissue injury continues after reperfusion. The observation of morphologic changes (cytosolic microvacuolation) seen in hippocampal hilar, CA1 pyramidal neurons, and cortical pyramidal neurons of layers 3 and 5 after reperfusion has led to the concepts of reperfusion injury and selective neuronal vulnerability.[21] As a result, much of the brain injury after even brief periods of anoxia is caused by the reperfusion injury after ROSC. Experimental studies have shown that these mechanisms can be minimized or prevented with the application of hypothermia.

Despite knowing the benefits of TH after experimental cardiac arrest for several decades,[22] it has only recently been studied extensively in humans. A decade has passed since the results of 2 randomized controlled trials provided evidence that TH (32°–34°C) for 12 to 24 hours is an effective treatment of patients who remain comatose after resuscitation from out-of-hospital cardiac arrest when the initial cardiac rhythm is ventricular fibrillation.[7,8] As with other therapeutic interventions after brain injury, time to treatment is important and this therapy should only be initiated within 6 hours of injury and without delay. In 2010, the American Heart Association recommended as part of routine post–cardiac arrest care that comatose adult patients surviving out-of-hospital ventricular fibrillation cardiac arrest should be cooled to 32°C to 34°C for 12 to 24 hours. Further, less robust recommendations were made for TH for comatose adult patients after in-hospital cardiac arrest of any initial rhythm or after out-of-hospital cardiac

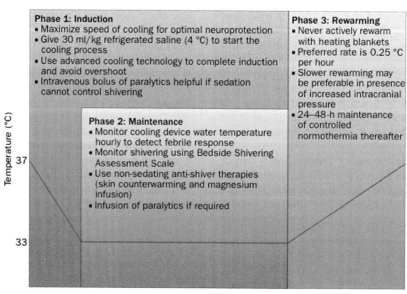

Fig. 1. Key management points during the 3 phases of TH.

arrest with an initial rhythm of pulseless electric activity or asystole.[23]

Traumatic Brain Injury

The application of hypothermia after traumatic brain injury (TBI) can have different effects based on patient selection as well as the timing, duration, and depth of cooling. Cooling within minutes to hours after the injury is designed to act as a neuroprotectant, mitigating many of the cellular mechanisms that eventually result in further damage. As hours and days after injury continue, the cumulative effect of these mechanisms is observed clinically, and TH can also be applied as an effective therapy for processes leading to increased ICP.

Thirteen controlled single-center studies conducted on adult patients with TBI showed significantly better outcomes associated with TH.[24] In contrast, 3 multicenter randomized controlled trials that tested early short-term (maximum 48 hours) TH[25–27] found no benefit with regard to survival and neurologic outcome.

The most recent study published is the National Acute Brain Injury Study: Hypothermia II (NABIS: H II), a multicenter trial including patients who were 16 to 45 years old after severe, nonpenetrating TBI, treated with TH.[27] The trial was stopped after inclusion of 108 patients, and no effect on outcome was seen. Subgroup analysis found that patients with surgically evacuated hematomas treated with TH had better outcomes, whereas those with diffuse brain injury treated with hypothermia had a trend to poorer outcome. The reasons for improvement in such a subpopulation may include the impact of temperature control on reperfusion injury–related spreading depolarizations, as recently reported by the Cooperative Study of Brain Injury Depolarizations (COSBID) study group.[28,29]

There are 17 controlled trials investigating the impact of hypothermia on outcome in patients with severe TBI and refractory intracranial hypertension and most of these studies show that hypothermia is an effective method for reducing ICP, although the data on outcome are inconsistent.[24] The magnitude of the effect of TH on ICP reduction is estimated to be approximately 10 mm Hg (range 5–23 mm Hg). Across the studies analyzed, the effect of TH on ICP reduction was superior to that achieved with moderate hyperventilation, barbiturates, and mannitol, but less effective than hemicraniectomy and hypertonic saline.[30]

The optimal target temperature of TH when used for ICP control is not well defined. There is experimental evidence that decreasing body temperature to between 35 and 35.5°C effectively treats intracranial hypertension, while maintaining sufficient cerebral perfusion pressure without cardiac dysfunction or oxygen debt.[31] Resting energy expenditure and cardiac output decreased progressively with hypothermia, reaching very low levels at temperatures less than 35°C.[31] At core temperatures less than 35°C there is a concomitant significant decrease brain tissue oxygenation.[32] Thus, 35 to 35.5°C may be the optimal temperature at which to treat patients with intracranial hypertension following severe TBI. However, instead of applying fixed temperature targets, TH may be better applied by titrating temperature to maintain ICP at less than 20 mm Hg. Although, from a meta-analysis, some have advocated that a duration of hypothermia of more than 48 hours may be beneficial,[33] the optimal duration of cooling is not known. Rather than focusing on optimal timing, a better target for cooling is ongoing efficacy for reduction of ICP weighed against the risk associated with deep sedation and impaired immune function that accompany prolonged cooling.

TH is effective in reducing increased ICP, and is therefore an appropriate option for reducing ICP after TBI. The Eurotherm3235 Trial, an international, multicenter, randomized controlled trial, will examine the effects of TH at 32 to 35°C as a treatment of increased ICP after TBI. The design of this study is adapted to overcome some of the failures of previous studies that have to do with patient selection, timing, and duration of treatment. Subjects are allowed to be enrolled up to 72 hours after TBI. The duration of cooling is titrated on the time to control ICP effectively (between 2 and 5 days), and rewarming is used at a rate of 0.25°C/h.[34]

Rewarming remains the most dangerous stage of hypothermia management. Large fluctuations in temperature can reverse the protective effects of cooling and aggravate secondary brain injury.[35,36] This is shown by impaired cerebrovascular vasoreactivity, hyperemia, and rebound intracranial hypertension.[37] Studies have documented rapid rewarming to be associate with increased episodes of rebound intracranial hypertension and worse outcomes.[27,38] A slow, controlled rewarming (0.1–0.2°C/h) should be used to reduce the risk of rebound cerebral edema and intracranial hypertension.

Subarachnoid Hemorrhage

The focus of TH in the acute phase of subarachnoid hemorrhage (SAH) is on mitigating the effect of the initial hemorrhage. Experimental studies have shown that mild to moderate hypothermia reverses acute cerebral perfusion pressure–independent hypoperfusion, enhances recovery of posthemorrhagic cerebral blood flow, and reverses edema formation. The vascular effects may be attributed to hypothermia-induced vasodilatory effects or to the prevention of autoregulatory impairment, whereas prevention of lactate accumulation may help reverse post-SAH cerebral edema.

In the clinical setting, few retrospective, nonrandomized studies have been reported examining the effect of mild hypothermia soon after SAH. Gasser and colleagues[39] reported the results of a study to evaluate the feasibility and safety of long-term hypothermia (>72 hours) in the treatment of severe brain edema after poor-grade SAH. Among 156 patients with SAH, 21 patients were treated with mild hypothermia and barbiturate coma. Of these, 9 patients were treated for less than 72 hours and 12 for longer than 72 hours. Functional independence at 3 months, defined as a Glasgow Outcome Scale (GOS) score of 4 or 5, was achieved in 48% of patients, but this was no different between the 2 groups. The most common form of complication was infection. Regardless of favorable results from case reports, conclusions regarding impact of TH on outcome are lacking, because there are no data from controlled prospective studies.

Intraoperative deep hypothermia (26°C) has been successfully used in patients undergoing high-risk cardiac and neurosurgical procedures requiring cardiopulmonary bypass and temporary circulatory arrest.[40] The Intraoperative Hypothermia for Aneurysm Surgery Trial[41] failed to show any improvement in mortality or functional or cognitive outcome, most likely because most subjects were in good clinical condition, with no acute brain injury and no temperature-modifiable brain injury (ie, temporary vessel occlusion) during surgery.

The application of hypothermia after parenchymal hemorrhage is understudied. Similar to SAH, clinical studies in intracranial hemorrhage have not been adequately designed to understand the impact of TH on outcome, although there has been a consistent demonstration of cooling to effectively reduce hemorrhage-related cerebral edema.[42,43]

Ischemic stroke

The perceived need for a secure airway, mechanical ventilation, and shivering control has limited the use of hypothermia as a therapeutic approach in patients after stroke. However, some studies have shown that it is possible to cool nonintubated patients after stroke, albeit with variable

success.[44–46] Schwab and Mayer[47] reported on 2 noncontrolled trials of induced hypothermia as salvage therapy for patients with established middle cerebral artery (MCA) infarction. Patients were admitted to an intensive care unit and hypothermia was achieved with surface cooling. ICP was monitored with intraparenchymal sensors placed ipsilateral to the infarct. In the first of these studies, published in 1998, hypothermia was induced in 25 malignant MCA infarct patients an average of 14 hours after stroke onset, and temperature was maintained at 33°C for 48 to 72 hours.[47] There was significant morbidity-associated cerebral edema caused by uncontrolled rewarming. Further data in patients with MCA infarct suggests that controlled rewarming rates of 0.1°C per hour or less allow for improved control of ICP compared with patients in whom rewarming is achieved in a passive, uncontrolled fashion.[47,48]

In a prospective randomized study, Els and colleagues[49] enrolled 25 consecutive patients with an ischemic infarction of more than two-thirds of 1 hemisphere to either hemicraniectomy alone, or in combination with hypothermia. Safety parameters were compared between both treatment groups and the clinical outcome was assessed at 6 months. Overall mortality was 12% (2 of 13 vs 1 of 12 in the 2 groups), but none of these three patients died because of treatment-related complications. There were no severe side effects of hypothermia. The clinical outcome showed a tendency for a better outcome in the hemicraniectomy plus moderate hypothermia group after 6 months. Delayed cooling for the treatment of cytotoxic brain edema does not provide definitive treatment of malignant cerebral edema, and should not be used as an alternative to the proven therapy for hemicraniectomy.[50,51] However, these results suggest that hypothermia may still be of benefit even in those patients who have undergone hemicraniectomy.

Many questions remain unanswered regarding the role of hypothermia as an adjunct to thrombolysis in the treatment of ischemic stroke. A trial sponsored by the National Institutes of Health is currently underway to evaluate the safety of a 6-hour window for intravenous thrombolytic therapy when coupled with hypothermia in the Intravascular Cooling in the Treatment of Stroke–Longer TPA Window trial. Other investigators are studying the effects of mild hypothermia combined with additional neuroprotective agents, such as caffeine and ethanol, in patients after ischemic stroke; however, until tested in a prospective controlled study, hypothermia therapy, either standalone or as an adjunct, remains experimental.[52,53]

Spinal Cord Injury

Approximately 11,000 to 12,000 individuals sustain a spinal cord injury (SCI) from motor vehicle accidents, sport-related injuries, and direct trauma.[54] Recent surgical advancements have reduced mortality and morbidity but long-term disability remains a significant problem.[55] There are currently no proven medical treatments that protect against the consequences of SCI. Experimental models have reliably shown a strong benefit of TH.[54] The only evidence thus far in the literature is a single-center study from the University of Miami that reported the results from 14 patients with an average age of 39.4 years (range, 16–62 years) with acute, complete (American Spinal Injury Association [ASIA] A) cervical SCIs using an intravascular cooling catheter to achieve modest (33°C) systemic hypothermia for 48 hours.[56] In this small series, the cooling approach was found to be feasible with no difference in rate of complications. Even though they noted that 6 of 14 patients converted from ASIA A status, large prospective studies are needed before TH can be considered as part of standard of care in this population.

Critical Care Management Issues of TH

Clinical management of hypothermia can be separated into 3 phases: induction, maintenance, and rewarming (**Fig. 2**). The widespread use of advanced temperature modulating devices has simplified bedside management of hypothermia. Each system works to induce and maintain core body temperature through conductive heat loss either by surface cooling or intravascular cooling. Surface cooling systems consist of pads that are applied to the skin of patients with circulating forced cold air or fluid,[57,58] whereas intravascular cooling systems consist of endovascular heat-exchange catheters that are placed via the femoral or subclavian vein to cool the blood.[59,60] Both methods can effectively induce and maintain

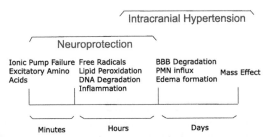

Fig. 2. Timeline for hypothermic protection. BBB, blood-brain barrier; PMN, polymorphonuclear leukocyte. (*From* Choi HA, Badjatia N, Mayer SA. Hypothermia for acute brain injury–mechanisms and practical aspects. Nat Rev Neurol 2012;8:214–22; with permission.)

hypothermia.[61] All of these devices work via a feedback loop that adjusts the temperature of the water circulating through the cooling system to maintain a constant target body temperature measured in the bladder or esophagus.[62]

When treating patients with hypothermia, induction should be as rapid as possible to reach the target temperature. Application of ice packs to a patient and the infusion of cold intravenous fluids (4°C normal saline or lactated ringers at 30–40 mL/kg over 1 hour) is the simplest and least expensive method of inducing hypothermia.[57,63–65] The use of large-volume (30 mL/kg) cold (4°C) fluid infusions has been well studied in postoperative and critical care settings and found to be an effective method to induce hypothermia. When used in conjunction with advanced temperature-modulating devices, a bolus of isotonic fluid can decrease core temperatures by 4°C/h. Even with large volumes administered, there seem to be no episodes of pulmonary edema or cardiac arrhythmia.[63] In addition to its rapid onset, the large volume of infusion can help offset the fluid imbalance that may be observed as a result of cold-induced diuresis during the induction of hypothermia.

During the maintenance period, advanced cooling technology can maintain core body temperature with only minor fluctuations (±0.5°C). Fever is the most frequent clinical sign of infection, but no longer occurs when hypothermia is induced. Monitoring the temperature of the circulating water in the cooling device can be used as a surrogate marker for increased heat production by the patient and may indicate a febrile response and possible infection.[66]

Rewarming is the most dangerous phase of hypothermia, particularly in patients with intracranial mass effect who are at risk of increased ICP. Rapid increases in body temperature can cause systemic vasodilation and hypotension, which in turn can trigger cerebral vasodilation and ICP plateau waves.[67–69] In general, rewarming should be performed as slowly as 0.1°C/h if increased ICP is a concern.[68,70] If ICP increase is observed, rewarming should be slowed or even halted. In most cases, a rewarming rate of 0.25°C/h is recommended, and in all cases rewarming should be performed in a controlled manner to avoid overshoot and hyperthermia.[71]

COMPLICATIONS AND ADVERSE EFFECTS

Shivering

Shivering is a thermoregulatory defense to maintain body temperature at the hypothalamic set point. In healthy humans, peripheral vasoconstriction is triggered at 36.5°C and shivering at

35.5°C.[72] Temperature thresholds for vasoconstriction and shivering are higher than normal in brain-injured patients; therefore, these thermoregulatory defenses may occur at higher temperatures.[73]

Control of shivering is essential for effective hypothermia, because shivering fights the cooling process and can trigger large increases in systemic and cerebral energy consumption and metabolic demand.[74,75] The first step in managing shivering is to have an effective tool for measurement. The Bedside Shivering Assessment Scale is a simple, validated, 4-point scale that enables repeated quantification of shivering at the bedside (**Table 1**).

Therapy for shivering should ideally stop or suppress the central thermoregulatory reflex rather than just uncoupling this response from skeletal muscle contraction, because this does not mitigate the ongoing cerebral and systemic stress response. Initial measures should focus on minimizing the use of high doses of analogosedatives, which can impair the ability to track neurologic examination changes and increase the risk for complications related to prolonged mechanical ventilation.[76]

The first step (**Table 2**) uses acetaminophen, buspirone, and magnesium infusion.[77–79] In addition, patients should be treated with forced warm-air skin counterwarming. An increase in mean skin temperature by 4°C, without affecting core body temperature, can increase the sensation of warmth

and blunt the shivering reflex by 1°C.[74,80] Approximately half of the patients who shiver in response to TH require additional pharmacologic therapy to prevent this response. Dexmeditomidine is a central-acting alpha-2 receptor agonist that has been shown to decrease the shivering threshold.[81] Propofol and the opioid meperidine is also effective at reducing shivering, but can cause oversedation and prolong the need for mechanical ventilation when given at high doses.[81,82] If all other options to prevent shivering are exhausted, paralysis (induced with vecuronium or cisatracurium) may be needed.[76]

Reduced Electrolyte Levels

In addition to decreased systemic and cerebral metabolism, other physiologic changes routinely occur in patients treated with hypothermia. Cooling drives electrolytes into the intracellular compartment and results in decreased levels of serum potassium, magnesium, and phosphate.[83] However, during rewarming these electrolytes are released from intracellular stores and move to the extracellular spaces. Care should therefore be taken to avoid excessive potassium replacement during the maintenance phase to avoid rebound hyperkalemia during rewarming.[84]

Acid-Base Status

As patients are cooled, carbon dioxide becomes more soluble, carbon dioxide partial pressure (Pco_2) levels decrease, and the pH rises. There are 2 ways to manage acid-base status during induced hypothermia: alpha-stat management refers to the practice of interpreting blood gas values at 37°C regardless of the patient's body temperature, and pH-stat management is correcting blood gas values to account for the colder body temperature. To maintain normal Pco_2 and pH levels with pH-stat management, a state of hypoventilation and hypercarbia is maintained, which results in cerebral vasodilation and could, in theory, lead to an increase in cerebral blood flow and ICP. Substantial controversy exists over which method of acid-base management, if either, is preferable.[21,85,86] In general, a given center should adopt 1 method and develop a protocol for respiratory management accordingly.

Insulin Resistance and Kidney Dysfunction

Insulin resistance occurs during hypothermia, which leads to hyperglycemia. During rewarming, insulin sensitivity may increase rapidly, and may lead to hypoglycemia if the insulin dose is not adjusted appropriately.[84] Peripheral vasoconstriction during hypothermia can cause a diversion of

Table 1		
The Bedside Shivering Assessment Scale (BSAS)		
Score	Shivering Status	Description
0	None	No shivering noted on palpation of the masseter, neck, or chest wall
1	Mild	Shivering localized to the neck and/or thorax only
2	Moderate	Shivering involves gross movement of the upper extremities (in addition to neck and thorax)
3	Severe	Shivering involves gross movements of the trunk and upper and lower extremities

The Bedside Shivering Assessment Scale is measured by palpating the temples and masseters, neck and shoulders, pectoralis muscles, biceps, and quadriceps.

Data from Lavinio A, et al. Cerebrovascular reactivity during hypothermia and rewarming. Br J Anaesth 2007;99(2):237–44.

Table 2
Antishivering protocol

Step	Level of Sedation	Intervention for Shivering	Dosage or Goal
0	Baseline	Acetaminophen	650–1000 mg Q 4–6 h
		Busiprone	30 mg Q 8 h
		Magnesium sulfate	0.5–1 mg/h IV; goal, 3–4 mg/dL
		Skin counterwarming	Maximum temperature, 43°C
1	Mild	Dexmedetomidine	0.2–1.5 µg/h
		Opioids	Meperidine 50–100 mg IM/IV
2	Moderate	Dexmedetomidine	0.2–1.5 µg/h
		Opioids	Meperidine 50–100 mg IM/IV
3	Deep	Propofol	50–75 µg/kg/min
4	Neuromuscular blockade	Vecuronium	0.1 mg/kg IV

Abbreviations: IM, intramuscular; IV, intravenous; Q, every.

blood to the kidneys, which can result in mild renal tubular dysfunction. The combination of cooling and kidney dysfunction causes a cold diuresis effect,[87–89] which can make fluid management during TH challenging.

Cardiac Function

Core body temperatures between 33 and 35°C are generally well tolerated by the heart. As long as shivering is well controlled, cooling results in bradycardia and reduced myocardial contractility, which causes reduced cardiac output and blood pressure. Temperatures less than 32°C can lead to serious cardiac arrhythmias such as atrial and ventricular tachycardia and fibrillation.[84,90] For this reason, 33°C is generally considered the safe lower limit of target temperature.

Impaired Immune Function

Cooling impairs leukocyte phagocytic function and immunosuppression, which explains the increased risk of pneumonia and other bacterial

Table 3
Evidence for the clinical usefulness of hypothermia in the NCCU

Clinical Scenario	Efficacy of TH	Type of Evidence	General Protocol	Level of Evidence
Cardiac arrest	Effective	2 phase III RCTs	32–34°C for 12–24 h	Level I
TBI	Ineffective	Multiple phase III RCTs, ongoing studies	32–34°C for 24 h	Level I
Cardiac arrest (PEA or asystolic)	Possible	Observational case series	32–34°C for 12–24 h	Level IIb
Increased ICP	Effective	Multiple RCTs and cohort studies	32–35°C titrated to ICP	Level II
Ischemic stroke	Feasible	Small feasibility trials, ongoing phase III trial	35.5°C for non–mechanically ventilated patients 32–35°C for mechanically ventilated patients	Level III
Intracerebral hemorrhage	Unknown	Observational case series	33–35°C	Level III
Subarachnoid hemorrhage	Unknown	Observational case series	33–35°C	Level III
Spinal cord injury	Feasible	Nonrandomized Prospective Study	33°C for 48 h	Level III

Abbreviations: PEA, pulseless electrical activity; RCTs, randomized controlled trials; TH, therapeutic hypothermia; VF, ventricular fibrillation; VT, ventricular tachycardia.

infections during hypothermia.[41,53,91] The risk for infectious complications seems to increase with prolonged hypothermia, although it is not clear at which time point the risk becomes universal. Tracking the development of infections can also be difficult in the absence of temperature increases and impaired white blood cell counts. Many of the temperature-modulating devices allow bedside clinicians to track the work of the device, which can be used as an indirect indicator of a mounting infection.

Hematologic Effects

Coagulopathy and thrombocytopenia seem to occur more frequently in spontaneous hypothermia after trauma than after medically induced hypothermia. Platelet dysfunction, increased fibrinolytic activity, and decreased activity of coagulation cascade enzymes all contribute to bleeding during hypothermia. Mild coagulopathy and platelet dysfunction also occur at temperatures of more than 35°C, but most trials have not shown an increased risk of serious bleeding, even in patients with preexisting intracranial hemorrhage.[92]

SUMMARY

Over the past decade, hypothermia has emerged as a mainstream intervention for many diseases seen in the NCCU. Studies in patients who have undergone cardiac arrest have unequivocally shown that the application of hypothermia to these individuals is safe and effective. However, the translation of neuroprotection with TH to other disease states has not been as successful (**Table 3**). Challenges in the safe and effective application of TH include adequately controlling shiver reflex and minimization of complications including infection, metabolic derangements, and cardiac arrhythmias. Many questions regarding the optimal timing, depth, and duration of cooling, and appropriate clinical management of the patient remain to be answered. Further prospective controlled studies focusing on the effects of TH on brain physiology and outcome in stroke, trauma, and other disease states in humans are needed before therapeutic hypothermia can be validated for use in these diseases in the NCCU.

REFERENCES

1. Bigelow WG, Lindsay WK, Greenwood WF. Hypothermia; its possible role in cardiac surgery: an investigation of factors governing survival in dogs at low body temperatures. Ann Surg 1950;132(5): 849–66.
2. Rosomoff HL, Holaday DA. Cerebral blood flow and cerebral oxygen consumption during hypothermia. Am J Physiol 1954;179(1):85–8.
3. Benson DW, Williams GR Jr, Spencer FC, et al. The use of hypothermia after cardiac arrest. Anesth Analg 1959;38:423–8.
4. Williams GR Jr, Spencer FC. The clinical use of hypothermia following cardiac arrest. Ann Surg 1958; 148(3):462–8.
5. Young RS, Zalneraitis EL, Dooling EC. Neurological outcome in cold water drowning. JAMA 1980; 244(11):1233–5.
6. Polderman KH. Induced hypothermia and fever control for prevention and treatment of neurological injuries. Lancet 2008;371(9628):1955–69.
7. Bernard SA, Gray TW, Buist MD, et al. Treatment of comatose survivors of out-of-hospital cardiac arrest with induced hypothermia. N Engl J Med 2002;346(8):557–63.
8. Hypothermia after Cardiac Arrest Group. Mild therapeutic hypothermia to improve the neurologic outcome after cardiac arrest. N Engl J Med 2002; 346(8):549–56.
9. Prakash O, Jonson B, Bos E, et al. Cardiorespiratory and metabolic effects of profound hypothermia. Crit Care Med 1978;6(5):340–6.
10. Oku K, Sterz F, Safar P, et al. Mild hypothermia after cardiac arrest in dogs does not affect postarrest multifocal cerebral hypoperfusion. Stroke 1993; 24(10):1590–7 [discussion: 98].
11. Baker AJ, Zornow MH, Grafe MR, et al. Hypothermia prevents ischemia-induced increases in hippocampal glycine concentrations in rabbits. Stroke 1991;22(5):666–73.
12. Feng JF, Zhang KM, Jiang JY, et al. Effect of therapeutic mild hypothermia on the genomics of the hippocampus after moderate traumatic brain injury in rats. Neurosurgery 2010;67(3):730–42.
13. Truettner JS, Alonso OF, Bramlett HM, et al. Therapeutic hypothermia alters microRNA responses to traumatic brain injury in rats. J Cereb Blood Flow Metab 2011;31(9):1897–907.
14. Kil HY, Zhang J, Piantadosi CA. Brain temperature alters hydroxyl radical production during cerebral ischemia/reperfusion in rats. J Cereb Blood Flow Metab 1996;16(1):100–6.
15. Olsen TS, Weber UJ, Kammersgaard LP. Therapeutic hypothermia for acute stroke. Lancet Neurol 2003;2(7):410–6.
16. van der Worp HB, Sena ES, Donnan GA, et al. Hypothermia in animal models of acute ischaemic stroke: a systematic review and meta-analysis. Brain 2007;130(Pt 12):3063–74.
17. Karibe H, Zarow GJ, Graham SH, et al. Mild intraischemic hypothermia reduces postischemic hyperperfusion, delayed postischemic hypoperfusion, blood-brain barrier disruption, brain edema, and

neuronal damage volume after temporary focal cerebral ischemia in rats. J Cereb Blood Flow Metab 1994;14(4):620–7.

18. Eguchi Y, Yamashita K, Iwamoto T, et al. Effects of brain temperature on calmodulin and microtubule-associated protein 2 immunoreactivity in the gerbil hippocampus following transient forebrain ischemia. J Neurotrauma 1997;14(2):109–18.

19. Xu L, Yenari MA, Steinberg GK, et al. Mild hypothermia reduces apoptosis of mouse neurons in vitro early in the cascade. J Cereb Blood Flow Metab 2002;22(1):21–8.

20. Lotocki G, Rivero Vaccari JP, Perez ER, et al. Alterations in blood-brain barrier permeability to large and small molecules and leukocyte accumulation after traumatic brain injury: effects of post-traumatic hypothermia. J Neurotrauma 2009;26(7):1123–34.

21. Polderman KH. Mechanisms of action, physiological effects, and complications of hypothermia. Crit Care Med 2009;37(7 Suppl):S186–202.

22. Stub D, Bernard S, Duffy SJ, et al. Post cardiac arrest syndrome: a review of therapeutic strategies. Circulation 2011;123(13):1428–35.

23. Peberdy MA, Callaway CW, Neumar RW, et al. Part 9: post-cardiac arrest care: 2010 American Heart Association Guidelines for Cardiopulmonary Resuscitation and Emergency Cardiovascular Care. Circulation 2010;122(18 Suppl 3):S768–86.

24. Polderman KH, Ely EW, Badr AE, et al. Induced hypothermia in traumatic brain injury: considering the conflicting results of meta-analyses and moving forward. Intensive Care Med 2004;30(10):1860–4.

25. Clifton GL, Miller ER, Choi SC, et al. Lack of effect of induction of hypothermia after acute brain injury. N Engl J Med 2001;344(8):556–63.

26. Shiozaki T, Hayakata T, Taneda M, et al. A multicenter prospective randomized controlled trial of the efficacy of mild hypothermia for severely head injured patients with low intracranial pressure. Mild Hypothermia Study Group in Japan. J Neurosurg 2001;94(1):50–4.

27. Clifton GL, Valadka A, Zygun D, et al. Very early hypothermia induction in patients with severe brain injury (the National Acute Brain Injury Study: Hypothermia II): a randomised trial. Lancet Neurol 2011;10(2):131–9.

28. Hartings JA, Bullock MR, Okonkwo DO, et al. Spreading depolarisations and outcome after traumatic brain injury: a prospective observational study. Lancet Neurol 2011;10(12):1058–64.

29. Hartings JA, Strong AJ, Fabricius M, et al. Spreading depolarizations and late secondary insults after traumatic brain injury. J Neurotrauma 2009;26(11):1857–66.

30. Schreckinger M, Marion DW. Contemporary management of traumatic intracranial hypertension: is there a role for therapeutic hypothermia? Neurocrit Care 2009;11(3):427–36.

31. Tokutomi T, Morimoto K, Miyagi T, et al. Optimal temperature for the management of severe traumatic brain injury: effect of hypothermia on intracranial pressure, systemic and intracranial hemodynamics, and metabolism. Neurosurgery 2007;61(1 Suppl):256–65 discussion 65–6.

32. Gupta AK, Al-Rawi PG, Hutchinson PJ, et al. Effect of hypothermia on brain tissue oxygenation in patients with severe head injury. Br J Anaesth 2002;88(2):188–92.

33. McIntyre LA, Fergusson DA, Hebert PC, et al. Prolonged therapeutic hypothermia after traumatic brain injury in adults: a systematic review. Jama 2003;289(22):2992–9.

34. Andrews PJ, Sinclair HL, Battison CG, et al. European society of intensive care medicine study of therapeutic hypothermia (32-35 degrees C) for intracranial pressure reduction after traumatic brain injury (the Eurotherm3235Trial). Trials 2011;12:8.

35. Suehiro E, Povlishock JT. Exacerbation of traumatically induced axonal injury by rapid posthypothermic rewarming and attenuation of axonal change by cyclosporin A. J Neurosurg 2001;94(3):493–8.

36. Ueda Y, Wei EP, Kontos HA, et al. Effects of delayed, prolonged hypothermia on the pial vascular response after traumatic brain injury in rats. J Neurosurg 2003;99(5):899–906.

37. Lavinio A, Timofeev I, Nortje J, et al. Cerebrovascular reactivity during hypothermia and rewarming. Br J Anaesth 2007;99(2):237–44.

38. Thompson HJ, Kirkness CJ, Mitchell PH. Hypothermia and rapid rewarming is associated with worse outcome following traumatic brain injury. J Trauma Nurs 2010;17(4):173–7.

39. Gasser S, Khan N, Yonekawa Y, et al. Long-term hypothermia in patients with severe brain edema after poor-grade subarachnoid hemorrhage: feasibility and intensive care complications. J Neurosurg Anesthesiol 2003;15(3):240–8.

40. Lougheed WM, Sweet WH, White JC, et al. The use of hypothermia in surgical treatment of cerebral vascular lesions; a preliminary report. J Neurosurg 1955;12(3):240–55.

41. Todd MM, Hindman BJ, Clarke WR, et al. Mild intraoperative hypothermia during surgery for intracranial aneurysm. N Engl J Med 2005;352(2):135–45.

42. Fingas M, Clark DL, Colbourne F. The effects of selective brain hypothermia on intracerebral hemorrhage in rats. Exp Neurol 2007;208(2):277–84.

43. Howell DA, Posnikoff J, Stratford JG. Prolonged hypothermia in treatment of massive cerebral haemorrhage; a preliminary report. Can Med Assoc J 1956;75(5):388–94.

44. Zweifler RM, Voorhees ME, Mahmood MA, et al. Induction and maintenance of mild hypothermia by surface cooling in non-intubated subjects. J Stroke Cerebrovasc Dis 2003;12(5):237–43.

45. Kammersgaard LP, Rasmussen BH, Jorgensen HS, et al. Feasibility and safety of inducing modest hypothermia in awake patients with acute stroke through surface cooling: A case-control study: the Copenhagen Stroke Study. Stroke 2000;31(9):2251–6.

46. Guluma KZ, Oh H, Yu SW, et al. Effect of endovascular hypothermia on acute ischemic edema: morphometric analysis of the ICTuS trial. Neurocrit Care 2008;8(1):42–7.

47. Schwab S, Georgiadis D, Berrouschot J, et al. Feasibility and safety of moderate hypothermia after massive hemispheric infarction. Stroke 2001; 32(9):2033–5.

48. Steiner T, Friede T, Aschoff A, et al. Effect and feasibility of controlled rewarming after moderate hypothermia in stroke patients with malignant infarction of the middle cerebral artery. Stroke 2001;32(12):2833–5.

49. Els T, Oehm E, Voigt S, et al. Safety and therapeutical benefit of hemicraniectomy combined with mild hypothermia in comparison with hemicraniectomy alone in patients with malignant ischemic stroke. Cerebrovasc Dis 2006;21(1-2):79–85.

50. Hofmeijer J, Kappelle LJ, Algra A, et al. Surgical decompression for space-occupying cerebral infarction (the Hemicraniectomy After Middle Cerebral Artery infarction with Life-threatening Edema Trial [HAMLET]): a multicentre, open, randomised trial. Lancet Neurol 2009;8(4):326–33.

51. Juttler E, Schwab S, Schmiedek P, et al. Decompressive Surgery for the Treatment of Malignant Infarction of the Middle Cerebral Artery (DESTINY): a randomized, controlled trial. Stroke 2007;38(9): 2518–25.

52. Abou-Chebl A, DeGeorgia MA, Andrefsky JC, et al. Technical refinements and drawbacks of a surface cooling technique for the treatment of severe acute ischemic stroke. Neurocrit Care 2004;1(2):131–43.

53. Hemmen TM, Raman R, Guluma KZ, et al. Intravenous thrombolysis plus hypothermia for acute treatment of ischemic stroke (ICTuS-L): final results. Stroke 2010;41(10):2265–70.

54. Dietrich WD, Levi AD, Wang M, et al. Hypothermic treatment for acute spinal cord injury. Neurotherapeutics 2011;8(2):229–39.

55. Fehlings MG, Vaccaro A, Wilson JR, et al. Early versus delayed decompression for traumatic cervical spinal cord injury: results of the Surgical Timing in Acute Spinal Cord Injury Study (STASCIS). PLoS One 2012;7(2):e32037.

56. Levi AD, Green BA, Wang MY, et al. Clinical application of modest hypothermia after spinal cord injury. J Neurotrauma 2009;26(3):407–15.

57. Kliegel A, Losert H, Sterz F, et al. Cold simple intravenous infusions preceding special endovascular cooling for faster induction of mild hypothermia after cardiac arrest–a feasibility study. Resuscitation 2005;64(3):347–51.

58. Mayer SA, Kowalski RG, Presciutti M, et al. Clinical trial of a novel surface cooling system for fever control in neurocritical care patients. Crit Care Med 2004;32(12):2508–15.

59. De Georgia MA, Krieger DW, Abou-Chebl A, et al. Cooling for Acute Ischemic Brain Damage (COOL AID): a feasibility trial of endovascular cooling. Neurology 2004;63(2):312–7.

60. Badjatia N, O'Donnell J, Baker JR, et al. Achieving normothermia in patients with febrile subarachnoid hemorrhage: feasibility and safety of a novel intravascular cooling catheter. Neurocritical Care 2004;1(2):145–56.

61. Hoedemaekers CW, Ezzahti M, Gerritsen A, et al. Comparison of cooling methods to induce and maintain normo- and hypothermia in intensive care unit patients: a prospective intervention study. Crit Care 2007;11(4):R91.

62. Moran JL, Peter JV, Solomon PJ, et al. Tympanic temperature measurements: are they reliable in the critically ill? A clinical study of measures of agreement. Crit Care Med 2007;35(1):155–64.

63. Rajek A, Greif R, Sessler DI, et al. Core cooling by central venous infusion of ice-cold (4 degrees C and 20 degrees C) fluid: isolation of core and peripheral thermal compartments. Anesthesiology 2000;93(3):629–37.

64. Bernard S, Buist M, Monteiro O, et al. Induced hypothermia using large volume, ice-cold intravenous fluid in comatose survivors of out-of-hospital cardiac arrest: a preliminary report. Resuscitation 2003;56(1):9–13.

65. Polderman KH, Rijnsburger ER, Peerdeman SM, et al. Induction of hypothermia in patients with various types of neurologic injury with use of large volumes of ice-cold intravenous fluid. Crit Care Med 2005;33(12):2744–51.

66. Oddo M, Frangos S, Maloney-Wilensky E, et al. Effect of shivering on brain tissue oxygenation during induced normothermia in patients with severe brain injury. Neurocrit Care 2010;12(1):10–6.

67. Jiang JY, Xu W, Li WP, et al. Effect of long-term mild hypothermia or short-term mild hypothermia on outcome of patients with severe traumatic brain injury. J Cereb Blood Flow Metab 2006; 26(6):771–6.

68. Linares G, Mayer SA. Hypothermia for the treatment of ischemic and hemorrhagic stroke. Crit Care Med 2009;37(7 Suppl):S243–9.

69. Clifton GL, Valadka A, Zygun D, et al. Very early hypothermia induction in patients with severe brain injury (the National Acute Brain Injury Study:

Hypothermia II): a randomised trial. Lancet Neurol 2011 Feb;10(2):131–9.

70. Polderman KH, Herold I. Therapeutic hypothermia and controlled normothermia in the intensive care unit: practical considerations, side effects, and cooling methods. Crit Care Med 2009;37(3):1101–20.

71. Badjatia N. Fever control in the neuro-ICU: why, who, and when? Curr Opin Crit Care 2009;15(2): 79–82.

72. Sessler DI. Defeating normal thermoregulatory defenses: induction of therapeutic hypothermia. Stroke 2009;40(11):e614–21.

73. Badjatia N. Hyperthermia and fever control in brain injury. Crit Care Med 2009;37(7 Suppl):S250–7.

74. Badjatia N, Strongilis E, Gordon E, et al. Metabolic impact of shivering during therapeutic temperature modulation: the Bedside Shivering Assessment Scale. Stroke 2008;39(12):3242–7.

75. Badjatia N, Strongilis E, Prescutti M, et al. Metabolic benefits of surface counter warming during therapeutic temperature modulation. Crit Care Med 2009;37(6):1893–7.

76. Choi HA, Ko SB, Presciutti M, et al. Prevention of Shivering During Therapeutic Temperature Modulation: The Columbia Anti-Shivering Protocol. Neurocrit Care 2011.

77. Zweifler RM, Voorhees ME, Mahmood MA, et al. Magnesium sulfate increases the rate of hypothermia via surface cooling and improves comfort. Stroke 2004;35(10):2331–4.

78. Mokhtarani M, Mahgoub AN, Morioka N, et al. Buspirone and meperidine synergistically reduce the shivering threshold. Anesth Analg 2001;93(5): 1233–9.

79. Kasner SE, Wein T, Piriyawat P, et al. Acetaminophen for altering body temperature in acute stroke: a randomized clinical trial. Stroke 2002; 33(1):130–4.

80. Lennon RL, Hosking MP, Conover MA, et al. Evaluation of a forced-air system for warming hypothermic postoperative patients. Anesth Analg 1990; 70(4):424–7.

81. Doufas AG, Lin CM, Suleman MI, et al. Dexmedetomidine and meperidine additively reduce the shivering threshold in humans. Stroke 2003;34(5): 1218–23.

82. Matsukawa T, Kurz A, Sessler DI, et al. Propofol linearly reduces the vasoconstriction and shivering thresholds. Anesthesiology 1995;82(5): 1169–80.

83. Polderman KH, Peerdeman SM, Girbes AR. Hypophosphatemia and hypomagnesemia induced by cooling in patients with severe head injury. J Neurosurg 2001;94(5):697–705.

84. Polderman KH. Application of therapeutic hypothermia in the intensive care unit. Opportunities and pitfalls of a promising treatment modality–Part 2: Practical aspects and side effects. Intensive Care Med 2004;30(5):757–69.

85. Bacher A. Effects of body temperature on blood gases. Intensive Care Med 2005;31(1):24–7.

86. Lay C, Badjatia N. Therapeutic hypothermia after cardiac arrest. Curr Atheroscler Rep 2010;12(5): 336–42.

87. Knight DR, Horvath SM. Urinary responses to cold temperature during water immersion. Am J Physiol 1985;248(5 Pt 2):R560–6.

88. Guluma KZ, Liu L, Hemmen TM, et al. Therapeutic hypothermia is associated with a decrease in urine output in acute stroke patients. Resuscitation 2010; 81(12):1642–7.

89. Zeiner A, Sunder-Plassmann G, Sterz F, et al. The effect of mild therapeutic hypothermia on renal function after cariopulmonary resuscitation in men. Resuscitation 2004;60(3):253–61.

90. Bergman R, Braber A, Adriaanse MA, et al. Haemodynamic consequences of mild therapeutic hypothermia after cardiac arrest. Eur J Anaesthesiol 2010;27(4):383–7.

91. Seule MA, Muroi C, Mink S, et al. Therapeutic hypothermia in patients with aneurysmal subarachnoid hemorrhage, refractory intracranial hypertension, or cerebral vasospasm. Neurosurgery 2009;64(1): 86–92 [discussion: 92–3].

92. Schefold JC, Storm C, Joerres A, et al. Mild therapeutic hypothermia after cardiac arrest and the risk of bleeding in patients with acute myocardial infarction. Int J Cardiol 2009;132(3):387–91.

Assessment of Brain Death in the Neurocritical Care Unit

David Y. Hwang, MD*, Emily J. Gilmore, MD*,
David M. Greer, MD, MA**

KEYWORDS

- Brain death • Intensive care unit • Organ donation • Ethics • Communication

KEY POINTS

- The concept of brain death developed in conjunction with the use of mechanical ventilators in modern intensive care units, and the guidelines for determining brain death have evolved over time.
- The most current American Academy of Neurology Practice Parameters for brain death determination emphasize 3 necessary clinical findings: coma (with a known irreversible cause), absence of brainstem reflexes, and apnea.
- Despite the availability of standardized guidelines, a large degree of practice variability exists, including the role of ancillary testing.
- Issues such as the relationship of brain death determination to organ donation and whether brain death represents "true death" have been debated in ethical, legal, and religious contexts, and special care should be taken when advising families of patients who may fulfill brain death criteria.

INTRODUCTION

The concept of brain death was born with the rise of modern intensive care medicine. When a lack of brain function precipitously leads to apnea, mechanical ventilation is the means by which patients can artificially maintain circulation and other bodily functions. Unfortunately, brain death is not a uniformly defined entity among institutions, states, countries, or religions. In addition, there is neither a universally accepted standard nor a consistently applied algorithm for its determination. It has been said, "if one subject in health and bioethics can said to be at once well settled and persistently unresolved, it is how to determine that death has occurred."[1]

HISTORICAL CONTEXT

The historical evolution of brain death as a concept has been reviewed in detail in the literature.[2–4]

Although Rabbi Moses Maimonides, in the Middle Ages, was among the first to suggest that the brain was of primary importance in life,[2] general medical opinion before the 1800s focused on the heart as the residence for a person's central and controlling "life force."[5] The advent of resuscitative measures in the mid-1970s, such as electroshock and artificial ventilation, forced the medical community to reconsider the location of "vital principles" as residing in a divine cardiac organ.[4]

As summarized by Machado and colleagues,[3] a number of experiments in the late 1800s demonstrated situations in which patients with high intracranial pressure ceased to have respirations but continued to have beating hearts shortly thereafter. Horsley,[6] Duckworth[7] and Cushing[8] noted in sequential and separate articles that patients with disease states such as intracerebral hemorrhage and brain tumors that increase intracranial pressure tended to pass away first from respiratory failure rather than circulatory arrest. These

Conflicts of Interest: The authors have no relevant conflicts of interest to declare.
Department of Neurology, Yale University School of Medicine, PO Box 208018, New Haven, CT 06520, USA
* Drs Hwang and Gilmore are co-first authors of this aiticle and contributed equally to its text.
** Corresponding author.
E-mail address: david.greer@yale.edu

Neurosurg Clin N Am 24 (2013) 469–482
http://dx.doi.org/10.1016/j.nec.2013.02.003
1042-3680/13/$ – see front matter © 2013 Elsevier Inc. All rights reserved.

reports include descriptions of patients who now fit widely accepted criteria for brain death; however, because they preceded the introduction of mechanical ventilation, the authors did not attempt to define death by neurologic criteria at that time.[3]

Leading up to the development and use of mechanical ventilators in intensive care units (ICUs) in the 1950s were important observations made regarding the use of ancillary testing in brain-injured patients.[3,4] Shortly after the first electroencephalogram was recorded by Berger[9] in 1929, Sugar and Gerard[10] were able to show in cats that an occlusion of a carotid artery resulted in the complete abolition of electric potentials in the brain—a real-time physiologic demonstration of cerebral blood flow, ischemia, and brain function. Another important report came in the 1950s, when Löfstedt and von Reis[11] described 6 patients with apnea and absent brainstem reflexes who showed no intracranial blood flow during cerebral angiography but who did not have subsequent cardiac arrest until 2 to 26 days afterward. Although autopsies showed advanced cerebral necrosis, no obstructions of the cerebral arteries were seen, a finding which led the investigators to conclude that increased intracranial pressure was the most probable explanation for the radiographic findings.[3,4,11]

One of the most seminal works with regard to the concept of brain death before the development of formal guidelines was authored by Mollaret and Goulon in 1959.[12] The authors coined the term "coma dépassé," meaning "a state beyond coma," to describe 23 ventilated patients in which loss of consciousness, brain stem reflexes, and spontaneous respirations were associated with absent encephalographic activity.[2] They argued that the patients' conditions were irreversible and that continuation of care in these cases was futile. This report coincided with a description of "death of the nervous system" by Wertheimer and colleagues[13] and Jouvet,[14] who proposed similar criteria to Mollaret and Goulon for stopping the ventilator in such cases.

CLINICAL DIAGNOSIS OF BRAIN DEATH
Guidelines Before American Academy of Neurology

In 1968, the Harvard Criteria, driven by the advances in critical care medicine, the advent of mechanical ventilation, and issues surrounding organ donation, were introduced in a landmark publication examining the definition of irreversible coma as a new criterion for death.[15] Coma in an individual with no discernible central nervous system activity was characterized by the following 4 features: unreceptivity and unresponsiveness, absent movements or breathing, absent reflexes, and a flat electroencephalogram.[15]

More than a decade later, the President's Commission put forth the Uniform Determination of Death Act (UDDA), which stated "an individual who has sustained either (1) irreversible cessation of circulatory and respiratory functions, or (2) irreversible cessation of all functions of the entire brain, including the brain stem, is dead. The determination of death must be made in accordance with accepted medical standards."[16] However, no definite criteria or algorithmic approach were delineated, thus allowing for continued variation in interpretation and practice.

It was not until 1995, when the American Academy of Neurology (AAN) set forth practice parameters on the determination of brain death, that there came a standard by which brain death could be algorithmically assessed.[17] Using principles from the definition provided by the UDDA, the AAN proposed "accepted medical standards" for the determination of brain death. Brain death was defined as "the irreversible loss of function of the brain, including the brainstem."[17] This was the first publication to not only give precise definitions but actually recommend a methodical approach to the clinical diagnosis of brain death, apnea testing, the use of ancillary tests, and the documentation of brain death in the medical record. The prerequisites for proceeding with the clinical diagnosis consisted of clinical and/or neuroimaging evidence of an acute central nervous system catastrophe compatible with the clinical diagnosis of brain death, the exclusion of complicating medical conditions (electrolyte, acid-base, or endocrine derangements), absence of drug intoxication or poisoning, and a core temperature of at least 32°C. This publication is the foundation for the current practice of declaring brain death in neurologically devastated patients.[17] See **Table 1** for a summary of the guidelines leading up to the AAN's practice parameter.

Current AAN Guidelines

In 2010, the AAN published an update to the 1995 guideline focusing on several clinical questions regarding the potential for misdiagnosis when using the criteria, adequate observation times, the implications of complex motor movements, and new ancillary tests.[18] The guidelines incorporated new evidence to date since the prior guidelines and provided a step-by-step approach to brain death determination (**Box 1**) that emphasized the 3 clinical findings necessary to declare brain death: coma (with a known irreversible cause), absence of brainstem reflexes, and apnea. The

Table 1
Summary of brain death determination leading up to the AAN practice parameter

Harvard Criteria (1968)	Minnesota Criteria (1971)	United Kingdom Criteria (1976)	President's Commission Criteria (1981)
• Unreceptivity and unresponsivity • No movements or breathing • No reflexes • Flat electroencephalogram • Exclusion of hypothermia (below 90°F or 32.2°C) and central nervous system depressants. *All the above tests shall be repeated at least 24 hours with no change.*	• No spontaneous movement • No spontaneous respirations when tested for a period of 4 min at a time • Absence of brain stem reflexes • A status in which all the findings above remain unchanged for at least 12 h • Electroencephalogram is not mandatory • Spinal reflexes have no bearing on the diagnosis of brain death *Brain death can be pronounced only if the pathologic process for the above are deemed irreparable with presently artificial means.*	• Establish etiology • Exclude mimicking conditions • Absent motor response • Absent brainstem reflexes • Apnea with a P_{CO_2} target of ≥50 mm Hg • Prolonged observation in anoxic-ischemic injury • Temperature should be ≥35°C	• Unreceptive and unresponsive coma • Absent papillary, corneal, oculocephalic, oculovestibular, oropharyngeal reflexes • Apnea with P_{CO_2} greater than 60 mm Hg • Absence of posturing or seizures • Irreversibility demonstrated by establishing cause and excluding reversible conditions (sedation, hypothermia, shock, and neuro muscular blockade) • Period of observation determined by clinical judgment • Use of cerebral flow tests when brainstem reflexes are not testable, sufficient cause cannot be established, or to shorten period of observation

Data from Wijdicks EF. Brain death. New York: Oxford University Press; 2011.

Box 1
Checklist for determination of brain death

Prerequisites (all must be checked)
- Coma, irreversible and cause known
- Neuroimaging explains coma
- Central nervous system (CNS) depressant drug effect absent (if indicated toxicology screen; if barbiturates given, serum level <10 g/mL)
- No evidence of residual paralytics (electrical stimulation if paralytics used)
- Absence of severe acid-base, electrolyte, endocrine abnormality
- Normothermia or mild hypothermia (core temperature $\geq$36°C)
- Systolic blood pressure $\geq$100 mm Hg
- No spontaneous respirations

Examination (all must be checked)
- Pupils nonreactive to bright light
- Corneal reflex absent
- Oculocephalic reflex absent (tested only if C-spine integrity ensured)
- Oculovestibular reflex absent
- No facial movement to noxious stimuli at supraorbital nerve, temporomandibular joint
- Gag reflex absent
- Cough reflex absent to tracheal suctioning
- Absence of motor response to noxious stimuli in all 4 limbs (spinally mediated reflexes are permissible)

Apnea testing (all must be checked)
- Patient is hemodynamically stable (even with the use of vasopressors)
- Ventilator adjusted to provide normocarbia ($Paco_2$ 34–45 mm Hg)
- Patient preoxygenated with 100% Fio_2 for $\geq$10 minutes to Pao_2 $\geq$200 mm Hg
- Patient well-oxygenated with a positive end-expiratory pressure (PEEP) of 5 cm of water
- Provide oxygen via a suction catheter to the level of the carina at 6 L/min or attach T-piece with continuous positive airway pressure (CPAP) at 10 cm H2O
- Disconnect ventilator
- Spontaneous respirations absent
- Arterial blood gas drawn at 8–10 minutes, patient reconnected to ventilator
- Pco_2 $\geq$60 mm Hg, or 20 mm Hg rise from normal baseline value
OR:
- Apnea test aborted

Ancillary testing (only 1 needs to be performed; to be ordered only if clinical examination cannot be fully performed because of patient factors, or if apnea testing inconclusive or aborted)
- Cerebral angiogram
- HMPAO single-photon emission computed tomography (SPECT)
- Electroencephalogram (EEG)
- Transcranial Doppler (TCD)

From Wijdicks EF, Varelas PN, Gronseth GS, et al. American Academy of Neurology. Evidence-based guideline update: determining brain death in adults: report of the Quality Standards Subcommittee of the American Academy of Neurology. Neurology 2010;74:1917; with permission.

AAN guidelines do not differentiate between a primary brainstem lesion ("brainstem" death) and a lesion of the cerebrum and brainstem ("whole brain" death) as long as the examination is consistent with brain death.[18] Guidelines in other countries vary in how they deal with patients with primary brainstem lesions (**Table 2**).

Variability Among Institutions

Because state law drives brain death policies on an institutional level, there remains significant practice variation despite the new detailed AAN Practice Parameter. Although most US state laws have adopted the UDDA and reference the AAN Practice Parameter, many have amendments addressing physician qualifications and the need for a second examination, as well as religious exemptions. Practice inconsistencies are evidenced both anecdotally through the personal experiences of providers who perform such declarations and systematically in relatively recent reviews of policies at esteemed institutions of neurology and neurosurgery across the country.[19] The disparity is widespread, ranging from which prerequisites should be met, what the lowest acceptable core temperature should be, how the apnea test should be performed, how many examiners should be required, and what and under which circumstances an ancillary test should be used.

The absence of federal or national standards and the vague policies adopted on a state and institutional level allow for tremendous liberty in interpretation, which contributes to the confusion for providers and mistrust among the public. There is room for misinterpretation and a grave potential for mistakes, of which the media never hesitates to take full advantage.[20] Most recently, a *New York Post* article highlighted several cases in which the motives of declaring brain death were called into question.[21] It is the variation in practice as well as on a state law level that in many ways adds further fuel to the fire. For example, New York State law requires that physicians consider accommodating families who, on religious or moral grounds, desire the maintenance of mechanical ventilation once a patient has been declared dead by neurologic criteria.[22] However, it is up to individual hospitals to establish written procedures on what constitutes reasonable accommodations in such circumstances. Because objections to the brain death standard based solely on psychological denial that death has occurred or on an alleged inadequacy of the brain death determination are not based on the individual's moral or religious beliefs, "reasonable accommodation" is not required in

such circumstances.[22] Unfortunately, such accommodations can send mixed messages to the public, particularly when there are publications of brain dead patients "surviving" for more than 14 years.[8] The ethical and legal controversies surrounding brain death will be touched on later in the article, but a comprehensive discussion is beyond the scope of this article.

With brain death guidelines falling under the jurisdiction of individual states' legislatures and ultimately at the discretion of institutions to formalize and implement, it will be difficult to reach conformity. This has led to an outcry from experts in the field to push for a national standard for the declaration of brain death, as well as advocate for a certification process, akin to Advanced Cardiac or Trauma Life Support (ACLS) training, for providers involved in the sensitive assessment of these patients.

Guidelines in Other Countries

Just as there is great variability across North America, there is great variability across the world with regard to the diagnosis of brain death. Until Wijdicks[23] published on the subject in 2002, the degree to which countries differed had not been formally characterized. Wijdicks[23] reviewed original brain death documents for 80 countries throughout the world; the differences were astounding. Although brainstem reflexes were consistently evaluated, there are marked differences in apnea test performance. A $Paco_2$ target value for the confirmation of apnea was used in only 59% of the guidelines, whereas 28% felt disconnecting a patient from the ventilator for 10 minutes after preoxygenation with 100% oxygen was sufficient. Additionally, the number of physicians required to diagnose brain death varied, with 44% of countries requiring 1 physician, 34% requiring 2 physicians, and 16% requiring more than 2 physicians. Forty percent of countries required ancillary testing, although the type varied considerably and appeared arbitrary. In one country surveyed, a cerebral angiogram was performed twice, separated by an "adequate" observation period to document the absence of cerebral blood flow. Half of countries surveyed require 2 or more physicians to confirm brain death. Most of Africa not only did not have legal provisions for organ transplantation but also could not perform brain death criteria testing simply because it was too difficult. In the Middle East, very few countries have official guidelines for determining brain death. Conceptually, brain death by neurologic criteria has not been accepted in Asia. China has no legal criteria for the determination of brain death. In countries that do have guidelines, there are often

Table 2
Differences in recommendations regarding clinical determination of brain death in Canada, the United Kingdom, and Germany

	Canada	United Kingdom	Germany
Definition of Neurologic determination of death (NDD)	The irreversible loss of the capacity for consciousness combined with the irreversible loss of all brainstem functions including the capacity to breathe.	The irreversible loss of the capacity for consciousness combined with the irreversible loss of the capacity to breathe due to the irreversible cessation of brainstem function. Does not entail the cessation of all neurologic activities in the brain.	Clinical determination of coma and loss of brainstem reflexes and apnea. Irreversibility established by repeat examination after 24 h.
Primary brainstem lesions	Death determined by neurologic criteria may be a consequence of intracranial hypertension or primary direct brainstem injury or both. No satisfactory ancillary tests for the confirmation of NDD in instances of isolated primary brainstem injury.	Primary brainstem lesions are sufficient to meet definition of NDD and ancillary testing is not required.	Must fulfill clinical criteria based on examination and in addition requires ancillary testing with electroencephalogram, evoked potentials, or absent cerebral blood flow in patients with primary brainstem lesions.
Global hypoxic-ischemic injury	Neurologic assessments unreliable in acute postresuscitation phase after cardiorespiratory arrest. Clinical evaluation for NDD should be delayed for 24 h after cardiorespiratory arrest or an ancillary test could be performed demonstrating absence of intracranial blood flow.	Acknowledges that in brain injury due to hypoxic-ischemic brain injury it may take longer to establish irreversibility of injury, although no specific observation period is stated.	Must wait at least 12 h to start brain death testing. Repeat examination after 24 h and requires ancillary testing to establish irreversibility.
Drug intoxications, including sedative and analgesic medications	Clinically significant drug intoxications may confound clinical NDD; however, therapeutic levels or therapeutic dosing of sedatives and analgesics do not preclude NDD. Under these circumstances, if patients fulfill minimal clinical criteria, NDD can be established by demonstration of absence of intracranial blood flow.	Acknowledges that actions of sedative and analgesic medications may confound NDD and that hypothermia may further prolong effects. Advises that length of time from discontinuation to exclude drug effects depends on multiple factors and should be based on pharmacokinetic principles. Recommends use of opioid and benzodiazepine antagonists and monitoring of specific drug levels with a threshold stated for thiopentone (95 mg/L) and midazolam (910 2 g/L). Acknowledges that ancillary tests may be required if drug effects cannot be completely excluded.	Must exclude potential confounders explaining clinical condition, including metabolic factors and sedative medications, but no specific recommendations regarding duration or drug levels.

Reprinted with permission from Webb A, Samuels O. Brain death dilemmas and the use of ancillary testing. Continuum. 2012;18:659-68.

panels of doctors who corroborate in order for the declaration of death to be made. Canada published criteria in 1999 that were quite similar to the AAN guidelines, differing only in that they did not require oculocephalic reflex testing, permitted hypothermia (Temperature ≥32.2°C) during apnea testing, as well as a variable interval between examinations depending on the etiology.[24]

Countries vary not only in their neurologic criteria for brain death but also in the way they approach primary brainstem lesions, global hypoxic-ischemic injury, and drug intoxications, including sedatives and analgesics. See **Table 2** for a comparison of the approach in Canada, the United Kingdom, and Germany to common clinical situations surrounding brain death.

Common Pitfalls

To our knowledge, there are no peer-reviewed reports in medical journals of conditions mimicking brain death that have detailed a complete brain death examination. The most-cited potential mimics are fulminant Guillain-Barre syndrome,[25–27] baclofen overdose,[28] barbiturate overdose,[29] delayed vecoronium clearance,[30] and hypothermia.[31] However, when the criteria for brain death are used correctly and corroborated with ancillary testing when necessary, there should be no concern for the misdiagnosis of brain death in such conditions.

On the other hand, there are several clinical signs or "red flags" that should caution one from moving forward with the assessment of brain death. These include, but are not limited to, a normal computed tomography (CT) scan, unsupported blood pressure, absence of diabetes insipidus, marked heart rate variations, fever or shock, marked metabolic acidosis, hypothermia lower than 32°C as this is often accidental and reversible, marked miosis (opiate or organophosphate toxicity), myoclonus (lithium or selective serotonin reuptake inhibitor [SSRI] toxicity), rigidity (SSRI or haloperidol toxicity), profuse diaphoresis, and positive urine or serum toxicology.[32]

The AAN guidelines recognize that "because there are deficiencies in the evidence base, clinicians must exercise considerable judgment when applying the criteria in specific circumstances" and that "ancillary tests can be used when uncertainty exists about the reliability of parts of the neurologic examination or when the apnea test cannot be performed."[18] There are conditions in which the diagnosis of brain death cannot be made on clinical grounds alone and confirmatory testing may be required. These include severe facial trauma preventing complete

brain stem reflex testing, preexisting pupillary abnormalities, and sleep apnea or severe pulmonary disease resulting in chronic retention of carbon dioxide.[18]

Patients who meet criteria for brain death are by definition motionless. However, there are a host of reflexes and movements that can cast doubt on the diagnosis and be alarming for the inexperienced examiner. Fortunately, many of these observations are well described phenomena in the literature and are entirely consistent with brain death.[33–35] In brain death, several functions, including temperature regulation, hypothalamic-pituitary-adrenal axis function, as well as spinal reflexes can be maintained for up to several hours/days. The presence of spinal reflexes is not surprising, given early twentieth century work showing retained forward location in cats and dogs with transected spinal cords.[36] It has been postulated that it is the absence of cortical inhibitory and modulatory afferents to spinal cord centers that allows for the activation of basic spinal cord sequences, causing the reflex movements commonly seen in brain death.[37] In addition to spinal reflexes,[38,39] movements after death have been described during apnea testing and during organ procurement, as well as in the morgue.[35,40,41] Movements can manifest in the head, neck, upper and lower extremities, and the trunk, and have been named "Lazarus signs" for their biblical connotation.[33,39,42] These movements range from neck, limb, and trunk flexion to facial twitches and finger jerks.[32]

In a recent publication describing a "new" spinal reflex observed in brain death, Mittal and colleagues[43] outline the following 5 aspects of the movements after brain death that may assist the clinician in differentiating spinal from postural responses:

1. There is no resemblance of a spinal response to the classic postural motor responses. These responses are recognized by synchronized decorticate (thumb folded under flexed fingers in a fist, pronated forearm, flexed elbow, and extended lower extremity with inverted foot) or decerebrate responses (pronated and extended upper and lower extremity).

2. Most often, the spinal responses are slow and short in duration. However, there can be some exceptions as follows: finger flexion can be seen as quick jerks with minimal excursions, and lower extremity responses are often more complex and can be wavy or shocklike.

3. The most common spinal response is triple flexion response (flexion in foot, knee, and hip) which may have variations, such as undulating toe sign or a Babinski sign.

4. Most movements are provoked and not spontaneous. The provocation can be movement during nursing care procedures of the patient, such as turning in bed or transfer from bed to a transport cart.

5. In some patients, spinal responses can be elicited by forceful neck flexion and by noxious stimuli below cervicomedullary junction. They are not seen with pressure at the supraorbital ridge or temporomandibular joint.

ANCILLARY BRAIN DEATH TESTING

Apnea testing is the final component in the clinical diagnosis of brain death. If for any reason apnea testing cannot be performed as discussed previously, then an ancillary test must be completed. It is not uncommon for providers to have concern about the safety of apnea testing. Some ICUs have published their experiences, but risks of reported complications are quite variable.[44–46] See **Box 1** for the prerequisites for proceeding with apnea testing. Identified factors associated with the early termination of apnea testing include insufficient preoxygenation, T-piece oxygen administration, high intratracheal flow of oxygen (>10 L/min), high A-a gradient (>300), hypotension (systolic blood pressure <90 mm Hg), mild acidosis (arterial pH <7.30), chest tube for pneumothorax, polytrauma, and younger age.[32]

In the United States, if apnea testing is performed and consistent with brain death, ancillary testing is not required. However, this is not the case worldwide. In 40% of 80 countries surveyed in 2002, an ancillary test was legally required.[23] When apnea testing cannot be performed or is aborted, there are several ancillary tests that can be used for the determination of brain death when an expert clinical neurologic examination is consistent with brain death. Ancillary tests measure a clinical state (cerebral circulatory arrest) that is closely related to the clinical determination of brain death.[47] Ancillary tests should never supersede the clinical examination and should never be performed on patients who do not meet neurologic criteria for brain death. Ancillary tests are divided into tests that assess the brain's electrical function and those that test the brain's blood flow.

The ancillary tests available often depend on institutional policies and resources. Validated tests include digital subtraction cerebral angiography, transcranial Doppler (TCD), electroencephalography (EEG), and nuclear cerebral blood flow scanning. Unfortunately, such tests are only as good as the technician performing them and the practitioner interpreting them. False-positive and false-negative ancillary tests are not uncommon.[47]

Digital subtraction cerebral angiography is the most invasive way of documenting cerebral circulatory arrest. Cerebral circulatory arrest is defined by a lack of opacification of the internal carotid arteries above the level of the petrous portion or of the vertebral arteries above the level of the atlanto-occipital junction. Some venous filling of the superior sagittal sinus may result from connections with the external carotid artery circulation. Specific criteria for confirmation of brain death by cerebral angiography have not been developed by neuroradiologic societies.[32] Another way to assess cerebral blood flow is with the use of TCDs. Unfortunately, TCDs are limited by one's ability to obtain a reliable signal, which is both operator and patient dependent. Approximately 10% to 20% of patients will not have an adequate bone window for ultrasound transmission.[18] However, when obtained, TCDs have a specificity of 98% to 100% and a sensitivity ranging from 88% to 99%.[32,48] Although EEG is quite simple to perform and provides insight into the cortical activity of the brain; it is often difficult to interpret secondary to artifact in either a positive or negative direction.[49] Electromyographic signal may produce a false-negative result, whereas sedation and hypothermia may produce a false-positive result. Cerebral scintigraphy, or nuclear cerebral blood flow scanning, is a frequently used method of determining cerebral circulatory arrest. After the intravenous administration of a tracer isotope, both dynamic and static images are taken with a gamma camera to detect cerebral blood flow. When uptake into the cerebral circulation is absent, the "hollow skull" or "empty light bulb" sign is present.[32] The Society of Nuclear Medicine has published detailed guidelines for scintigraphy for brain death determination.[50] See **Box 2** for the AAN's summary of ancillary tests.

At this time, magnetic resonance angiography, CT angiography, somatosensory evoked potentials and the bispectral index are not accepted ancillary tests because of insufficient evidence to support their use as part of a brain death evaluation.

ORGAN DONATION

Although it is important that both the medical community and the lay public recognize that the concept of irreversible brain death did not evolve solely to benefit organ transplants but rather inevitably developed out of the advancement of critical care,[3,51] donation after brain death is currently a principal source of transplant organs in Western countries.[52] If a patient in the ICU who has been declared brain dead has also been identified as a potential organ donor, the goals of care for the

Box 2
Methods of ancillary testing for the determination of brain death

Cerebral angiography

- The contrast medium should be injected in the aortic arch under high pressure and reach both anterior and posterior circulations.
- No intracerebral filling should be detected at the level of entry of the carotid or vertebral artery to the skull.
- The external carotid circulation should be patent.
- The filling of the superior longitudinal sinus may be delayed.

Electroencephalography

- A minimum of 8 scalp electrodes should be used.
- Interelectrode impedance should be between 100 and 10,000 Ω.
- The integrity of the entire recording system should be tested.
- The distance between electrodes should be at least 10 cm.
- The sensitivity should be increased to at least 2 μV for 30 minutes with inclusion of appropriate calibrations.
- The high-frequency filter setting should not be set below 30 Hz, and the low-frequency setting should not be above 1 Hz.
- Electroencephalography should demonstrate a lack of reactivity to intense somatosensory or audiovisual stimuli.

Transcranial Doppler ultrasonography

- TCD is useful only if a reliable signal is found. The abnormalities should include either reverberating flow or small systolic peaks in early systole. A finding of a complete absence of flow may not be reliable owing to inadequate transtemporal windows for insonation. There should be bilateral insonation and anterior and posterior insonation. The probe should be placed at the temporal bone, above the zygomatic arch and the vertebrobasilar arteries, through the suboccipital transcranial window.
- Insonation through the orbital window can be considered to obtain a reliable signal. TCD may be less reliable in patients with a prior craniotomy.

Cerebral scintigraphy (technetium Tc 99m exametazime [HMPAO])

- The isotope should be injected within 30 minutes after its reconstitution.
- Anterior and both lateral planar image counts (500,000) of the head should be obtained at several time points: immediately, between 30 and 60 minutes later, and at 2 hours.
- A correct intravenous injection may be confirmed with additional images of the liver demonstrating uptake (optional).
- No radionuclide localization in the middle cerebral artery, anterior cerebral artery, or basilar artery territories of the cerebral hemispheres (hollow skull phenomenon).
- No tracer in superior sagittal sinus (minimal tracer can come from the scalp).

From Wijdicks EF, Varelas PN, Gronseth GS, et al. American Academy of Neurology. Evidence-based guideline update: determining brain death in adults: report of the Quality Standards Subcommittee of the American Academy of Neurology. Neurology 2010;74:1917; with permission.

patient should transition toward optimal preservation of as many organs as possible. Although hospital systems may have dedicated organ bank teams who can help dictate the care plans for brain-dead patients who are donors, it is important for all involved physicians and staff to be aware of special considerations that these patients warrant,

especially with regard to widespread physiologic changes that regularly occur during brain death.[53] The presence of an intensivist comanaging these patients with an organ bank team has been shown to improve organ recovery for transplantation.[54]

The most common physiologic dysfunctions that are associated with brain-dead patients have been the subject of multiple recent reviews.[52,53,55] A predictable pattern of hemodynamic compromise begins with systemic hypertension induced by an attempt to maintain cerebral perfusion, followed by a transient "autonomic storm" with massive catecholamine release from brainstem dysfunction. A subsequent catecholamine insufficiency then results in marked vasodilation and hypotension, which may require treatment with a combination of vasopressin and catecholamines, such as dopamine.[56,57] The initial rise in systemic vascular resistance and rise in cardiac afterload may also increase hydrostatic pressure across the capillary membranes of the lungs, a phenomenon resulting in "neurogenic pulmonary edema."[58] Maintenance of adequate of oxygenation and avoidance of barotrauma with low tidal volume ventilation apply to the potential organ donor as they do to other patients in the ICU.[59]

Posterior pituitary dysfunction is seen in up to 90% of patients after brain death, which leads to central diabetes insipidus and requires hypotonic volume replacement and exogenous replacement of antidiuretic hormone, usually with vasopressin or desmopressin.[60] Dysfunction of the anterior pituitary hormones is more variable, but may involve the "sick euthyroid" syndrome, insulin resistance, and adrenal insufficiency.[52] Hypothalamic damage may manifest itself as hypothermia.[53] Generalized tissue factor release may cause disseminated intravascular coagulation and/or coagulopathy.[53]

A wide variation in the treatment of brain-dead organ donors has led to the development of some goal-driven protocols for standardized management in the literature,[61,62] most notably with the introduction of the United Network for Organ Sharing (UNOS) Critical Pathway for the Organ Donor.[63] These protocols are essentially geared toward keeping physiologic parameters as close to normal as possible. However, it is important to note that much of the data for developing such protocols are from retrospective studies, and the field of medical management of brain-dead patients currently has few randomized control trials as guides.[64] Care of the potential multi-organ donor often involves prioritization of salvageable organs, which may complicate management.[52] Special situations, such as pregnant brain-dead women who are identified as organ donors, require further strategies to achieve a balance of competing outcome goals.[65]

It is important to be aware as well that controversy exists over the timing between brain death determination and organ retrieval, given that the physiologic changes of brain death may promote ongoing donor organ injury. Various reports have been geared toward demonstrating this effect, notably in the cardiac literature,[66] as heart transplants are not available by any other means aside from donation after brain death. A number of recent studies from the neurology literature have argued that requiring a second brain death examination for formal declaration—no longer mandated by the American Academy of Neurology[18] —is not only redundant but also negatively affects the recovery of donor organs.[67,68] Conversely, other studies have argued that the length of time from the declaration of brain death to the procurement of organs is less important than the optimization of critical care for these patients.[69–71]

ETHICAL AND RELIGIOUS CONCERNS

Following the publication of the 1968 Harvard Committee report and other more recent criteria, neurologic determination of death has largely become accepted in societies around the world, with widespread consensus among medical professionals and lawmakers.[23,72] Understandably, the logic and coherence of "brain death" as a concept, in and of itself, has nonetheless generated controversy over the past half-century, not only seen in books intended for laypeople[46,73] but also throughout formal bioethical circles.

Arguments regarding the incoherence of defining death by neurologic criteria have been repeatedly reviewed and debated in academic forums over decades.[74–77] Recently, these arguments have been advocated ardently by Truog in multiple articles,[78–80] among others. Among the major points made are that patients determined to be brain "dead" but who remain on life support maintain a variety of integrative bodily functions, such as "circulating blood, maintaining respiration and body temperature, regulating salt and water homeostasis, digesting food, healing wounds, fighting infections… even gestating fetuses successfully."[81] It is possible that a patient who fulfills all criteria for brain death may in fact survive with mechanical ventilation for extended periods of time.[82] Miller and Truog write, "All neurologic conceptions of death… fail to capture a critical feature of what we mean by 'death'— that is, a dead human body is a corpse."[80] This viewpoint—the so-called "circulatory formulation"[83] —has in part been tied to the idea that perhaps it may be ethically sound for donors to not necessarily be "dead" at the time of organ procurement for transplantation, but that this "dead donor rule" should instead be abandoned and that patients who have suffered severe and irreversible brain damage should simply be allowed to donate organs despite the fact that are not yet dead.[84]

Bernat[83] has written extensively in defense of the ethics regarding current conceptions of brain death, stating that whereas many of these arguments against death by neurologic criteria have logical merit, a purely circulatory formulation of death is "unnecessarily conservative." Championing a "whole-brain formulation" of death, Bernat states that "the cessation of the organism as a whole requires only that all clinical brain functions cease."[83] This formulation makes "intuitive and practical sense" and, perhaps most importantly, "can be translated into successful public policy that is… acceptable and maintains… the integrity of the organ procurement enterprise."[85] The ethics of brain death determination were officially reviewed by the US President's Council on Bioethics, and, in a subsequent white paper,[86] the status quo of medical and public policy was upheld. However, in an effort to address ongoing controversies, the Council suggested "total brain failure" as an alternative to the phrase "brain death," while maintaining that, regardless of the name attached to the process, fulfilling the associated criteria does in fact mean that a given patient fulfills the criteria for "death."[86]

It should be noted that whereas the debate over the legitimacy of brain death has also continued among religious communities, the concept has mostly been accepted by the world's major belief systems.[87,88] Protestantism,[89] Catholicism,[90] and Reform and Conservative Judaism[91] have for the most part accepted brain death as a concept.[83] Notably, divergent views on whether death by neurologic criteria does in fact represent death exist within Orthodox Judaism[91] and Islam.[92] Brain death determination is practiced in Hindi societies[93] and in Confucian-Shinto Japan,[85] although the latter of which has had a protracted nationwide debate for decades and has instituted a law where a patient's family can veto a diagnosis of brain death if it is not consistent with their beliefs.[94]

DISCUSSION WITH PATIENTS' FAMILIES

Discussing brain death with the families of patients who may fulfill the neurologic criteria has the understandable potential to raise questions: "What is death? When does it happen? And does life linger on after a diagnosis of brain death?"[95] Multiple studies, reviewed by Long and colleagues,[95] have demonstrated that many family members of (1) patients who have been declared brain dead and (2) living patients who are potential future organ donors are unable to describe the medicolegal definition of brain death accurately. Of note, in a single survey study of 403 family members

of brain-dead patients who either did or did not donate organs, Siminoff and colleagues[96] found that whereas the 95% of respondents were at least able to give a partially correct definition of brain death, only 15.8% of these respondents equated brain death with actual death. Furthermore, almost one-third of the participants in the study agreed with the statement that a person is dead only when the heart has stopped beating,[96] reflecting the aforementioned academic debate in the literature.[95]

Various strategies for helping families best understand and cope with the determination of brain death for a loved one have been proposed. Giving a family adequate time to process and accept the meaning of brain death is important,[97] especially because in most situations the associated neurologic catastrophe was unexpected.[98] In certain situations, families may find it useful to review neuroimaging with the physician team.[99] It is also generally accepted as appropriate that families be given a choice as to whether to observe the brain death testing process.[100] Some families may find that, given that their loved one may appear to be breathing on a ventilator, witnessing brain death testing may help them rationalize emotional and cognitive conflict.[100,101] To remove distrust on the part of the family that a patient's physician may have vested interest in organ donation, multiple studies have now advocated that the topic of organ donation be first brought up by a nonphysician health care worker, followed by a more detailed discussion with an organ bank coordinator. "Decoupling" of the news of brain death from the request for organ donation has been shown to increase consent rates for organ donation.[102,103]

SUMMARY

Defining death by neurologic criteria is not without controversy, but having a consensus for what criteria constitute brain death and how best to evaluate for those criteria is a necessity in our current era of intensive care medicine and organ donation. Future directions for this field must include efforts to decrease practice variability among institutions in North America and worldwide, so as to decrease confusion, avoid pitfalls, and further solidify the conceptual and ethical legitimacy of brain death.

REFERENCES

1. Rosenbaum SH. Ethical conflicts. Anesthesiology 1999;91:3–4.
2. Baron L, Shemie SD, Teitelbaum J, et al. Brief review: history, concept and controversies in the

neurological determination of death. Can J Anaesth 2006;53:602–8.

3. Machado C, Kerein J, Ferrer Y, et al. The concept of brain death did not evolve to benefit organ transplants. J Med Ethics 2007;33:197–200.

4. Powner DJ, Ackerman BM, Grenvik A. Medical diagnosis of death in adults: historical contributions to current controversies. Lancet 1996;348:1219–23.

5. Pernick MS. Back from the grave: recurring controversies over defining and diagnosing death in history. In: Zaner RM, editor. Death: beyond whole brain criteria. Dordrecht (The Netherlands): Kluber Academic Publishers; 1988. p. 17–74.

6. Horsley V. On the mode of death in cerebral compression and its prevention. Q Med J 1894;2:306–9.

7. Duckworth D. Some cases of cerebral disease in which the function of respiration entirely ceases for some hours before that of the circulation. Edinb Med J 1898;3:145–52.

8. Cushing H. Some experimental and clinical observations concerning states of increased intracranial tension. Am J Med Sci 1902;124:375–400.

9. Berger H. On the electroencephalogram of man. Electroencephalogr Clin Neurophysiol 1969;(Suppl 28):37–73.

10. Sugar O, Gerard RW. Anoxia and brain potentials. J Neurophysiol 1938;1:558–72.

11. Löfstedt S, von Reis G. Intracranial lesions with abolished passage of x-ray contrast through the internal carotid arteries. Opusc Med 1956;4:345–60.

12. Mollaret P, Goulon M. The depassed coma (preliminary memoir). Rev Neurol 1959;101:3–15 [in French].

13. Wertheimer P, Jouvet M, Descotes J. A propos du diagnostic de la mort du systeme nerveux - dans les comas avec arret respiratoire traites par respiration artificielle. Presse Med 1959;67:87–8.

14. Jouvet M. Diagnostic electro-sous-cortico-graphique de la mort du systeme nerveux central au cours de certains comas. Electroencephalogr Clin Neurophysiol 1959;11:805–8.

15. A definition of irreversible coma. Report of the Ad Hoc Committee of the Harvard Medical School to Examine the Definition of Brain Death. JAMA 1968;205:337–40.

16. Guidelines for the determination of death. Report of the medical consultants on the diagnosis of death to the President's Commission for the Study of Ethical Problems in Medicine and Biomedical and Behavioral Research. JAMA 1981;246:2184–6.

17. Wijdicks EF. Determining brain death in adults. Neurology 1995;45:1003–11.

18. Wijdicks EF, Varelas PN, Gronseth GS, et al. Evidence-based guideline update: determining brain death in adults: report of the Quality Standards Subcommittee of the American Academy of Neurology. Neurology 2010;74:1911–8.

19. Greer DM, Varelas PN, Haque S, et al. Variability of brain death determination guidelines in leading US neurologic institutions. Neurology 2008;70:284–9.

20. Bartscher JF, Varelas PN. Determining brain death—no room for error. Virtual Mentor 2010;12:879–84.

21. Schram J. Organs taken from patients that doctors were pressured to declare brain dead: suit. New York Post 2012.

22. Guidelines for determining brain death. 2005. Available at: http://www.health.ny.gov/professionals/doctors/guidelines/determination_of_brain_death/docs/determination_of_brain_death.pdf. Accessed December 7, 2012.

23. Wijdicks EF. Brain death worldwide: accepted fact but no global consensus in diagnostic criteria. Neurology 2002;58:20–5.

24. Guidelines for the diagnosis of brain death. Canadian Neurocritical Care Group. Can J Neurol Sci 1999;26:64–6.

25. Bakshi N, Maselli RA, Gospe SM Jr, et al. Fulminant demyelinating neuropathy mimicking cerebral death. Muscle Nerve 1997;20:1595–7.

26. Hassan T, Mumford C. Guillain-Barre syndrome mistaken for brain stem death. Postgrad Med J 1991;67:280–1.

27. Joshi MC, Azim A, Gupta GL, et al. Guillain-Barre syndrome with absent brainstem reflexes—a report of two cases. Anaesth Intensive Care 2008;36:867–9.

28. Ostermann ME, Young B, Sibbald WJ, et al. Coma mimicking brain death following baclofen overdose. Intensive Care Med 2000;26:1144–6.

29. Kirshbaum RJ, Carollo VJ. Reversible iso-electric EEG in barbiturate coma. JAMA 1970;212:1215.

30. Kainuma M, Miyake T, Kanno T. Extremely prolonged vecuronium clearance in a brain death case. Anesthesiology 2001;95:1023–4.

31. Fischbeck KH, Simon RP. Neurological manifestations of accidental hypothermia. Ann Neurol 1981;10:384–7.

32. Wijdicks EF. Brain death. New York: Oxford University Press; 2011.

33. Ropper AH. Unusual spontaneous movements in brain-dead patients. Neurology 1984;34:1089–92.

34. Saposnik G, Bueri JA, Maurino J, et al. Spontaneous and reflex movements in brain death. Neurology 2000;54:221–3.

35. Han SG, Kim GM, Lee KH, et al. Reflex movements in patients with brain death: a prospective study in a tertiary medical center. J Korean Med Sci 2006;21:588–90.

36. Saposnik G, Basile VS, Young GB. Movements in brain death: a systematic review. Can J Neurol Sci 2009;36:154–60.

37. Tresch MC, Saltiel P, d'Avella A, et al. Coordination and localization in spinal motor systems. Brain Res Brain Res Rev 2002;40:66–79.

38. Jorgensen EO. Spinal man after brain death. The unilateral extension-pronation reflex of the upper limb as an indication of brain death. Acta Neurochir 1973;28:259–73.

39. Mandel S, Arenas A, Scasta D. Spinal automatism in cerebral death. N Engl J Med 1982;307:501.

40. Rodrigues W, Vyas H. Movements in brain death. Eur J Neurol 2002;9:687–8.

41. Dosemeci L, Cengiz M, Yilmaz M, et al. Frequency of spinal reflex movements in brain-dead patients. Transplant Proc 2004;36:17–9.

42. Heytens L, Verlooy J, Gheuens J, et al. Lazarus sign and extensor posturing in a brain-dead patient. Case report. J Neurosurg 1989;71:449–51.

43. Mittal MK, Arteaga GM, Wijdicks EF. Thumbs up sign in brain death. Neurocrit Care 2012;17:265–7.

44. Goudreau JL, Wijdicks EF, Emery SF. Complications during apnea testing in the determination of brain death: predisposing factors. Neurology 2000;55:1045–8.

45. Jeret JS, Benjamin JL. Risk of hypotension during apnea testing. Arch Neurol 1994;51:595–9.

46. Foley EP. The law of life and death. Cambridge (MA): Harvard University Press; 2011.

47. Wijdicks EF. The case against confirmatory tests for determining brain death in adults. Neurology 2010;75:77–83.

48. de Freitas GR, Andre C. Sensitivity of transcranial Doppler for confirming brain death: a prospective study of 270 cases. Acta Neurol Scand 2006;113:426–32.

49. Buchner H, Schuchardt V. Reliability of electroencephalogram in the diagnosis of brain death. Eur Neurol 1990;30:138–41.

50. Donohoe KJ, Frey KA, Gerbaudo VH, et al. Procedure guideline for brain death scintigraphy. J Nucl Med 2003;44:846–51.

51. Machado C. A definition of human death should not be related to organ transplants. J Med Ethics 2003;29:201–2 [author reply: 2].

52. Dare AJ, Bartlett AS, Fraser JF. Critical care of the potential organ donor. Curr Neurol Neurosci Rep 2012;12:456–65.

53. McKeown DW, Bonser RS, Kellum JA. Management of the heartbeating brain-dead organ donor. Br J Anaesth 2012;108(Suppl 1):i96–107.

54. Singbartl K, Murugan R, Kaynar AM, et al. Intensivist-led management of brain-dead donors is associated with an increase in organ recovery for transplantation. Am J Transplant 2011;11:1517–21.

55. Wood KE, Becker BN, McCartney JG, et al. Care of the potential organ donor. N Engl J Med 2004;351:2730–9.

56. Pennefather SH, Bullock RE, Mantle D, et al. Use of low-dose arginine-vasopressin to support brain-dead organ donors. Transplantation 1995;59:58–62.

57. Schnuelle P, Berger S, de Boer J, et al. Effects of catecholamine application to brain-dead donors on graft survival in solid organ transplantation. Transplantation 2001;72:455–63.

58. Bittner HB, Kendall SW, Chen EP, et al. The effects of brain-death on cardiopulmonary hemodynamics and pulmonary blood-flow characteristics. Chest 1995;108:1358–63.

59. Mascia L, Pasero D, Slutsky AS, et al. Effect of a lung protective strategy for organ donors on eligibility and availability of lungs for transplantation a randomized controlled trial. JAMA 2010;304:2620–7.

60. Novitzky D, Cooper DK, Rosendale JD, et al. Hormonal therapy of the brain-dead organ donor: experimental and clinical studies. Transplantation 2006;82:1396–401.

61. Hagan ME, McClean D, Falcone CA, et al. Attaining specific donor management goals increases number of organs transplanted per donor: a quality improvement project. Prog Transplant 2009;19:227–31.

62. Rosendale JD, Chabalewski FL, McBride MA, et al. Increased transplanted organs from the use of a standardized donor management protocol. Am J Transplant 2002;2:761–8.

63. Franklin GA, Santos AP, Smith JW, et al. Optimization of donor management goals yields increased organ use. Am Surg 2010;76:587–94.

64. Ware LB, Koyama T, Billheimer D, et al. Advancing donor management research: design and implementation of a large, randomized, placebo-controlled trial. Ann Intensive Care 2011;1:20.

65. Esmaeilzadeh M, Dictus C, Kayvanpour E, et al. One life ends, another begins: management of a brain-dead pregnant mother—A systematic review. BMC Med 2010;8:74.

66. Ramjug S, Hussain N, Yonan N. Prolonged time between donor brain death and organ retrieval results in an increased risk of mortality in cardiac transplant recipients. Interact Cardiovasc Thorac Surg 2011;12:938–42.

67. Lustbader D, O'Hara D, Wijdicks EF, et al. Second brain death examination may negatively affect organ donation. Neurology 2011;76:119–24.

68. Varelas PN, Rehman M, Abdelhak T, et al. Single brain death examination is equivalent to dual brain death examinations. Neurocrit Care 2011;15:547–53.

69. Nijboer WN, Moers C, Leuvenink HG, et al. How important is the duration of the brain death period for the outcome in kidney transplantation? Transpl Int 2011;24:14–20.

70. Wauters S, Verleden GM, Belmans A, et al. Donor cause of brain death and related time intervals: does it affect outcome after lung transplantation? Eur J Cardiothorac Surg 2011;39:e68–76.

71. Inaba K, Branco BC, Lam L, et al. Organ donation and time to procurement: late is not too late. J Trauma 2010;68:1362–6.

72. Freeman RB, Bernat JL. Ethical issues in organ transplantation. Prog Cardiovasc Dis 2012;55:282–9.

73. Teresi D. The undead: organ harvesting, the ice-water test, beating heart cadavers: how medicine is blurring the line between life and death. 1st edition. New York: Pantheon Books; 2012.

74. Veatch RM. The whole-brain-oriented concept of death: an outmoded philosophical formulation. J Thanatol 1975;3:13–30.

75. Green MB, Wikler D. Brain death and personal identity. Philos Public Aff 1980;9:105–33.

76. Youngner SJ, Bartlett ET. Human death and high technology: the failure of the whole-brain formulations. Ann Intern Med 1983;99:252–8.

77. Halevy A, Brody B. Brain death: reconciling definitions, criteria, and tests. Ann Intern Med 1993;119:519–25.

78. Truog RD. Is it time to abandon brain death? Hastings Cent Rep 1997;27:29–37.

79. Truog RD. Brain death—too flawed to endure, too ingrained to abandon. J Law Med Ethics 2007;35:273–81.

80. Miller FG, Truog RD. The incoherence of determining death by neurological criteria: a commentary on controversies in the determination of death, a white paper by the President's Council on Bioethics. Kennedy Inst Ethics J 2009;19:185–93.

81. Shah SK, Truog RD, Miller FG. Death and legal fictions. J Med Ethics 2011;37:719–22.

82. Shewmon DA. Chronic "brain death": meta-analysis and conceptual consequences. Neurology 1998;51:1538–45.

83. Bernat JL. Contemporary controversies in the definition of death. Prog Brain Res 2009;177:21–31.

84. Collins M. Reevaluating the dead donor rule. J Med Philos 2010;35:154–79.

85. Bernat JL. The whole-brain concept of death remains optimum public policy. J Law Med Ethics 2006;34:35–43, 3.

86. Controversies in the determination of death: a white paper by the President's Council on Bioethics. Washington, DC: 2009.

87. Veith FJ, Fein JM, Tendler MD, et al. Brain death. I. A status report of medical and ethical considerations. JAMA 1977;238:1651–5.

88. Tonti-Filippini N. Religious and secular death: a parting of the ways. Bioethics 2012;26:410–21.

89. Campbell CS. Fundamentals of life and death: Christian fundamentalism and medical science.

In: Youngner SJ, Arnold RM, Schapiro R, editors. The definition of death: contemporary controversies. Baltimore (MD): Johns Hopkins University; 1999. p. 194–209.

90. Furton EJ. Brain death, the soul, and organic life. Natl Cathol Bioeth Q 2002;2:455–70.

91. Rosner F. The definition of death in Jewish law. In: Youngner SJ, Arnold RM, Schapiro R, editors. The definition of death: contemporary controversies. Baltimore (MD): Johns Hopkins University Press; 1999. p. 210–21.

92. Randhawa G. Death and organ donation: meeting the needs of multiethnic and multifaith populations. Br J Anaesth 2012;108(Suppl 1):i88–91.

93. Jain S, Maheshawari MC. Brain death—the Indian perspective. In: Machado C, editor. Brain death. Amsterdam (The Netherlands): Elsevier; 1995. p. 261–3.

94. Aita K. Japan approves brain death to increase donors: will it work? Lancet 2009;374:1403–4.

95. Long T, Sque M, Addington-Hall J. What does a diagnosis of brain death mean to family members approached about organ donation? A review of the literature. Prog Transplant 2008;18:118–25 [quiz: 26].

96. Siminoff LA, Mercer MB, Arnold R. Families' understanding of brain death. Prog Transplant 2003;13:218–24.

97. Ormrod JA, Ryder T, Chadwick RJ, et al. Experiences of families when a relative is diagnosed brain stem dead: understanding of death, observation of brain stem death testing and attitudes to organ donation. Anaesthesia 2005;60:1002–8.

98. Coolican MB. Families: facing the sudden death of a loved one. Crit Care Nurs Clin North Am 1994;6:607–12.

99. Pearson IY, Bazeley P, Spencer-Plane T, et al. A survey of families of brain dead patients: their experiences, attitudes to organ donation and transplantation. Anaesth Intensive Care 1995;23:88–95.

100. Doran M. The presence of family during brain stem death testing. Intensive Crit Care Nurs 2004;20:32–7.

101. Long T, Sque M, Addington-Hall J. Conflict rationalisation: how family members cope with a diagnosis of brain stem death. Soc Sci Med 2008;67:253–61.

102. Siminoff LA, Arnold RM, Hewlett J. The process of organ donation and its effect on consent. Clin Transplant 2001;15:39–47.

103. Helms AK, Torbey MT, Hacein-Bey L, et al. Standardized protocols increase organ and tissue donation rates in the neurocritical care unit. Neurology 2004;63:1955–7.

Index

Note: Page numbers of article titles are in **boldface** type.

Neurosurg Clin N Am 24 (2013) 483–490
http://dx.doi.org/10.1016/S1042-3680(13)00048-X
1042-3680/13/$ – see front matter © 2013 Elsevier Inc. All rights reserved.

Moving?

Make sure your subscription moves with you!

To notify us of your new address, find your **Clinics Account Number** (located on your mailing label above your name), and contact customer service at:

Email: journalscustomerservice-usa@elsevier.com

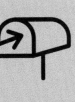

800-654-2452 (subscribers in the U.S. & Canada)
314-447-8871 (subscribers outside of the U.S. & Canada)

Fax number: 314-447-8029

Elsevier Health Sciences Division
Subscription Customer Service
3251 Riverport Lane
Maryland Heights, MO 63043

*To ensure uninterrupted delivery of your subscription, please notify us at least 4 weeks in advance of move.

Printed and bound by CPI Group (UK) Ltd, Croydon, CR0 4YY

03/10/2024

01040347-0019